Introduction to Occupational Therapy

Introduction to Occupational Therapy

4th Edition

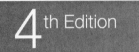

Jane Clifford O'Brien, PhD, OTR/L
Associate Professor and Program Director
Occupational Therapy Department
Westbrook College of Health Professions
University of New England
Portland, Maine

Susan M. Hussey, MS, OT/L
Professor and Coordinator
Sacramento City College
Science and Allied Health Division
Sacramento, California

Barbara Sabonis-Chafee, MS, OTR/L
Editor Emeritus

ELSEVIER
MOSBY

3251 Riverport Lane
St. Louis, Missouri 63043

Library of Congress Cataloging-in-Publication Data
O'Brien, Jane Clifford.
  Introduction to occupational therapy / Jane Clifford O'Brien, Susan M. Hussey, Barbara Sabonis-Chafee — 4th ed.
    p. ; cm.
  Rev. ed. of: Introduction to occupational therapy / Susan Hussey, Barbara Sabonis-Chafee, Jane Clifford O'Brien. 3rd ed. c2007.
  Includes bibliographical references and index.
  ISBN 978-0-323-08465-9 (pbk. : alk. paper)
  I. Hussey, Susan M.   II. Sabonis-Chafee, Barbara.   III. Sabonis-Chafee, Barbara. Introduction to occupational therapy.   IV. Title.
  [DNLM: 1. Occupational Therapy. WB 555]
  LC classification not assigned
  615.8'515–dc23   2011030755

Publishing Director: Linda Duncan
Executive Editor: Kathy Falk
Managing Editor: Jolynn Gower
Publishing Service Manager: Julie Eddy
Senior Project Manager: Andrea Campbell
Project Manager: Kamatchi Madhavan
Design Direction: Amy Buxton

Printed in the United States of America

Last digit is the print number: 9 8 7 6 5 4 3

In memory of Dr. Gary Kielhofner, whose life work and dedication to the occupational therapy profession made a difference in the lives of persons with disabilities. He inspired and mentored OT practitioners around the world and in so doing improved the quality of life for those in need of occupational therapy services.

JOB

Preface

It has been more than 20 years since the first edition of *Occupational Therapy: Introductory Concepts* was published (1989) by Barbara Sabonis-Chafee. This fourth edition of *Introduction to Occupational Therapy* encompasses many of the ideas and concepts from that first text and reinforces Ms. Sabonis-Chafee's feelings about occupational therapy's uniqueness in the health field as she reflects below.

"An occupational therapist is a facilitator of the patient/client's struggle toward independence—of however much or little that person is capable. . . The occupational therapy profession functions from a mindset that is different from technical specialties. The concern for the whole person is expected in every individual intervention plan. The practitioner is not the repository of some 'cure' but the link in assisting a person in finding his or her own abilities or capacities. The profession's philosophical base emphasizes that health involves body, mind, and spirit—in total integration. Dysfunction in any part affects the whole person. If a person loses the ability to walk, it is not only his or her legs that are deficient; the entire being is profoundly affected!"

This edition is written for those studying occupational therapy at either the professional level (occupational therapist) or the technical level (occupational therapy assistant) or for those who are exploring the profession to determine whether this is the field for them. *Introduction to Occupational Therapy* gives readers a solid overview of the important concepts of occupational therapy. This edition incorporates the *Occupational Therapy Practice Framework* and the basics of evidence-based practice. Numerous case studies are presented to help illustrate the concepts.

The text is divided into three sections. The first section introduces the reader to the field of occupational therapy by providing the history and philosophy of occupational therapy, current issues, and future trends in the profession. Section 2 focuses on the occupational therapy practitioner, educational requirements to practice, roles and responsibilities of practitioners, ethical and legal dimensions of practice, and the professional organizations. Section 3 concentrates on the practice of occupational therapy by describing the practice framework and the process of occupational therapy practice; settings of practice; intervention approaches; and special skills required by OT practitioners, including establishing therapeutic relationships, selecting therapeutic activities, and developing clinical reasoning.

This edition of *Introduction to Occupational Therapy* has been organized to make learning easy for the reader. Each chapter begins with a testimonial written by an occupational therapist or an occupational therapy assistant about his or her experiences in occupational therapy. These personal accounts highlight the humanistic nature of the profession and they relate theories and concepts to the real world of occupational therapy. Each chapter includes objectives outlining the main points and key terms, which are typeset in boldface throughout the text. Case studies are interwoven throughout the chapters, and a summary at the end of each chapter provides a synopsis of the material covered. Learning activities and review questions provide ways to apply the information and concepts covered in the chapter.

Teachers and students may find it useful to supplement textbook reading with materials available on the Evolve website, which includes separate instructor and student sites that contain the following:
- Review questions
- Student learning exercises
- Suggested activities
- Individual and group classroom exercises
- Crossword puzzles
- Case studies (some specific to Instructor only)
- Multiple choice questions (Instructor site only)
- PowerPoint slides (Instructor site only)

The suggested activities can be easily incorporated into class planning. Many of the activities require that students present to the class as a way to reinforce learning and help the students be active. The review questions at the end of each chapter serve as guides for class discussion and learning.

Acknowledgments

I would like to acknowledge my mentors Anita Bundy, Anne Fisher, and the late Gary Kielhofner for their guidance and knowledge. A special thanks to my family—Mike, Scott, Alison, and Molly—whose support, laughter, play, creativity, and interesting stories energize me every day. My fellow University of New England colleagues and students deserve recognition for their support. I would like to acknowledge Kate Loukas, Nancy MacRae, and Renee Taylor for their input throughout the process. Thank you to future practitioner Kate Hanrahan (MSOT 2012) who verified references and completed research for this text. The American Occupational Therapy Association provided various materials for this book. A special thanks to Susan Hussey and Barbara Sabonis-Chaffee for all of their excellent work on earlier editions of this text. Finally, thank you to Kathy Falk, Jolynn Gower, and Andrea Campbell for their support, guidance, gentle reminders, and professionalism. It is always a joy to work with them.

JOB

Contents

xii Contents

SECTION I

Occupational Therapy
The Profession

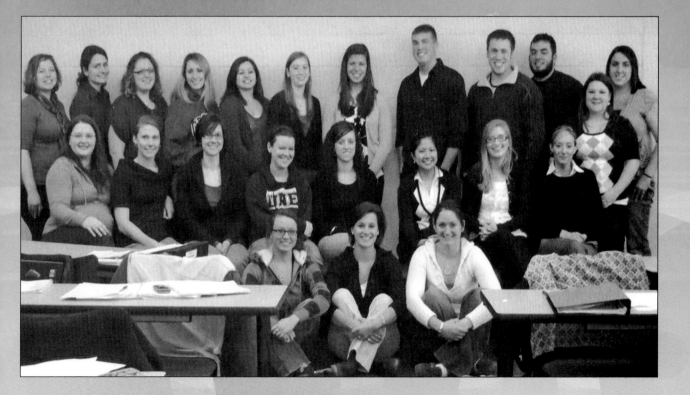

For many years, I believed that I first became interested in occupational therapy when I worked as a research assistant in a psychiatric hospital. The occupational therapy clinic was a few doors from my office, and I had a first-hand view of the patients' responses to creating tie-dyed T-shirts and scented candles. Defeat and uneasiness were replaced by smiles and confidence, all in a matter of hours.

The activities reminded me of my childhood. My mother patiently taught me and my six younger sisters and brothers many different arts and crafts. More importantly, she let us loose in the "playroom," where we spent endless hours with glue, scissors, bits of wire, yarn, plastic lace, found objects, and scraps of paper from my father's office, making whatever we pleased. I learned needle crafts from my mother, and my grandmother taught me cross-stitch embroidery when I was 8 years old. Throughout these formative years, a consistent theme was there—activities are fun and important; they can be lifelong companions and sources of joy and self-esteem.

The link between my own childhood experiences of working through activities and the reactions of patients to occupational therapy grew stronger as I watched from my office. It wasn't long before I applied and was accepted into occupational therapy school. In the more than 20 years since I graduated, I never regretted my career decision, and I often look back with some amazement to the coincidences that led me to it. I love teaching people, especially those who fear they cannot learn or cannot do—because, of course, they can learn and can do. To me, it is the greatest pleasure to witness the "ah-hah!" look and the triumphant expression that comes with accomplishment in the face of fear.

It soon became obvious that my ties to occupational therapy predated my research assistant job. It wasn't until after I graduated from school and had been working several years and after one of my younger sisters also graduated from occupational therapy school that my mother revealed that she, too, had also been studying occupational therapy but left school to raise her family after meeting and marrying my father. Now, when I think of the playroom of my childhood, I remember my mother—the almost-occupational therapist—quietly and secretly passing the message and mission to her children.

MARY BETH EARLY, MS, OTR/L
Professor
Occupational Therapy Assistant Program
LaGuardia Community College
City University of New York
Long Island City, New York

Key Terms

Activity
Areas of occupation
Client
Contrived activities
Function
Goal
Independence
Media
Occupation
Occupation-centered activities
Occupational performance
Occupational therapist
Occupational therapy
Occupational therapy assistant
Occupational therapy practitioner
Patient
Preparatory activities
Purposeful activity
Therapy

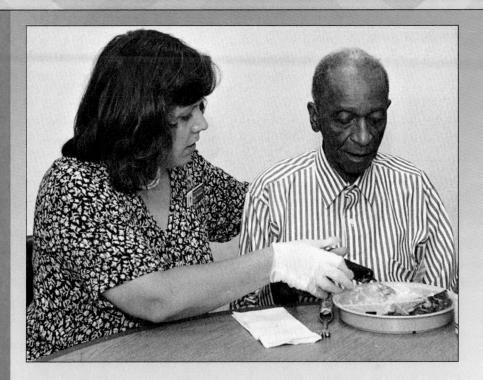

Objectives

After reading this chapter, the reader will be able to do the following:

- Understand the basic terminology used in occupational therapy
- Describe the nature and scope of the practice of occupational therapy
- Identify personality characteristics fitting for a career in occupational therapy
- Describe levels of occupational therapy personnel
- Identify types of activities used in occupational therapy intervention

This chapter provides an overview of the occupational therapy profession, beginning with answers to questions that someone new to the profession may ask. Compare your current knowledge with new insights that may arise while reflecting on the answers to these questions.

What Is Occupational Therapy?

The *Merriam-Webster's Collegiate Dictionary*® provides definitions for six words that help one to understand occupational therapy[9]:

Occupation: Activity in which one engages

Therapy: Treatment of an illness or disability

Goal: End toward which effort is directed

Activity: State or condition of being involved

Independence: State or condition of being self-reliant (independent)

Function: Action for which a person is specifically fitted

These terms provide a skeletal definition. **Occupational therapy** is a practice that uses goal-directed activity to promote independence in function. The *Occupational Therapy Practice Framework: Domain and Process*, from the American Occupational Therapy Association (AOTA), provides more specificity to the above definition[4]:

Areas of occupation: Various life activities, including activities of daily living (ADL), instrumental activities of daily living, education, work, play, leisure, and social participation[4,7]

Occupational performance: The ability to carry out activities of daily life (including activities in the areas of occupation)[4,7]

Purposeful activity: An activity used during intervention that is goal-directed and may or may not be viewed as meaningful to the client.[4,8] These activities typically involve an end product and are goal-directed.

American Occupational Therapy Association (AOTA) defines occupational therapy (Box 1-1) for professionals and consumers as a profession that uses therapeutic activities to help persons engage in meaningful activities.[3]

Are There Different Levels of the Occupational Therapy Practitioner?

Occupational therapy practitioner refers to two different levels of clinicians: an **occupational therapist** (OT) or an **occupational therapy assistant** (OTA). The OT has more extensive education and training in theory and evaluation than the OTA, who works under the supervision of an OT. Often, the OT is referred to as performing at the "professional" level, while the OTA performs at the "technical" level of practice. As of 2007, OTs must successfully graduate with a Master's degree; OTAs must successfully complete a two-year associate's degree program. Herein, OT practitioner refers to those within the field at either level. These two roles are discussed in greater depth in Chapters 5 and 7.

Box 1-1

AOTA's Definition of Occupational Therapy for the Model Practice Act

"… the therapeutic use of everyday life activities (occupations) with individuals or groups for the purpose of participation in roles and situations in home, school, workplace, community, and other settings. Occupational therapy services are provided for the purpose of promoting health and wellness and to those who have or are at risk for developing an illness, injury, disease, disorder, condition, impairment, disability, activity limitation, or participation restriction. Occupational therapy addresses the physical, cognitive, psychosocial, and other aspects of performance in a variety of contexts to support engagement in everyday life activities that affect health, well-being, and quality of life."

From *American Occupational Therapy Association: Definition of occupational therapy practice for the AOTA Model Practice Act*, Bethesda, MD, 2004, American Occupational Therapy Association. (Available from the State Affairs Group, American Occupational Therapy Association, 4720 Montgomery Lane, PO Box 31220, Bethesda, MD, 20824-1220.)

What Does an Occupational Therapy Practitioner Do?

OT practitioners work with clients of all ages and diagnoses. The goal of occupational therapy intervention is to increase the ability of the client to participate in everyday activities, including feeding, dressing, bathing, leisure, work, education, and social participation. The OT practitioner interacts with a client to assess existing performance, set therapeutic goals, develop a plan, and implement intervention to enable the client to function better in his or her world. OT practitioners may advocate for clients, make or modify equipment, and/or provide hands-on experiences to help people reengage in life. The OT practi-tioner records progress and communicates intervention specifics to others (e.g., professionals, families, insurance agencies). However, the OT practitioner does not simply do something to or for the client; rather, the OT practitioner guides the person to actively participate in intervention. Therefore, it is important for the OT practitioner to establish rapport (a relationship of mutual trust) with the client. The therapeutic relationship has value and plays a key role in the intervention process. Section III provides a detailed description of the practice of occupational therapy.

Do Occupational Therapy Practitioners Help People Get Jobs?

Although the term *occupation* commonly refers to jobs in which individuals get paid, it also encompasses the many things people do that are meaningful to them. OT practitioners help clients engage in **occupations** (e.g., activities that have meaning and give people identity). For example, being a mother is an occupation for many clients. This occupation requires that a person complete many activities and tasks. Mothers shop for food and cook meals. Cooking is an **activity** associated with the occupation of being a mother. Cooking may be performed at a much different level for the mother who finds meaning and identity in cooking for her family. **Tasks** refer to the basic units of action (e.g., mixing the batter is a task associated with cooking).

OT practitioners analyze clients' occupations so that they may help clients return to occupations they value. The following example illustrates the distinction between these terms. Gardening is an occupation for Beth; she loves spending time picking out plants, designing layouts, and caring for the garden. She attends many gardening events with friends who have similar interests. However, she does not necessarily enjoy weeding on hot summer days and finds this to be a chore. Therefore, weeding is an activity. She understands the importance of weeding but does not find it essential to her identity. It simply is something she must do within her occupation of gardening. The task involved in weeding involves grasping and pulling. Conversely, Jackie does not find gardening enjoyable at all. However, she wants her home to look nice, and, consequently, she plants flowers for this reason. For Jackie, gardening is an activity; her occupation is a homeowner.

Why Refer to Both "Patient" and "Client"?

Occupational therapy services are provided to people in many different settings. Professionals working in various settings use different terms to refer to those served. For example, in a hospital or rehabilitation setting, professionals use the term **patient,** but they use the term **client** when working in a mental health facility or training center. Individuals receiving services may also be referred to as *residents, participants, consumers,* or by their names, according to the setting's policies. In this text, the term client is used and is meant to include all settings.

Are There Personality Characteristics Best Suited for a Career Choice in Occupational Therapy?

OT practitioners have differing interests, personalities, and backgrounds. However, all practitioners possess a desire to help others; they genuinely like people, and they are able to relate to both individuals and small groups. OT practitioners appreciate diversity and value people's ability to change. Generally, OT practitioners are creative thinkers who enjoy hands-on work and are skilled problem solvers. As with any member of the health care professions, those interested in occupational therapy demonstrate the ability to handle their own personal problems and feelings before trying to help others. To support improved engagement in occupation, the OT practitioner empathizes with clients yet expects and demands effort from them. Because OT practitioners must educate and instruct clients and caregivers, an interest in teaching is also desirable. Practitioners use creative problem solving; they need the ability to find new ways of doing things and flexibility in approaching situations. Occupational therapy is a lifelong profession; therefore, commitment and dedication are important. As in other professions, the OT practitioner is never *finished* with education but must always invest in growing with the field and continually maintaining competency.

What Does an Occupational Therapy Educational Program Cover?

Because of the broad scope of the profession, the knowledge base for students in occupational therapy represents several scientific areas, including biological and behavioral sciences, sociology, anthropology, and medicine.[1,6] The student gains an understanding of normal human development and pathological conditions that affect normal development and function. With these sciences as a foundation, the student learns the theory and processes related to occupational therapy. Educational programs focus on helping students develop an attitude and

awareness that enable the new professional to be sensitive to the various needs of those seeking treatment. Occupational therapy education is aimed not only at developing specific skills, but it also seeks to develop the student's way of thinking. A problem-solving approach that relies on critical thinking is necessary to evaluate function, analyze activities, and design intervention that facilitates engagement in occupations.

Programs provide specific skills training for those techniques most widely used in the profession, although students continue to learn techniques once engaged in clinical practice. All educational programs include a clinical training phase (referred to as *fieldwork*). The student's clinical experiences help integrate the elements of theory and practice. Upon completion of the educational and fieldwork programs, students are prepared to practice in an entry-level position.

What Is the Main Emphasis of Occupational Therapy Curricula?

Both the OT (professional) and OTA (technical) educational programs are accredited by the Accreditation Council for Occupational Therapy Education (ACOTE), which is a part of AOTA. Programs are designed to conform to a series of guidelines, called *standards*.[1,2] The course of study features general theory, skills training, and the foundation for clinical reasoning. Occupational therapy curricula have a strong science base and include a focus on human development across the life span.[1,2] Curricula promote professionalism and engagement in occupation through a holistic approach to practice (including the psychological, neurological, and musculoskeletal aspects of occupations). Occupational therapy education is designed to teach the student problem-solving techniques and skills.

Who Are the People Served and What Kinds of Problems or Disabilities are Addressed by Occupational Therapy?

The mandate of the occupational therapy profession is to help clients engage in occupations, and the recipients of therapy include people who have problems that interfere with their ability to engage in everyday activities. Clients present with a range of problems, including genetic, neurological, orthopedic, musculoskeletal, immunological, and cardiac dysfunctions, as well as psychological, social, behavioral, or emotional disorders. OT practitioners help clients who have functional disabilities by increasing their abilities to do the everyday things they wish to do.

OT practitioners serve all ages (infants to older adults) and clients with physical, cognitive, psychological, and/or psychosocial impairments, which may be the result of an accident or trauma, disease, conflict or stress, social deprivation, genetics, or congenital anomalies (birth defects).

For example, an OT practitioner working with children may treat a 2-pound newborn infant in a hospital neonatal unit, a preschool child in an early intervention program, or a child who has cerebral palsy and attends public school. An

OT practitioner may work with an adolescent in a drug treatment center or an adolescent in a rehabilitation center who has cognitive limitations as a result of a brain injury. A client may have experienced physical limitations from spinal cord injury after an automobile accident and need to learn to adjust to living with a disability. OT practitioners may teach a homemaker who has had a stroke, resulting in the lack of use of one side of her body, how to manage her home and care for her family again. A client who experiences disability or trauma must learn to establish and embrace his new identity. OT practitioners may help with this aspect of disability. A client with a psychological diagnosis, such as schizophrenia, may need help from an OT practitioner to learn skills such as shopping, keeping a checkbook, and using public transportation, or to regain everyday tasks that many take for granted. An OT practitioner might make a splint for a client with a hand injury or work with an older adult in a skilled nursing facility; an OT practitioner may work in a program that helps an individual learn to use assistive technology and train for a new job after an injury. The common goal of all occupational therapy intervention is to improve the person's ability to participate in daily living. (See the photographic essay at the end of this chapter.)

How Are These Services Delivered and in What Kinds of Settings?

OT personnel work in hospitals, clinics, schools, clients' homes, community settings, and even prisons. Some practitioners consult or work in the workplace or in specialty settings (e.g., assistive technology centers). OT practitioners may work in inpatient settings (i.e., clients stay in the setting overnight) or outpatient settings (i.e., clients sleep at home and attend during the day). Acute care settings provide care immediately after trauma and typically involve short hospital stays. Rehabilitation settings provide longer care and intensive therapy from a variety of professionals. Frequently, OT practitioners consult with other team members, who may include physicians, physical therapists, speech therapists, social workers, nutritionists, case managers, nurses, educators, and family members.

OT practitioners evaluate a client's abilities and areas of weakness to develop an intervention plan, which is based on the client's interests, motivations, and goals. Intervention services may be provided in individual or group sessions, depending upon the specific needs of the clients. Typically, OT practitioners provide home programs for clients and their families so that therapy goals may be addressed even when the client is not receiving direct service. Further discussion of the intervention process may be found in Section III.

What Kinds of Activities are Used by the Occupational Therapy Practitioner During Intervention?

OT practitioners use purposeful activity (e.g., activities that are meaningful to clients) to help clients regain skills and abilities or compensate for changes in abilities so that they may engage in occupations. Adaptations or modifications may be used to change the way a certain activity is performed so that the client can be successful. For example, clients may use a built-up–handled spoon to compensate for a weak hand grasp. The goal of therapy sessions is to help clients do the things they wish to do again. Thus, OT practitioners analyze the desired occupations and determine the skills and abilities necessary for successful performance.

Intervention may begin with **preparatory activities,** which help get the client ready for the purposeful activity.[4,5] Such things as range of motion (e.g., moving the limbs through a range), exercise, strengthening, or stretching are considered preparatory activities. **Contrived activities** are made-up activities that may include some of the same skills required for the occupation.[5] These activities are used to help simulate the actual activity and may help get the client ready. For example, a client may work on tying shoes by using a doll to simulate this activity before actually tying her own shoes. Or a client may practice the components required to spread jelly before actually preparing a sandwich for lunch. Purposeful activities are generally meaningful to the client but may be one task of the occupation.[4] For example, making a sandwich is only part of making lunch. Purposeful activities have an end product and involve allowing the client to have choice. Fisher advocates that OT practitioners facilitate **occupation-centered activities.**[5] In fact, clients retain skills better and are more motivated when performing the actual occupation.[5] Occupation-centered activities are performed in the natural setting (physical, social, and temporal). For example, preparing lunch at home at noon using one's own kitchen supplies is occupation-centered therapy.

OT practitioners develop goals for each client, based upon the client's strengths (abilities) and weaknesses. The practitioner selects activities using a variety of therapeutic **media.** Media refers to the objects and materials the practitioner uses to facilitate change. Media may include games, toys, activities, dressing or self-care activities, work activities, arts, crafts, computers, industrial activities, sports, music and dance, role-playing and theater, yoga, gardening, homemaking activities, magic, pet care, and creative writing. Activities may also include the use of assistive technology, aquatics, animal-assisted therapy, ergonomics, and community integration. OT practitioners use their creativity and problem-solving skills to design therapy to meet the needs of the client.

Occupational Therapy Intervention Across the Life Span: A Photographic Essay

The following photographic essay illustrates (see Figures 1-1 to 1-11) the wonderful diversity of occupational therapy and is a visual answer to the question, "What types of people will I work with as an OT practitioner?"

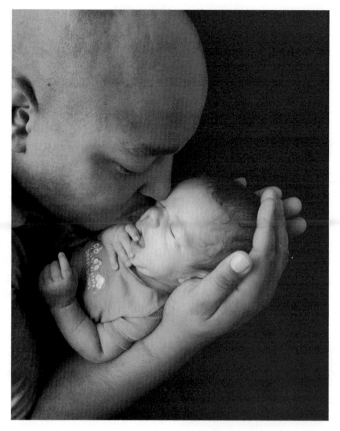

Figure 1-1 Premature and at-risk infants may have difficulty calming. OT practitioners working with infants coach families on the application of touch and calming techniques. © iStockphoto.com

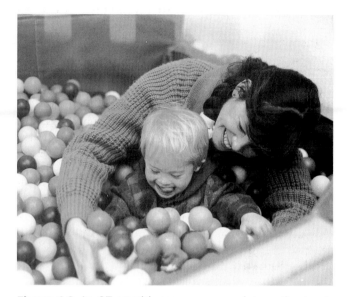

Figure 1-2 An OT practitioner uses sensory integration treatment to provide a variety of sensory experiences. Immersion in a pool of balls presents challenges to a child with a sensory disorder. (From Case-Smith J, O'Brien JC: *Occupational Therapy for Children,* ed 6, St. Louis, 2010, Elsevier.)

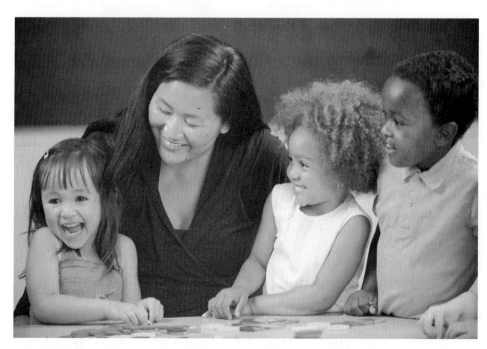

Figure 1-3 OT practitioners working in early intervention or school settings engage children in play. (Courtesy of Shay McAtee. IN Case-Smith J, O'Brien JC: *Occupational therapy for children,* ed 6. St. Louis, 2010, Elsevier.)

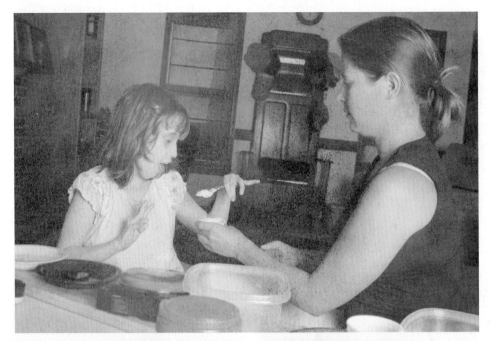

Figure 1-4 An OT practitioner helps a young girl who has difficulty with hand skills and movement learn to feed herself. © iStockphoto.com

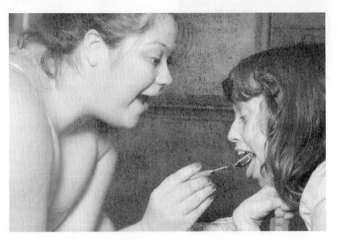

Figure 1-5 The practitioner provides special feeding techniques to help the young girl develop skills to chew and swallow food. © iStockphoto.com

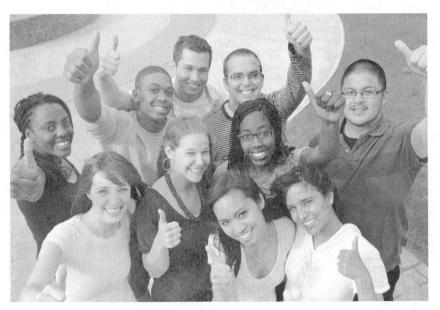

Figure 1-6 OT practitioners help teens develop their identity skills for the future and leisure interests. OT practitioners may help teens develop self-confidence through success in a variety of activities.

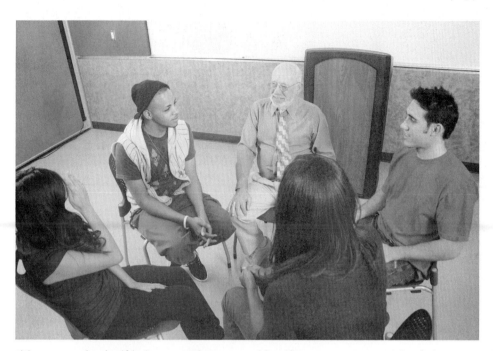

Figure 1-7 OT practitioners may lead self-help groups for teens to identify support systems and to help teens explore and develop coping and performance skills in a variety of areas. © iStockphoto.com

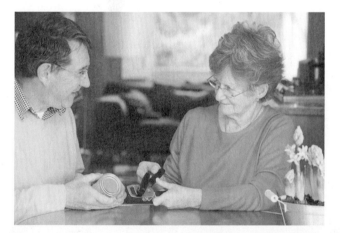

Figure 1-8 The OT practitioner shows a woman, who has arthritis resulting in difficulty holding objects, how to use an adaptive utensil and protect her hand. Practitioners help adults adjust to physical and psychological challenges. © iStockphoto.com

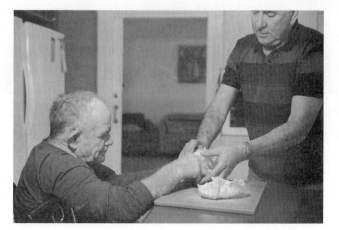

Figure 1-9 An OT practitioner helps a man make a salad. This helps the man develop hand skills and independence. Preparing a meal is an everyday activity that allows the man to return to his occupations. © iStockphoto.com

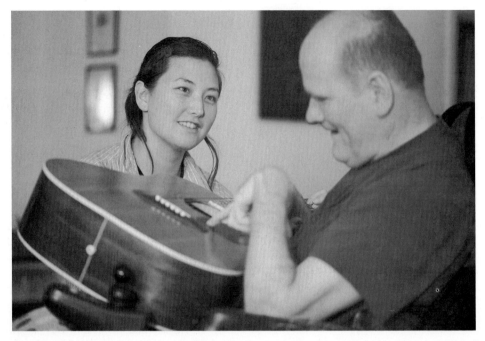

Figure 1-10 An OT practitioner engages an adult, who had a stroke, in playing his guitar. The OT practitioner is enabling this man to return to an activity that is meaningful and gives him a sense of self. © iStockphoto.com

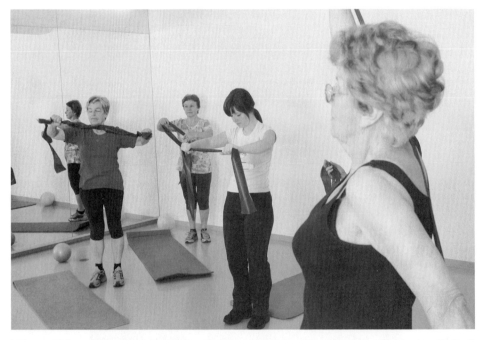

Figure 1-11 The OT practitioner leads a physical activity group for older women. Physical activity has many benefits. © iStockphoto.com

Summary

A person pursuing a career in occupational therapy must be ready to seek solutions to help clients engage in everyday living. OT practitioners work with diverse clients who have varying abilities, limitations, and desires. Creative persons who have an interest in science and health care and who like working with clients of all ages and abilities will find the career of occupational therapy rewarding.

Review Questions

1. What is occupational therapy?
2. What type of education is required to become an OT or OTA?
3. What types of things do OT practitioners do?
4. In what kinds of settings do OT practitioners work?
5. What is the difference between preparatory, purposeful, contrived, and occupation-based activity?

References

1. Accreditation Council for Occupational Therapy Education: *Accreditation standards for a master's-degree level educational program for the occupational therapist*, Bethesda, MD, January 2008, American Occupational Therapy Association.

2. Accreditation Council for Occupational Therapy Education: *Accreditation standards for an educational program for the occupational therapy assistant*, Bethesda, MD, January 2008, American Occupational Therapy Association.

3. American Occupational Therapy Association: *Definition of occupational therapy practice for the AOTA Model Practice Act*, Bethesda, MD, 2004, American Occupational Therapy Association. (Available from the State Affairs Group, American Occupational Therapy Association, 4720 Montgomery Lane, PO Box 31220, Bethesda, MD, 20824-1220.) [revision in progress].

4. American Occupational Therapy Association: Occupational therapy practice framework: Domain and process, ed 2, *Am J Occup Ther* 62:625–683, 2008.

5. Fisher AG: Uniting practice and theory in an occupational framework, *Am J Occup Ther* 52(7):509–521, 1998.

6. Larson E, Wood W, Clark F: Occupational science: Building the science and practice of occupation through an academic discipline. In Crepeau EB, Cohn ES, Schell BAB, editors: *Willard and Spackman's Occupational Therapy*, ed 10, Philadelphia, 2003, Lippincott Williams & Wilkins, pp 15–26.

7. Law M, Cooper B, Strong S, et al: Person-environment-occupation model: A transactive approach to occupational performance, *Can J Occup Ther* 63:9–23, 1996.

8. Low JE: Historical and social foundations for practice. In Trombly CA, Radomski MV, editors: *Occupational Therapy for Physical Dysfunction*, ed 5, Philadelphia, 2002, Lippincott Williams & Wilkins, pp 17–30.

9. Mish F, editor: *Merriam-Webster's Collegiate Dictionary*®, ed 11, Springfield, MA, 2004, Merriam-Webster.

Years ago, I chose to become an occupational therapist after observing other therapists at work. I was impressed by their creativity and people orientation. Back then and today, if you were to ask me what I like most about being an occupational therapist, I would list two reasons. Since my education, I have learned to appreciate our holistic roots, which are based on some of the principles of the Moral Treatment Movement. I have also recognized that our profession's meaningful beginning and most of our current literature and research come from this theme. Intrinsic to our field is the emphasis on function and the promotion of client independence. I have tried to incorporate these central themes in my practice over the years, and I could cite many examples of how I have applied them. Although the field continues to grow and change with the times, I have always recognized our roots, which continue to remain inherent to practice.

HELENE LOHMAN, MA, OTR/L
Assistant Professor
Department of Occupational Therapy
School of Pharmacy and Allied Health Professions
Creighton University
Omaha, Nebraska

CHAPTER 2

Looking Back: A History of Occupational Therapy

Key Terms

Adolf Meyer
Americans with Disabilities Act of 1990
American Occupational Therapy Association (AOTA)
Arts and Crafts Movement
Balanced Budget Act of 1997
Benjamin Rush
Civilian Vocational Rehabilitation Act
Deinstitutionalism
Education of All Handicapped Children
Eleanor Clarke Slagle
Gary Kielhofner
George Edward Barton
Habit training
Handicapped Infant and Toddlers Act
Herbert Hall
Holistic
Individuals with Disabilities Education Act (IDEA)
Medicare
Moral Treatment
National Society for the Promotion of Occupational Therapy
Philippe Pinel
Prospective Payment System
Reconstruction Aides
Reductionistic
Rehabilitation Act of 1973
Rehabilitation Movement
Soldier's Rehabilitation Act
Susan Cox Johnson
Susan Tracy
Technology Related Assistance for Individuals with Disabilities Act of 1988
Thomas Kidner
William Rush Dunton
William Tuke
World War I

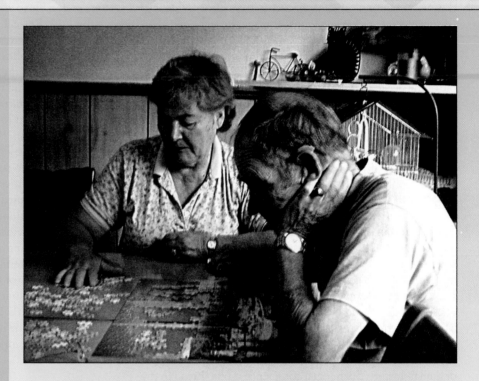

Objectives
After reading this chapter, the reader will be able to do the following:

- Identify major social influences that gave rise to the field of occupational therapy
- Name individuals who were involved in the inception of occupational therapy
- Recognize how societal influences shaped the field of occupational therapy
- Describe the concepts that have persisted throughout the history of occupational therapy
- Describe the influence of historical concepts on the current practice of occupational therapy
- Identify and describe key pieces of federal legislation that have influenced the practice of occupational therapy

Robert Bing, an occupational therapist, advises, "We exist in the present, yet are future oriented. To make sense of the present or future, we must have knowledge about and an appreciation of the past."[5]

To understand the occupational therapy profession today, it is necessary to examine the past and understand how the profession originated and developed. The history of occupational therapy can be traced with two threads that are intertwined. The social, political, and cultural thread identifies the many currents of human events that have influenced the development of occupational therapy through time. This includes legislative history that has influenced the delivery of health care services in general and occupational therapy services in particular. The second thread represents the people of the occupational therapy profession and how they have influenced the direction of the profession. This chapter provides an overview of the social, political, and cultural events that influenced occupational therapy and introduces key individuals who developed and shaped today's profession.

Eighteenth and Nineteenth Centuries

The late 1700s and early 1800s can be distinguished by an awakening of a social consciousness, an awareness that social structures lead to vast inequities. People began to believe that a measure of life's goodness should be available to all people. Evidence of this awakening is found in the novels of Charles Dickens and in the founding of various welfare organizations. This new sense of social conscience gave rise to the Civil War, which eliminated the practice of slavery in America, a previously accepted practice that extended back through all of human history. Such social conscience is one thread in the course of human history.

This awakening brought many previously ignored and cruel practices to light, one of which was the treatment of those with mental disorders. Thought to be possessed by the devil, the "insane" were feared by society; locked away like criminals; and often chained, abused, and ignored. The concept of Moral Treatment developed from this focus on the group of suffering humanity.

Moral Treatment

Moral Treatment was grounded in the philosophy that all people, even the most challenged, are entitled to consideration and human compassion. Whereas previously the "insane" were confined and frequently abused, the Moral Treatment Movement sought ways to make the existence of those confined more bearable. One of the ways was involvement in purposeful activity.

Two men from different parts of the world are credited with conceiving the Moral Treatment Movement: **Philippe Pinel** and **William Tuke.**[4] Philippe Pinel, a physician in France, introduced "work treatment" for the "insane" in the late 1700s. He used occupation to divert the patients' minds away from their emotional disturbances and toward improving their skills.

He used physical exercise, work, music, and literature in his treatment. In addition, he introduced farming as an important element of institutional life.[4]

The Society of Friends, also known as Quakers, had a great influence in England. An English Quaker and wealthy merchant, William Tuke, became aware of the terrible conditions in an asylum in York, England, and he suggested establishing the York Retreat.[4] Tuke and Thomas Fowler, the appointed visiting physician, believed that Moral Treatment methods were preferable to using restraint and drugs. The environment at the York Retreat was like that of a family in which the patients were approached with kindness and consideration.[4]

After the publication of Pinel's work in 1801 and Tuke's work in 1813 on the use of Moral Treatment, many hospitals in both Europe and the United States implemented reforms.[4] In the United States, a Quaker named **Benjamin Rush** was the first physician to institute Moral Treatment practices.

Participants in the Moral Treatment Movement demonstrated that establishing a structure and having the patients engage in simple work tasks promoted better health. Organizing activities for the patients brought order and purpose to unstructured confinement. For these persons, whose day-to-day functioning fell outside the bounds of socially acceptable behavior, there was an individualized routine of personal caretaking and productive involvement.

Though the term *Moral Treatment* began to fade by the mid-1800s, many of the concepts initiated by this movement continued. The practice of occupational therapy eventually emerged from this humanitarian concern for each human being and from the use of structured activity that simulated a more normal life for asylum inmates.

Early Twentieth Century and the Beginning of the Occupational Therapy Profession

Changes in science, technology, medicine, and industry toward the end of the nineteenth century and into the beginning of the twentieth century, including new modes of communication and transportation, accelerated the pace of everyday life. Machines were first used in the production of goods; Henry Ford developed the moving assembly line for the production of automobiles in 1913.

In reaction to the expanding use of tools and machines, a contingency of proponents of the arts and crafts developed. Led by John Ruskin and William Morris, the **Arts and Crafts Movement** was started in England. Ruskin was an English author, poet, artist, and art critic. Morris was an English poet, designer, and socialist reformer. Proponents of the Arts and Crafts Movement in both England and America were opposed to the production of items by machine, believing that this alienated people from nature and their own creativity. They sought to restore the ties between beautiful work and the worker, by returning to high standards of design and craftsmanship not found in mass-produced items. They believed that using one's hands to make items connected people to their work, physically and mentally, and thus was healthier.[17] Arts and crafts societies were created to allow people to experience the pleasure of making practical and beautiful items for everyday use. These societies had a long-lasting effect on communities.

At the turn of the twentieth century, some members of society became concerned for those who were taken from the mainstream of life by injury or illness and thereafter expected to sit on the sidelines. Until this time, a person with a disability either "got better" or was denied competitive involvement in life. The time came to look beyond these two alternatives; there was a need and desire for other options. An awareness that a "handicapped" person is still productive surfaced in sanitariums and hospitals for convalescent individuals. These events influenced the development of the occupational therapy profession.

Founders of the Profession

These events brought together several individuals who all had a shared belief in the benefits of occupation as treatment and were influential in the founding of the profession in the United States. These individuals had backgrounds in a variety of disciplines that included psychiatry, medicine, architecture, nursing, arts and crafts, rehabilitation, teaching, and social work. Their backgrounds served to enrich the depth and breadth of the profession of occupational therapy.[17] This fledgling form of treatment was called by various names during this period of development, including *ergotherapy*, *activity therapy*, *occupation treatment*, *moral treatment*, and *the work cure*. The origination of the term *occupation therapy* is ascribed to William Rush Dunton. Later, George Barton recommended that the term be changed to *occupational therapy*.

Herbert Hall

At the turn of the century, chronic illness and disability, such as tuberculosis, neurasthenia, and industrial accidents, were on the rise as people became victims of the urban and industrial life. Adapting the Arts and Crafts Movement for medical purposes was a treatment concept developed by **Herbert Hall,** a physician who graduated from Harvard Medical School. He worked with invalid patients, providing medical supervision of crafts for the purpose of improving their health and financial independence.[17]

In 1904, he established a facility at Marblehead, Massachusetts, where patients with neurasthenia worked on arts and crafts as part of treatment. Neurasthenia, a disorder that was commonly seen in women, caused severe weakness during the performance of work activities. The treatment usually prescribed at the time was total rest. Hall's alternative to the "rest cure" was arts and crafts activities, beginning with participation on a limited basis from bed and gradually increasing the level of activity until the patient went to the workshop, in which she worked on weaving looms, ceramics, and other crafts.[17] He called this approach the "work cure." In 1906, he received a grant of $1000 to study the "treatment of neurasthenia by progressive and graded manual occupation." Hall was also a prolific writer.

Even though Hall was not present at the founding meeting, his work with occupation was widely recognized by the other founders. He also took on a leadership role in the early history of the Society by serving as the President of the National Society for the Promotion of Occupational Therapy from 1920 to 1923.

George Edward Barton

George Edward Barton was a dynamic and resourceful architect who studied in London under William Morris, one of the leaders of Britain's Arts and Crafts Movement. Later, he returned to Boston to incorporate the Boston Society of Arts and Crafts. After personally experiencing a number of disabling conditions—tuberculosis, foot amputation, and paralysis of the left side of his body—Barton was determined to improve the plight of convalescent individuals. In 1914, Barton opened Consolation House for convalescent patients in Clifton Springs, New York, where occupation was used as a method of treatment.

Barton studied rehabilitation courses available at the time and made contact with people dedicated to reforming the conditions in asylums, many of whom were influenced by the Moral Treatment Movement. Among those whom Barton established contact with were Dr. William R. Dunton, Jr., Eleanor Clarke Slagle, Susan Tracy, and Susan Cox Johnson.

Dr. William Rush Dunton, Jr.

William Rush Dunton, Jr., considered the father of occupational therapy, was a psychiatrist who spent his career treating psychiatric patients. In 1891, he was hired as the assistant staff physician at the Sheppard Asylum (later named the Sheppard and Enoch Pratt Hospital) in Towson, Maryland. Having studied the treatment programs of Pinel and Tuke, he was interested in implementing a similar program at the Sheppard Asylum.

In the early 1910s, the hospital introduced a regimen of crafts for its patients. While hospital staff performed necessary medical procedures and provided a structured environment, the patients were expected to actively participate in their rehabilitation by working in the workshop.[17] Dunton was known for his writings on the value of occupation for treatment. In 1915, he published *Occupational Therapy: A Manual for Nurses*. It describes simple activities that the nurse can use or adapt in the treatment of patients. Dunton served as Treasurer and President of the National Society for the Promotion of Occupational Therapy and edited the association's journal for 21 years.

Eleanor Clarke Slagle

Often referred to as the mother of occupational therapy,[17] **Eleanor Clarke Slagle** began her career as a student in social work (Figure 2-1). She attended training courses in curative occupations in 1908 at the Chicago School of Civics and Philanthropy, which was affiliated with Hull House and Jane Addams. After this training, she worked at state hospitals in

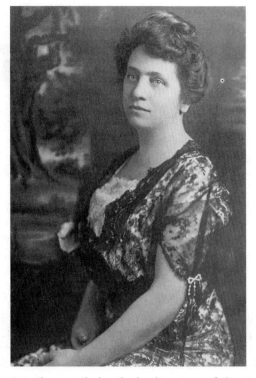

Figure 2-1 Eleanor Clarke Slagle. (Courtesy of the Archives of the American Occupational Therapy Association, Inc., Bethesda, MD.)

Michigan and New York. In 1912, she was asked by Adolf Meyer to direct a new occupational therapy department at the Henry Phipps Psychiatric Clinic of Johns Hopkins Hospital in Baltimore, Maryland. It was at this time that Slagle developed the area of work for which she is most noted, "habit training." **Habit training** is described as a "re-education program designed to overcome disorganized habits, to modify other habits, and to construct new ones, with the goal of restoring and maintaining health."[5,6] Habit training involved all hospital personnel and took place 24 hours a day. Slagle summarized it as a "directed activity, and [it] differs from all other forms of treatment in that it is given in increasing doses as the patient improves."[11]

In 1914, Slagle returned to Chicago, where she lectured at the Chicago School of Civics and Philanthropy and started a workshop for the chronically unemployed.[17] Soon after, she organized the first professional school for OT practitioners, the Henry B. Favill School of Occupations.

Slagle's dedication to the profession can be illustrated by the fact that her home was the Association's first unofficial headquarters. During her lifetime, she held each office within the Association and served as Executive Secretary for 14 years. In 1953, the American Occupational Therapy Association (AOTA), formerly known as the National Society for the Promotion of Occupational Therapy, established the Eleanor Clarke Slagle Lectureship Award, named in her honor. Today, the AOTA awards this prestigious honor to occupational therapists (OTs) who have made significant contributions to the profession.

Susan Tracy

Susan Tracy was a nursing instructor involved in the Arts and Crafts Movement and in the training of nurses in the use of occupations. She was hired in 1905 to work at the Adams Nervine Asylum, a small mental institution in Jamaica Plain, Massachusetts. While at this institution, she supervised the nursing school, developed the occupations program, and conducted postgraduate courses for nurses.[17] Tracy's book, *Studies in Invalid Occupations*,[21] is the first-known book written on occupational therapy. In it she describes the selection and practical use of arts and crafts activities for patients. Throughout her career, Tracy was involved in teaching many training courses. She believed only nurses were qualified to practice occupations, and she tried to make patient occupations a nursing specialty. Tracy was involved with her work and not able to attend the first meeting of the National Society for the Promotion of Occupational Therapy, but she actively served as Chair on the Committee of Teaching Methods.

Susan Cox Johnson

Susan Cox Johnson was a designer and arts and crafts teacher from Berkeley, California. She later became the Director of Occupations at the New York State Department of Public Charities. In this position, she sought to demonstrate that occupation could be morally uplifting, that it could improve the mental and physical state of patients and inmates in public hospitals and almshouses, and that these individuals could contribute to their self-support.[13] Following her work in this capacity, she joined the faculty of Teachers College in the Department of Nursing and Health, where she taught occupational therapy. She was an advocate for high educational standards and for the training of competent practitioners versus training large numbers of practitioners.

Thomas Kidner

Thomas Kidner was a friend and fellow architect-teacher of George Barton. He was influential in establishing a presence for occupational therapy in vocational rehabilitation and tuberculosis treatment. In 1915, he was appointed Vocational Secretary of the Canadian Military Hospitals Commission. In this position, he was responsible for developing a system of vocational rehabilitation for disabled Canadian veterans from World War I. As a Canadian architect, he was recognized for constructing institutions for individuals with physical disabilities. In many of his architectural drawings for these facilities, he included workshops for occupational therapy. When the United States passed the Vocational Rehabilitation Act in 1920 (see the following section), Kidner encouraged OTs to capitalize on this opportunity. He became very interested in tuberculosis when he realized that many men disabled in World War I were diagnosed with the disease. He helped promote the movement to hospitalize individuals with the disease and designed hospitals in both Canada and the United States for the treatment of tuberculosis patients.[17] At one point, he served as Secretary of the National Tuberculosis Association.

National Society for the Promotion of Occupational Therapy

The formal "birth" of the profession of occupational therapy can be traced to a specific event. On March 15, 1917, a small group of people from varied backgrounds convened the initial organizational meeting and produced the Certificate of Incorporation of the **National Society for the Promotion of Occupational Therapy,** in Clifton Springs, New York. Included in this group were George Barton, William Dunton, Eleanor Clark Slagle, Susan Cox Johnson, Thomas Kidner, and Isabel Newton, who attended in the capacity as Barton's secretary (later his wife) and was, in fact, made Secretary of the new organization. Reportedly, George Barton rejected William Rush Dunton's nomination of Hall for inclusion at the founding meeting.[13] Miss Tracy could not attend but was made a charter member of the Association. The object of the Association as set forth in its Constitution was "to study and advance curative occupations for invalids and convalescents; to gather news of progress in occupational therapy and to use such knowledge to the common good; to encourage original research, to promote cooperation among occupational therapy societies, and with other agencies of rehabilitation."[1]

In September 1917, 26 men and women held the first annual meeting of the organization. Early in these formative years, a set of principles was developed (Box 2-1). Dunton presented the principles in 1918 at the second annual meeting of the National Society for the Promotion of Occupational Therapy.

Philosophical Base: Holistic Perspective

There was another person whose influence helped shape the emerging profession of occupational therapy, though he was not present at the first organizational meeting. **Adolf Meyer,** a

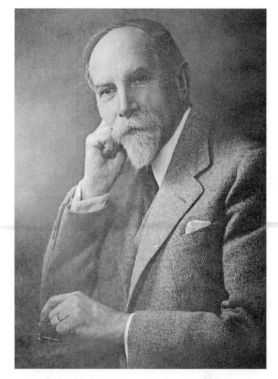

Figure 2-2 Adolf Meyer. (Courtesy of the Archives of the American Occupational Therapy Association, Inc., Bethesda, MD.)

Swiss physician who immigrated to the United States in 1892 and later became a professor of psychiatry at Johns Hopkins University, expressed a point of view that eventually formed the philosophical base of the profession (Figure 2-2).

Meyer was committed to a **holistic** perspective and developed the psychobiological approach to mental illness. He advocated that each individual should be seen as a complete and unified whole, not merely a series of parts or problems to be managed. He maintained that involvement in meaningful activity was a distinct human characteristic. Further, he believed that providing an individual with the opportunity to participate in purposeful activity promoted health.

In 1921 at the fifth annual meeting of the National Society for the Promotion of Occupational Therapy in Baltimore, Meyer delivered the keynote address. "The Philosophy of Occupational Therapy" was later published in the organization's first journal in 1922. In his keynote address he stated that:

There are many . . . rhythms which we must be attuned to: the larger rhythms of night and day, of sleep and waking hours . . . and finally the big four—work and play and rest and sleep, which our organism must be able to balance even under difficulty.
The only way to attain balance in all this is actual doing, actual practice, a program of wholesome living as the basis of wholesome feeling and thinking and fancy and interests.[15]

Adolph Meyer provided the initial foundational philosophical statement for the profession. Examination of political, social, and cultural events that shaped the profession follows.

Box 2-1

Dunton's Principles of Occupational Therapy

Any activity should have a cure as its objective.
The activity should be interesting.
There should be a useful purpose other than to merely gain the patient's attention and interest.
The activity should preferably lead to an increase in knowledge on the patient's part.
Activity should be carried on with others, such as a group.
The occupational therapist should make a careful study of the patient and attempt to meet as many needs as possible through activity.
Activity should cease before the onset of fatigue.
Genuine encouragement should be given whenever indicated.
Work is much to be preferred over idleness, even when the end product of the patient's labor is of poor quality or is useless.

From Dunton WR: The principles of occupational therapy. In Proceedings of the National Society for the Promotion of Occupational Therapy: Second annual meeting, Catonsville, MD, 1918, Spring Grove State Hospital Press.

World War I

Along with the use of occupations for the "insane" and the early sheltered workshops for convalescent individuals, such as Barton's Consolation House, **World War I** and the creation of **reconstruction aides** served to influence the profession.

In May 1917, 1 month following President Woodrow Wilson's declaration of war, the U.S. military initiated a reconstruction program. The purpose of the program was to rehabilitate soldiers who had been injured in the war so that they could either return to active military duty or be employed in a civilian job. The program was placed under the direction of orthopedic professionals and included occupational therapy aides, as well as physiotherapy aides and vocational evaluators. In early 1918 on a trial basis, the program began at Walter Reed Hospital in Washington, DC, with a group of physiotherapy aides and occupational therapy aides who were civilian women with no military ranking.[9] The physiotherapy aides used techniques such as massage and exercise in their therapy, and they worked primarily with orthopedic patients, whereas the occupational therapy aides used arts and crafts to treat the mind and the body.[17] OTs worked with both orthopedic and psychiatric patients.

Several training programs were implemented, and hundreds of women were trained to be practitioners. The program was also implemented overseas when the first group of reconstruction aides was sent to France to assist in the rehabilitation of soldiers. Under appalling working conditions—no rank, no uniforms, no materials or equipment, no prepared working areas—the reconstruction aides demonstrated to the Army that involvement in activities had a beneficial effect on hospitalized soldiers suffering from "shell shock."[14] The approach proved to be beneficial to the Army, and the demand for the aides' services increased throughout the war.

As the need for reconstruction aides increased, so did the need for training. Not only did existing schools and hospitals add quick training courses, but also new schools were created to meet the need. Typically, the programs consisted of instruction in arts and crafts, medical lectures, and hospital etiquette, as well as practical experience in a hospital or clinic. Although only a high school diploma was required, many of the women accepted into these programs had previous training in social work, in teaching, or in the arts.[17] Many supporters of occupational therapy viewed this as an opportunity to expand the field. Others (including Susan Cox Johnson) felt that the training programs were hastily developed in response to the war, and they were concerned about the proficiency of the newly trained practitioners.

The war ended in November 1918, and many of the women who trained to become reconstruction aides left the field. Only a small percentage of the aides were actually OTs. Others eventually became OTs, and some went back to their prior roles (e.g., artist, teacher).[14] Many of the training programs closed.

Reconstruction aides showed the validity of activity as therapy and linked occupational therapy with physical disabilities.

Post–World War I Through the 1930s

Rehabilitation remained important after the war. Two pieces of federal legislation provided the impetus for the development or expansion of vocational rehabilitation programs that often included OT practitioners. The Smith-Sears Veterans Rehabilitation Act of 1918, also known as the **Soldier's Rehabilitation Act,** established a program of vocational rehabilitation for soldiers disabled on active duty. Injured soldiers returned home, and OT practitioners had a role helping soldiers adjust to their "industrial responsibilities" in civilian life. OT practitioners focused on rehabilitating the soldiers so they could return to productive living.

In 1920, Congress passed the Smith-Fess Act, also known as the **Civilian Vocational Rehabilitation Act** (PL 66-236). This act provided federal funds to states on a 50-50 matching basis to provide vocational rehabilitation services to civilians with physical disabilities. To be eligible for benefits, applicants for the program had to be unable, because of their disability, to engage "successfully" in "gainful employment." Funds were provided for vocational guidance, training, occupational adjustment, prosthetics, and placement services. The passage of the Smith-Hughes and Smith-Sears Acts was the beginning of the federal government's involvement in funding health care services. Occupational therapy became valued as a provider of some of these prevocational and rehabilitation services.

Another important area of growth for occupational therapy during this time was in treating and caring for patients with tuberculosis. Thomas Kidner was instrumental in promoting occupational therapy services for vocational rehabilitation and tuberculosis treatment. Tuberculosis sanatoriums employed OTs all across the country.

The Great Depression, from 1930 to 1939, affected all aspects of society, including the health care fields. It slowed the development of occupational therapy, bringing department closures and reductions of occupational therapy staff positions. Schools closed, and membership in the association decreased. Attention to rehabilitative care, which began with World War I, did not reemerge until World War II brought new and similar needs.

Progress of the Profession

In 1921, the membership voted to change the name of the National Society for the Promotion of Occupational Therapy to the **American Occupational Therapy Association (AOTA).** The profession continued to grow and evolve under this new name.

Minimum Standards Adopted for Training

Several of the emergency schools set up to provide training during the war remained open in the 1920s and attempted to recruit practitioners to the new profession. The training courses varied considerably from one another. Furthermore, the heterogeneous nature of the existing workforce (arts and crafts instructors, reconstruction aides, and some college-educated practitioners) called for the development of a workforce that was uniform so that occupational therapy could advance as a profession.[17] At the time, there were eight occupational therapy schools in the United States. The first *Minimum Standards for Courses of Training in Occupational Therapy* was adopted in 1923 by the membership of AOTA. The standards included prerequisites for admission into training programs, length of courses, and content of courses. The standards stipulated that courses of training for OTs needed to be a minimum of 1 year, with 8 or 9 months of medical and craft training and 3 or 4 months of clinical work in hospitals. Lacking any legal ability to close schools that did not meet the standards, the association endorsed those schools that met the standards. These standards were revised twice by AOTA during the 1920s, with each revision requiring more training.

In 1929, AOTA decided to establish a national registry that identified practitioners who had graduated from schools that the association endorsed.[1] The registry began on January 1, 1931. In 1935, the American Medical Association (AMA), at the request of AOTA, assumed the inspection and accreditation of occupational therapy schools. Five schools were accredited in 1938. This collaboration with the AMA continued until 1994, when it was determined that the profession of occupational therapy should be responsible for accrediting and monitoring its own educational programs.

Growth Through Publication

An emphasis upon publication shaped the profession of occupational therapy and continued to mold its emerging character. Within 5 years of the organization's founding, it published a journal devoted to the profession. Dunton, who published on the use of occupation for treatment purposes, served as the editor for the *Archives of Occupational Therapy* from 1922–1947. The journal name changed to *Occupational Therapy and Rehabilitation* in 1925 and *American Journal of Occupational Therapy* in 1947.[18] The journal has become known informally as *AJOT* (pronounced a-jot). Since, 1925 membership in the national organization has included a journal subscription.

The postwar period allowed occupational therapy to became closely coupled with medicine and the medical model of education. This led to the beginning of specialization and of a more scientific approach. It set the stage for attempts by physical medicine to control the developing profession of occupational therapy. On one hand, the support occupational therapy had received from physicians was instrumental in the growth of the profession. On the other hand, the profession's unique philosophy based on occupation and a holistic perspective was threatened by the **reductionistic** views of medicine at the time.

World War II: 1940-1947

World War II created a new demand for more OTs. Because they had not achieved military status during World War I, few OTs were employed in the Army or in Army hospitals when World War II broke out.[10] Initially, the War Department required OTs to be graduates of an accredited school. However, the educational requirements took 18 months to complete, which was too long for the Army to wait to get trained OTs.[10] Once again, War Emergency Courses were implemented to quickly train needed OTs. As a result, the number of employed practitioners increased significantly. AOTA data indicate that in 1945 there were 2177 members.

Beginning in 1945, successful completion of an examination became a requirement for registering as an OT practitioner. The examination was initially in essay format; in 1947, it adopted the format of in objective test.

Post–World War II: 1950s-1960s

The occupational therapy profession changed quickly and in numerous ways after WWII. Overall, there was a continued shift away from a generalist approach to one of specialization in physical rehabilitation.

New Drugs and Technology

The discovery of neuroleptic drugs (tranquilizers and antipsychotics) in the mid-1950s changed the course of psychiatric treatment. As psychotic behavior yielded to chemical control, it became possible to discharge many people, eventually leading to a national plan to release clients—the national **Deinstitutionalization** Plan. In anticipation of local care needs, community mental health programs were developed.

New technologies were developed, such as splinting materials, wheelchairs, and more advanced prosthetics and orthotics. Special training was required for OT practitioners who would be using this new therapeutic material and equipment.

Rehabilitation Movement

The time from 1942 to 1960 is often called the period of the **Rehabilitation Movement.**[16] The Veterans Administration (VA) hospitals increased in size and number to handle the casualties of war and continued care of veterans. The VA hospitals, which had employed OTs in psychiatric and tuberculosis units since its beginnings in 1921, developed physical medicine and rehabilitation departments to serve veterans with physical disabilities. OTs were employed in these departments. After the war, in 1947, the U.S. Army established the Women's Medical Specialist Corps. Women in the fields of occupational therapy, physical therapy, and dietetics, who had been classified as civilian employees during the war, were commissioned as officers of the Army. The Corps later became the Army Medical Specialist Corps to allow men and women to serve as commissioned officers in the military. The Korean War that began in 1950 called for the continuation of Army hospitals with active occupational therapy departments.

Growth in health care was not limited to the Veterans Administration. Due to the polio epidemic and new medical procedures and antibiotics that were saving lives, more individuals were living with disabilities. Facilities and services were needed to meet the needs of individuals with disabilities. The Hill-Burton Act assisted states in determining what hospitals and health care facilities were needed and provided grants to states to construct these facilities. OTs were hired as one type of rehabilitation professional. They were teaching patients activities of daily living, designing orthotic devices, training patients how to use prosthetics, using progressive resistive exercise, introducing muscle reeducation techniques, and evaluating patients' vocational aptitudes and abilities.[16]

Federally Mandated Health Care

Medicare (PL 89-97) was enacted in 1965, and it increased the demand for occupational therapy services. Under Medicare guidelines, those who are 65 years of age or older or those who are permanently and totally disabled receive assistance in paying for their health care. It covers occupational therapy services in the inpatient setting and limited coverage for outpatient services. Initially, this legislation did not provide for services provided by OT practitioners in independent practice settings. In 1988, legislation granted OTs the right to Medicare provider numbers, permitting direct reimbursement for occupational therapy services.

Changes in the Profession

The 1950s and 1960s brought organizational changes to AOTA to improve both the overall function of and the membership representation in the ever-growing and expanding organization. The American Occupational Therapy Foundation (AOTF) was founded in 1965 to promote research in occupational therapy through financial support.[1] AOTA and AOTF are discussed further in Chapter 6.

A shift in practice to physical rehabilitation and working with individuals with severe disabilities required practitioners to expand their knowledge. Services that were once based on occupation and arts and crafts changed to a more technical focus, using modalities particular to the area of specialization. OT faculty decreased the emphasis on teaching of arts and crafts and focused on a medical and scientific approach. Leaders of the profession spoke out against specialization and encouraged the profession to return to its roots of occupation. However, the trend toward the reductionistic model and specialization would continue through the 1960s.

New Level of Practitioner: The Occupational Therapy Assistant

With an increasing number of OTs practicing in medical and rehabilitation facilities, there was a shortage of therapists working in psychiatric settings. Aides and technicians working under OT practitioners in psychiatric settings became knowledgeable in the intervention techniques used.

As Shirley Holland Carr reports, "Supportive personnel knew how to do things, but lacked goal-oriented intervention methods necessary to work without immediate supervision."[7]

This led to the development of a new level of practitioner, the occupational therapy assistant (OTA). The first 3-month educational program for OTAs began in 1958 in psychiatry, and a second course for general practice was offered in 1960. Initially, these training programs were based in hospitals. Later, the programs were offered in technical schools and community colleges. The first directory of OTAs was published in 1961 and listed 553 names.[3] Although the introduction of this new level of practitioner was a major milestone for the profession, there was a lack of agreement as to the appropriate roles of the OT and the OTA.

1970s Through 1980s

This period of time included the introduction of personal computers, a substantial increase in drug and alcohol abuse, and the appearance of a new disease with no known cure, acquired immune deficiency syndrome (AIDS). The Deinstitutionalization Plan gained acceptance and was implemented across the United States. Consequently, individuals who previously resided in mental hospitals and facilities for the developmentally delayed were transferred from these institutions to smaller community facilities. Many of the large state institutions closed. Some services were developed in communities to support these individuals, but overall there was a lack of services to support these individuals. As a result, many individuals with chronic mental illness and intellectual deficits (previously referred to as mental retardation) ended up homeless, which remains an issue today.

Several important pieces of legislation for persons with disabilities were passed by the U.S. Congress in the 1970s and 1980s: the Rehabilitation Act of 1973, the Education for All Handicapped Children Act of 1975, the Handicapped Infants and Toddlers Act of 1986, and the Technology Related Assistance for Individuals with Disabilities Act of 1988.

The **Rehabilitation Act of 1973** came during a time of great social change and unrest. Persons with disabilities, inspired by the civil rights movement of the 1960s, became a new force and exerted significant influence on rehabilitation legislation. The Rehabilitation Act of 1973 established several important principles. First, the Act emphasized priority service for persons with the most severe disabilities and mandated that state agencies establish an order of selection that would place the most severely disabled person first for service. Second, under the Act, every client accepted for services participates in the service planning process by completing an Individualized Written Rehabilitation Program (IWRP) that specifies their vocational goal and key supporting objectives, such as physical restoration, counseling, educational preparation, work adjustment, and vocational training. Third, the Act called for the development of a set of standards by which the impact of rehabilitation services could be assessed. Fourth, the Act emphasized the need for rehabilitation research. Finally, it included civil rights provisions that gave equal opportunity for people with disabilities. It prohibited discrimination in employment or in admissions criteria to academic programs solely on the basis of a disabling condition.

OT practitioners' work with children in schools emerged during this time as another specialty area, aided in part by the passage of the **Education for All Handicapped Children Act of 1975** (PL 94-142). This act establishes the right of all children to a free and appropriate education, regardless of handicapping condition. This law includes occupational therapy as a related service. Before the passage of PL 94-142, many children with disabilities did not attend school or receive therapy services. This law requires a written individual education plan (IEP) for each student, that describes the student's specialized program and measurable goals. The **Handicapped Infants and Toddlers Act** (PL 99-457) was passed in 1986 as an amendment to the Education for All Handicapped Children Act. The amendment extends the provision of PL 94-142 to include children from 3 to 5 years of age and initiates new early intervention programs for children from birth to 3 years of age. Occupational therapy is considered a primary service. These two laws increased occupational therapy services provided to children and the number of OT personnel employed within the school environment.

The **Technology Related Assistance for Individuals with Disabilities Act of 1988** (PL 100-407) addresses the availability of assistive technology devices and services to individuals with disabilities. Many OT practitioners are involved in providing these services.

These pieces of legislation increased the demand for occupational therapy services. However, the 1970s also saw rises in the cost of health care. The 1980s brought about changes in the health care system in an attempt to contain health care costs.

Prospective Payment System

In 1983, President Reagan made a fundamental change to the way in which health care dollars were dispersed by signing the **Social Security Amendments** into law. Up until this point, hospitals were reimbursed based on the actual cost of services provided. With the implementation of the Medicare **Prospective Payment System (PPS)** created by these amendments, a nationwide schedule was established that delineated what the government would pay for each inpatient stay of a Medicare beneficiary. The level of payment is set by descriptive categories according to the individual's diagnosis, called diagnosis-related groupings, or DRGs. In this system of fixed payment for DRGs, massive changes in hospital organization and care delivery occurred. Most notably, patient length of stay in acute care hospitals was shortened, and there was an increased use of long-term care facilities and home health services.

Gary Kielhofner: Return to Occupation

"Life takes on meaning in the minute-by-minute reality in which experience ourselves achieving the ordinary things."

Dr. Gary Kielhofner (February 15, 1949–September 2, 2010) developed the Model of Human Occupation (MOHO) as a graduate student under the supervision of Dr. Mary Reilly, a professor of occupational therapy at the University of Southern California. (See Figure 2-3.) Over 30 years, Dr. Kielhofner further developed and refined this model.[12,23] Dr. Kielhofner was a prolific scholar who published 19 textbooks and over 150 journal articles. He listened to feedback from students, colleagues, and clinicians to develop a model that would allow OT practitioners at all levels to better address the important issues concerning their clients. In so doing, Dr. Kielhofner provided the profession with evidence to support occupation-based practice and tools (21 assessments) to evaluate clients. MOHO is the most evidence-based model of practice in occupational therapy.[12,24,25] At the time of this writing, there were over 254 research-based articles published on MOHO. Dr. Kielhofner never lost sight of his goal to make a difference in the lives of those with disabilities. He was a visionary who promoted the field of occupational therapy through the quality of his scholarship.

Dr. Kielhofner received his bachelors degree in psychology from St. Louis University. He earned his Master's degree in occupational therapy and doctoral degree in public health from the University of Southern California.

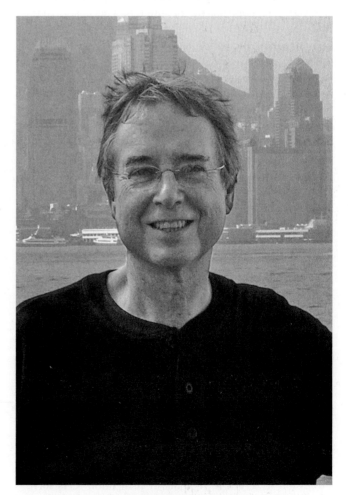

Figure 2-3 Gary Kielhofner, DrPH, OTR/L, FAOTA.

He held faculty appointments at Boston University, and Virginia Commonwealth University, and most recently University of Illinois at Chicago, where he served as Professor and Wade Meyer Chair for 30 years. Dr. Kielhofner furthered the scholarship of practice model to bridge the gap between practice and academics, by engaging in participatory research work with the community. The *Scholarship of Practice* model helped develop effective programming and research supporting the use of MOHO in practice and making a difference in many clients' lives. Notably, Dr. Kielhofner worked to help persons with HIV/AIDS re-engage in meaningful occupations and experience quality of life. With colleagues from around the world, he designed programs to help those with mental illness, children, and adults with physical disabilities. He was a dynamic leader who encouraged all to achieve. Dr. Kielhofner mentored numerous students, practitioners, and faculty around the world, always encouraging and inspiring others to excel. His creativity, passion, and energy helped move the profession forward to benefit clients. His legacy will continue as the profession embodies occupation-based practice.

Advances at AOTA

AOTA expended great efforts to ensure that occupational therapy would be appropriately included in the onslaught of new federal governmental legislation directed at the delivery of health care. Lobbying for the interests of occupational therapy became a function of AOTA during the 1970s and 1980s and remains an important aspect of the association's role.

In the 1980s, AOTA moved into its own building, thus signifying a new era that began to yield results of AOTA's long-standing emphasis on research. This decade witnessed a wealth of new books and publications, including a new research journal, the *Occupational Therapy Journal of Research*. There was also growth in the number of educational programs that offered a graduate degree.

In 1986, AOTA separated professional membership and certification procedures by declaring the association no longer responsible for board certification. Instead, on completion of all requirements, an OT practitioner is certified through the National Board for Certification in Occupational Therapy (NBCOT®), subject to certification regulations; AOTA membership is separate and voluntary.

State Regulation of Occupational Therapy

State regulatory legislation became a controversial issue of the 1970s. Individual states began to introduce laws requiring that OT practitioners become licensed in order to practice. AOTA's Representative Assembly supported state licensing to ensure quality occupational therapy services in 1975. (Regulation and licensure are discussed in detail in Chapter 6.)

A Return to the Roots of the Profession: Occupation

By the 1970s, there was a large contingent of OTs urging the profession to return to its roots in occupation. OTs such as Mary Reilly, Elizabeth Yerxa, Phil Shannon, and Gail Fidler

called upon therapists to reject the practices of reductionism and return to the principles of moral treatment and occupation. Shannon described the "derailment of occupational therapy."[20] He observed that there were two philosophies in conflict with each other. One, based on the philosophy of moral treatment, held a holistic and humanistic view of the individual. The other saw the individual as a "mechanistic creature susceptible to manipulation and control via the application of techniques."[20] He further noted that "If OT persists in this direction, what was once and still is one of the great ideas of 20th century medicine will be swept away by the tide of technique philosophy."[20]

There was growing realization that something needed to be done. Occupational therapy was lacking a science unique to occupation, theories of practice, and research that demonstrated the effectiveness of occupational therapy. It was during this time that different theories and models for occupational therapy started to emerge. One such model is the Model of Human Occupation that was developed by Kielhofner and his associates.[12] Occupational science, a basic science that supports occupational practice, also emerged.[23]

1990s to the Present

The Information Age, characterized by technologies, including cell phones, faxes, personal computer applications, and the networking of computers, allows individuals to have immediate access to news and world events without leaving the chair. In occupational therapy, computer technology is used as an intervention modality, such as the use of computer software that is used to retrain cognitive skills. Billing and documentation of services are typically done on a computer. The overall effects of the Information Age on society in general, and health care in particular, are yet to be seen.

The societal climate includes two-income families as the norm. The number of individuals living with disabilities is increasing, as is the number of individuals over 65 years of age. The population in the United States is becoming ever more culturally diverse, and many individuals and families cannot afford the cost of health care.

One of the most significant pieces of legislation to pass during the 1990s was the **Americans with Disabilities Act of 1990** (ADA) (PL 101-336). The ADA provides civil rights to all individuals with disabilities. It guarantees equal access to and opportunity in employment, transportation, public accommodations, state and local government, and telecommunications for individuals with disabilities. OT personnel provide consultation to private and public agencies to assist them in meeting these guidelines.

The Education for All Handicapped Children Act, Public Law 94-142 (1975), was reauthorized and renamed the **Individuals with Disabilities Education Act (IDEA)** in 1991. IDEA requires school districts to educate students with disabilities in the least restrictive environment (LRE). Specifically, the IDEA requires states to establish procedures assuring that students with disabilities are educated, to the maximum extent appropriate, with students without disabilities. IDEA also mandates that the local school district is responsible for providing assistive technology devices and related services as deemed appropriate to the child's education. In 1997, the president signed the Individuals with Disabilities Education Act Amendments of 1997, Public Law 105-17. The Individuals with Disabilities Education Act Amendments of 1997 (IDEA 97) further improves the educational opportunities for children with disabilities. The focus of IDEA 97 is on improving educational results for children with disabilities. The law stipulates that the assistive technology needs of children with disabilities must be considered along with other special factors by the Individualized Education Plan (IEP) team in formulating the child's IEP. IDEA 97 also strengthens the role of parents in educational planning and decision-making on behalf of their children. IDEA defines occupational therapy as a related service that can be provided to a student to enable him or her to participate in and benefit from the educational process.

In the medical arena, occupational therapy services are restricted by what insurance companies will cover, and managed care continues in efforts to contain spiraling health care costs. OTs and OTAs have had to continuously adapt to the regulations and reimbursement limitations affecting the health care environment. Furthermore, health care practitioners struggle on a daily basis with ethical questions related to the allocation of health care services.

The intent of the **Balanced Budget Act of 1997 (BBA)** was to reduce Medicare spending, create incentives for the development of managed care plans, encourage enrollment in managed care plans, and limit fee-for-service payment and programs. Under Medicare Part B Outpatient Rehabilitation Benefit, there is an annual $1500 cap per person receiving occupational therapy services, and a separate $1500 cap per person for physical therapy and speech-language pathology services combined. Currently, AOTA is working to extend the moratorium.

The uncertainty around the BBA has forced practitioners to broaden their horizons and look beyond traditional areas of practice. More therapists are working in community-based programs, and the job market is on the upswing. The Bureau of Labor Statistics (BLS) predicts that employment for OTs is projected to increase faster than the average for all occupations (21% to 35%). Employment of OTAs is expected to grow much faster than average (increase 36% or more) through 2012. The BLS expects the demand of OT practitioners to rise due to growth in the number of individuals with disabilities or limited function, the baby-boom generation's movement into middle age (when incidence of heart attacks and stroke increases), and growth in the population 75 years of age and older. All of these populations will require therapy services.[22] To help meet the challenges associated with the costs of providing services to an aging population, the Centers for Disease Control has encouraged community organizations and public health agencies to include health promotion among older adults, prevention of disability, maintenance of capacity, and enhancement of quality of life in

their scope.[8] These are all areas in which occupational therapy can have a role.

Occupational Therapy Entry-Level Education, Continuing Competence, and Recertification

Ongoing issues for the profession include the need to develop scientists in the profession to conduct research, the need for gathering and disseminating occupational therapy research, the application of evidence-based knowledge in practice, and continuing competency of practitioners.

Baccalaureate programs in occupational therapy will be phased out by 2017, and students will be required to have a graduate degree to be eligible to take the certification exam. This requirement will result in the training of OTs who have the knowledge and skills to be competent in today's practice environment and to be consumers of research. As of December 2010, the Accreditation Council for Occupational Therapy Education listed 153 accredited occupational therapy programs and 129 (160) accredited OTA programs.[25]

State licensure laws typically require evidence that the practitioner is keeping current in the field. The Commission on Continuing Competence and Professional Development (CCCPD) was put in place by AOTA in May 2002 to recommend standards for continuing competence and to develop strategies for communicating information to OT practitioners and consumers about issues of continuing competency affecting occupational therapy. NBCOT® also recently implemented recertification, which requires the completion of professional development units to maintain certification as an OT or OTA.

Occupation-Based Practice

It is an exhilarating time to be practicing in occupational therapy. The richness and complexity of occupation and evidence of its impact on clients are documented through research. Academic leaders in the profession are creating a science of occupation, developing theories to guide practice, identifying best practices by examining evidence-based practice, and generating research that demonstrates the effectiveness of occupational therapy.[19]

In May 2008, the AOTA adopted a revised framework of practice for the profession. The *Occupational Therapy Practice Framework: Domain and Process*[2] delineates language and concepts that describe the focus of the profession. The document is meant to be used by OT practitioners to examine current practice and to consider emerging practice areas. It was also written to assist external audiences, such as third-party payers, in understanding occupational therapy's unique focus on supporting function and health and the process by which that is achieved. The new practice framework reflects a return to our roots because it is centered on the use of occupation to support participation in life.

As history demonstrates, occupational therapy is a dynamic and ever-evolving profession. Many of the issues that have been identified in this final period will continue to evolve. The profession and practice of occupational therapy will remain responsive to societal, cultural, and political needs.

Summary

By studying the history of occupational therapy, we gain knowledge that will enhance our current practice. Occupational therapy grew out of the rising social consciousness of the early twentieth century and became a profession in March 1917. It evolved out of Moral Treatment in psychiatric facilities, rehabilitation in sanitariums, and restoration for soldiers injured in battle. The profession views the use of occupation as a course of treatment. Changes in society have often meant changes in the profession. Occupational therapy has evolved through merging theory and research while focusing on health and function. As a field of practice, occupational therapy's history of a holistic approach and use of occupation make it unique from other health care services.

Learning Activities

1. Refer to Box 2-1 and Dunton's Principles of Occupational Therapy. How could you update these principles to reflect current occupational therapy practice?
2. Research and write a short paper on the Moral Treatment Movement of the 1800s.
3. Compile short biographies on the founders of occupational therapy by reading three or four sources.
4. Search back volumes of the *American Journal of Occupational Therapy* (and the older *Archives of Occupational Therapy* and *Occupational Therapy and Rehabilitation*, if available).
5. Use lists of article titles to show the changes in emphasis from decade to decade.
6. Research and write a short paper on any single social influence, legislation, or technical development. Elaborate on how the event affected the practice and profession of occupational therapy.
7. Research and make a wall chart with a time line that depicts significant events and changes in AOTA since its inception.

Review Questions

1. What major social influences gave rise to the field of occupational therapy?
2. Who are some of the key people involved in the evolution of the occupational therapy profession?
3. What key concepts have persisted throughout the history of occupational therapy?
4. How has the profession changed over time?
5. What are some key pieces of federal legislation that have influenced the practice of occupational therapy?

References

1. American Occupational Therapy Association: *History of AOTA accreditation*. Retrieved January 25, 2011, from http://www.aota.org/Educate/Accredit/Overview/38124.aspx.
2. American Occupational Therapy Association: Occupational therapy practice framework: Domain and process, ed 2, *Am J Occup Ther* 62:625–683, 2008.
3. American Occupational Therapy Association: *Directory Certified Occupational Therapy Assistants for the Year 1961*, New York, 1961, American Occupational Therapy Association.
4. Bing R: Looking back, living forward: Occupational therapy history. In Sladyk K, Ryan SE, editors: *Ryan's Occupational Therapy Assistant: Principles, Practice Issues and Techniques*, ed 4, Thorofare, NJ, 2005, Slack.
5. Bing R: Living forward, understanding backward. In Ryan S, editor: *The Certified Occupational Therapy Assistant: Principles, Concepts, and Techniques*, ed 2, Thorofare, NJ, 1993, Slack.
6. Bing R: Occupational therapy revisited: A paraphrasatic journey, *Am J Occup Ther* 35(8):499, 1981.
7. Carr SH: The COTA heritage: Proud, practical, stable, dynamic. In Sladyk K, Ryan SE, editors: *Ryan's Occupational Therapy Assistant: Principles, Practice Issues and Techniques*, ed 4, Thorofare, NJ, 2005, Slack.
8. Centers for Disease Control and Prevention: Public health and aging: Trends in aging—United States and worldwide, *Morb Mortal Wkly Rep* 52(6):101–106, 2003. Retrieved January 25, 2011, from http://www.cdc.gov/mmwr/preview/mmwrhtml/mm5206a2.htm.
9. Gutman SA: Looking back—influence of the US military and occupational therapy reconstruction aides in World War I on the development of occupational therapy, *Am J Occup Ther* 49:256, 1995.
10. The Historical Unit, U.S. Army Medical Department: *Medical Department, United States Army Medical Training in World War II*, Washington, D.C., Office of the Surgeon General, Department of the Army, 1974. Retrieved January 25, 2011, from http://history.amedd.army.mil/booksdocs/wwii/medtrain/default.htm.
11. Kidner TJ: Occupational therapy: Its development, scope, and possibilities, *Occup Ther Rehabil* 10:3, 1931.
12. Kielhofner G: *A Model of Human Occupation*, Baltimore, MD, 1985, Williams & Wilkins.
13. Licht S: The founding and founders of the American Occupational Therapy Association, *Am J Occup Ther* 21:269, 1967.
14. Low JF: The reconstruction aides, *Am J Occup Ther* 46:38, 1992.
15. Meyer A: The philosophy of occupation therapy, *Arch Occup Ther* 1:1, 1922. (Reprinted in *Am J Occup Ther* 31:10, 1977.)
16. Punwar AJ, Peloquin SM: *Occupational Therapy Principles and Practice*, ed 3, Baltimore, 2000, Lippincott Williams & Wilkins.
17. Quiroga V: *Occupational Therapy: The First 30 Years 1900 to 1930*, Bethesda, MD, 1995, American Occupational Therapy Association.
18. Reed KL, Sanderson SR: *Concepts of Occupational Therapy*, ed 4, Philadelphia, 1999, Lippincott Williams & Wilkins.
19. Schwartz KB: History of occupation. In Kramer P, Hinojosa J, Royeen CB, editors: *Perspectives in Human Occupation: Participation in Life*, Baltimore, 2003, Lippincott Williams & Wilkins.
20. Shannon PD: The derailment of OT, *Am J Occup Ther* 31(229):1977.

21. Tracy SE: *Studies in Invalid Occupation* reprint. Charleston, SC, 2010, BiblioBazaar.
22. Yerxa E: An introduction to occupational science: A foundation for OT in the 21st century, *OT Health Care* 6(4):3, 1989.
23. Kielhofner G: *A Model of Human Occupation: Theory and application*, ed 4, Baltimore, 2008, Lippincott Williams & Wilkins.
24. Haglund L, Ekbladh E, Thorell LH, et al: Practice models in Swedish psychiatric occupational therapy, *Scand J Occup Ther* 7:107–113, 2000.
25. National Board for Certification in Occupational Therapy: A practice analysis study of entry-level occupational therapist registered and certified occupational therapy assistant practice, *Occup Ther J Res: Occup, Particip, and Health* 24(Suppl 1):S1–S31, 2004.

Occupational therapy is by far the most unique of allied health care professions. The delicate balance of art, science, and human interaction on which the profession is based contributes not only to this uniqueness but also to the obvious effectiveness of occupational therapy intervention throughout the life span.

GLEN GILLEN, EdD, OTR, FAOTA
Assistant Professor in Clinical Occupational Therapy
Columbia University
New York, New York

CHAPTER 3

Philosophical Principles and Values in Occupational Therapy

Key Terms

Active being
Activity
Adaptation
Altruism
Axiology
Client-centered approach
Dignity
Epistemology
Equality
Freedom
Holistic approach
Humanism
Justice
Metaphysical
Occupation
Occupation as a means
Occupation as an end
Occupational performance
Phenomenological
Professional philosophy
Prudence
Quality of life
Role
Reductionistic
Task
Truthfulness

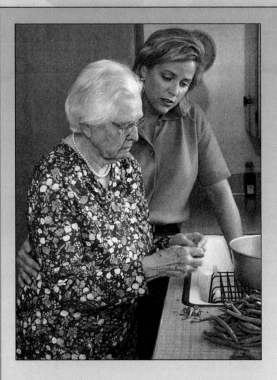

Objectives

After reading this chapter, the reader will be able to do the following:

- Understand the importance of a profession's philosophical base
- Describe the general components of a philosophy
- Describe the philosophy of occupational therapy (OT)
- Articulate occupational therapy's view of humankind
- Explain the meaning of *occupation* in the context of the profession and understand its role in occupational performance and well-being
- Name the values of the profession
- Describe adaptation as used in occupational therapy
- Distinguish between occupation as a means and occupation as an end
- Describe the client-centered approach and its relevance to occupational therapy

Students in occupational therapy (OT) or occupational therapy assistant (OTA) programs will better understand the profession when they are familiar with its philosophical base. A **professional philosophy** refers to the set of values, beliefs, truths, and principles that guide the practitioner's actions. As such, the OT philosophy defines the nature of the profession, guides the actions of practitioners,

and supports the profession's domains. Theories, models of practice, frames of reference, and intervention approaches that guide OT practice are derived from the profession's philosophy.

This chapter begins with a general description of philosophy before examining OT philosophy and describing the core concepts of occupational therapy practice.

Understanding Philosophy

Philosophy refers to a set of basic principles or concepts underlying somebody's practice or conduct.[20] Philosophy of a profession can be divided into three areas of concern—metaphysical, epistemology, and axiology—which seek to address questions concerning the values and beliefs of the profession.[16] **Metaphysical** refers to questions concerned with the nature of humankind. **Epistemology** is related to the "nature, origin, and limits of human knowledge"[16] and investigates questions such as "How do we know things?" and "How do we know that we know? **Axiology** is concerned with the study of values. Therefore, this area explores questions of desirability and questions of ethics (e.g., "What are the standards and rules of right conduct?").[16] Using these questions as guidelines and the core concepts of occupational therapy as guidelines, the philosophical base of the occupational therapy profession can be examined.

Philosophical Base of Occupational Therapy

The philosophical base of occupational therapy was adopted in 1979 and reaffirmed in 2004 (Box 3-1). Examining occupational therapy in terms of the metaphysical, epistemology, and axiology components provides a framework to understand the philosophical base of occupational therapy (Figure 3-1). The core concepts of occupational therapy operationalize the philosophy of the profession (Box 3-2).

Box 3-1

The Philosophical Base of Occupational Therapy

Man is an active being whose development is influenced by the use of purposeful activity. Using their capacity for intrinsic motivation, human beings are able to influence their physical and mental health and their social and physical environment through purposeful activity. Human life includes a process of continuous adaptation. Adaptation is a change in function that promotes survival and self-actualization. Biological, psychological, and environmental factors may interrupt the adaptation process at any time throughout the life cycle. Dysfunction may occur when adaptation is impaired. Purposeful activity facilitates the adaptive process.

Occupational therapy is based on the belief that purposeful activity (occupation), including its interpersonal and environmental components, may be used to prevent and mediate dysfunction and to elicit maximum adaptation. Activity as used by the therapist includes both an intrinsic and a therapeutic purpose.

From American Occupational Therapy Association: The philosophical base of occupational therapy, *Am J Occup Ther* 49:1026, 1995. Reviewed by COE and COP in 2004.

What Is Humankind?

The metaphysical component of philosophy examines the question, "What is humankind?" This philosophical question becomes the basis for a profession designed to enhance a person's ability to engage in life.

Occupational Therapy Views Humans Holistically

The U.S. health care system uses a **reductionistic** approach, wherein humankind is reduced to separately functioning body parts. Professionals specialize in specific areas and treat these body functions independently for greater expediency and efficiency; their purpose is to isolate, define, and treat body functions and to focus on a specific problem. The reductionistic approach has been successful in producing cures and technological developments. However, clients remain frustrated with health care systems that are inefficient and costly. Therefore, many medical practitioners are returning to approaches that allow them to address all of the bodily functions of the client (i.e., the family practitioner approach).

Since its beginning, occupational therapy has adhered to a **holistic approach.** The holistic perspective can be traced to Adolf Meyer. In *The Philosophy of Occupation Therapy*, he states, "Our body is not merely so many pounds of flesh and bone figuring as a machine, with an abstract mind or soul added to it. [Rather, it is a live organism acting] in harmony with its own nature and the nature about it."[10] The holistic approach emphasizes the organic and functional relationship between the parts and the whole being. This approach maintains that a person is a whole—an interaction of biological, psychological, sociocultural, and spiritual elements. If any element (or subsystem) is negatively affected, a disruption or disturbance will be reflected throughout the whole.

Belief in a holistic approach is a core concept of the OT profession. This means that evaluations and intervention plans should reflect the needs of the whole person. OT practitioners treating only the body (or parts of the body) or only the mind, are not following the commitment to holism.[2,10,12] In such cases, the consumer is denied one of the unique aspects of occupational therapy: the holistic approach.

Occupational Therapy Views Humans as Active Beings for Whom Occupation Is Critical to Well-Being

Occupational therapy views humans as **active beings.** Humans are actively involved in controlling and determining their own behavior and are capable of changing behavior as desired.[12] Furthermore, humans are viewed as open systems in which there is continuous interaction between the person and the environment. The person's behaviors influence the physical and social environment; in turn, the person is affected by changes in the environment.

Occupation refers to "the ordinary and familiar things that people do every day."[1] It is the term used to "capture the breadth and meaning of 'everyday life activity.'"[1]

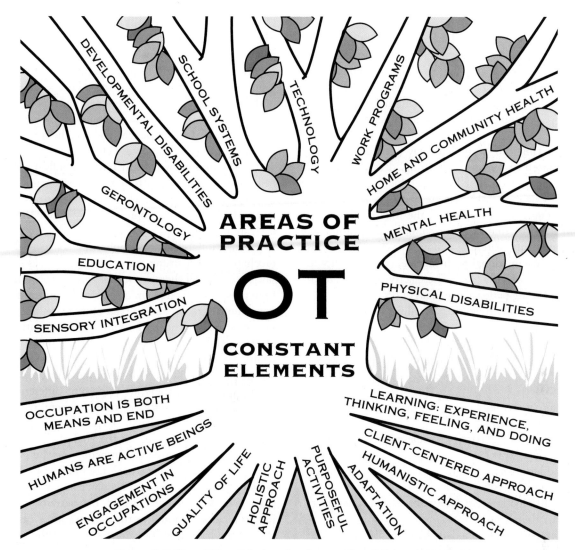

Figure 3-1 The philosophical roots of occupational therapy practice.

Core Concepts of Occupational Therapy

- Occupational therapy views humans holistically.
- Occupational therapy views humans as active beings wherein occupation is critical to well-being.
- Occupational therapy classifies occupations under activities of daily living, instrumental activities of daily living, self-care, education, work, play and leisure, and participation in social activities.
- Human learning entails experience, thinking, feeling, and doing.
- The profession views occupation as both a means and an end.
- Every human being has the potential for adaptation.
- Occupational therapy is based on humanism wherein the values of altruism, equality, freedom, justice, dignity, truth, and prudence are central to the profession.
- The client, family, and significant others are active participants throughout the therapeutic process in what is referred to as a client-centered approach.

Each person performs certain occupations (e.g., feeding, dressing, bathing, social participation, work, education, leisure). Occupations also fulfill each individual's need for security, belonging, physiological esteem, and self-actualization.[13] Occupational therapy practitioners believe that engagement and participation in occupations are essential to one's identity and well-being.

Occupational Therapy Classifies Occupations

Occupational therapy classifies occupations under activities of daily living, instrumental activities of daily living, self-care, education, work, play and leisure, and participation in social activities. OT practitioners explore many aspects of occupations in practice including (1) the range of occupations and activities that make up people's lives (performance in areas of occupation); (2) the skills used by people to perform occupations and activities (performance skills); (3) the habits, routines, and roles that are assumed by individuals in carrying out occupations or activities (performance patterns); (4) the internal or external context, or conditions, in which occupation occurs and influences performance (cultural, personal, physical, social, temporal, and virtual); (5) the demands of the activity which affect skill and success of performance; and (6) the factors that reside within the client and influence performance such as physiological and psychological body functions and anatomical body structures (organs and limbs).[1] These various dimensions of occupation all make up occupational therapy's domain of concern and are described in detail in Chapter 9.

At a given time, an individual may be occupied with caring for himself or herself by bathing, dressing, or eating. A person may be occupied with productive tasks, such as paid employment or tasks that are necessary for the care of his or her family. At other times, the individual may be involved in activities that he or she simply finds pleasurable, such as playing cards, watching a movie, or exercising. This is referred to as **occupational performance,** or "the ability to carry out activities of daily life."[1] These activities are categorized in the following performance areas of occupation[1]:

- Activities of daily living (e.g., feeding, dressing, bathing, toileting, hygiene)
- Instrumental activities of daily living (e.g., meal preparation, budgeting, homemaking, care for pets, care for others)
- Rest and sleep
- Education activities (e.g., going to school, studying, formal or informal)
- Work activities (e.g., activities related to employment and volunteer work)
- Play and leisure activities (e.g., activities that promote pleasure and diversion)
- Social participation (e.g., activities related to interacting with others)

Occupations performed on a daily basis are also influenced by individual occupational roles. Christiansen and Townsend define **role** as "a pattern of behavior that involves certain rights and duties that an individual is expected, trained, and often encouraged to perform in a particular social situation."[6] Role has also been defined as "a culturally defined pattern of occupation that reflects particular routines and habits."[5] Expectations of the individual's culture provide subtle messages about which roles to adopt and when.[6] The duration of roles varies, depending upon the role. For example, it may be a long-term role, such as a parent or spouse, or a short-term role, such as a patient in a hospital. A specific occupation may also be carried out in different roles and contexts, which will influence how that occupation is performed. For example, the activity of reading may be carried out in the role of a parent reading a story to a child at home, in the role of a student reading a textbook in the library, or in the role of a consumer reading food labels in the grocery store. The role in which the activity is being performed gives meaning to it as an occupation.[6]

How Does a Person Know What He Knows?

Epistemology investigates the nature, origin, and limits of human knowledge.[16] This component of philosophy provides a base for understanding motivation, change, and learning.

Human Learning Entails Experience, Thinking, Feeling, and Doing

Occupational therapy believes that humans learn through experience—thinking, feeling, and doing. This principle is found in many of the early writings of the founding members of the profession.[10,15,17] Humans are unique in that they have a sense of time—past, present, and future. This enables humans to remember past experiences and use them for present and future knowing. For example, a child who touches a hot stove and burns himself will learn rather rapidly (and painfully) from this experience not to touch a stove again. Past experiences also play a role in what the person finds meaningful. A child who likes the sound of a toy may be motivated to activate it again.

Occupational therapy emphasizes *doing* as the primary mechanism for learning and relearning various skills. Meyer saw occupational therapy's role as "giving *opportunities* rather than prescriptions." He saw a need for "opportunities to work, opportunities to do and to plan and create, and to learn to use material."[10] The philosophical base mentions the use of purposeful activity (occupation) to improve or maintain health. On a broad level, OT practitioners use both the terms *occupation* and *activity* to describe participation in daily life pursuits. However, there are important differences in these terms. The term **activity** describes a general class of human actions that are goal directed.[11] Goal-directed behavior implies that the person is focused on the goal of the activity rather than the processes involved in achieving the goal.[3] AOTA in the *Occupational Therapy Practice Framework* delineates an activity from an occupation as something an individual may participate in to achieve a goal, but activity may not have importance or meaning in the person's life.[1] **Tasks** are considered the basic units of behavior and are the simplest form of an action (i.e., reaching for a ball).

The Profession Views Occupation as Both a Means and an End

Through the therapeutic use of occupation and activity, the client is involved on many levels. Coordination between the person's sensorimotor, cognitive, and psychosocial systems is necessary and elicited when an individual engages in occupations and activities.[3] OT practitioners use occupation and activity as a means to help a client learn a new skill, restore a deficient ability, compensate in the presence of a functional disability, maintain health, or prevent dysfunction.[3] Mary Reilly summarizes this concept in her Eleanor Clarke Slagle lectureship when she states, "Man, through the use of his hands as they are energized by mind and will, can influence the state of his own health."[14]

In the practice of occupational therapy, occupation is seen as both a means and an end. **Occupation as a means** is the use of a specific occupation to bring about a change in the client's performance. When occupation is used as a means, it may be equivalent to activity. **Occupation as an end** is the desired outcome or product of intervention (i.e., the performance of activities or tasks that the person deems as important to life), and it is derived from the person's values, experiences, and culture.[18]

The therapeutic use of occupation and activity requires that the OT practitioner analyze both of these professional tools from multiple perspectives. Analysis of occupation and activity is a skill specific to occupational therapy and is discussed in detail in Chapter 15.

Every Human Being Has the Potential for Adaptation

Through this "knowing by doing," a human learns to adapt. A child who wants a toy on a table may initially cry to obtain it. Eventually, the child will learn to pull up to a standing position to reach for the toy. When he is successful at getting the object, he will stand to get the toy more frequently. This is one example of adaptation. The philosophical base of occupational therapy defines individual **adaptation** as "a change in function that promotes survival and self-actualization."[4] The concept of adaptation can be traced back to Adolph Meyer, who stated that diseases in psychiatry are "largely problems of adaptation" and that "psychiatry was among the first disciplines to recognize the need for adaptation and the value of work as a help in the problems of adaptation."[10] Adaptation takes place as part of the normal developmental process, in the process of adjusting to stress or change.[9]

In occupational therapy, occupation and activity are used to promote adaptation. Through occupation and activity, the individual achieves mastery over the environment, which contributes to the individual's feeling of competency.[7] Gail Fidler and Jay Fidler describe the development of competence. They write, "The ability to adapt, to cope with the problems of everyday living, and to fulfill life roles requires a rich reservoir of experiences gathered from direct engagement with both human and non-human objects in one's environment." They continue, "It is through such action with feedback from both human and non-human objects that an individual comes to know the potential and limitations of self and the environment and achieves a sense of competence and intrinsic worth."[8]

The process of adaptation is viewed as coming from within the individual. The client is actively involved in creating the change. The role of the OT or OTA in this process is to arrange the surroundings, materials, and demands of the environment to facilitate a specific adaptive response.[9] Practitioners of occupational therapy are optimistic that each and every individual has the potential to grow, adapt, and change.[19]

What Is Desirable?

Axiology examines the values of a profession and what is considered just and right in terms of the profession. For occupational therapy, the concepts of client-centered care, quality of life, and ethics fall under axiology.

The Client, Family, and Significant Others Are Active Participants

The profession understands the importance of having the client, family, and significant others as active participants throughout the therapeutic process. The client is actively involved, not only in the modality itself but also in identifying personal goals and preferences for treatment. This allows the practitioner to understand the individual's idea of what constitutes quality of life. Occupational therapy believes that **quality of life** is important. What is meaningful and that which provides satisfaction to an individual is **phenomenological;** that is, it is determined by the experience of that individual.[19] Therefore, the OT practitioner involves the client, family, and significant others in the occupational therapy process to assure they are addressing concerns that improve the client's quality of life.

Occupational therapy seeks to improve the quality of life for any person whose functional ability is impaired or limited. This goal is achieved by helping the client develop greater independence in the performance of any area of occupational behavior. For example, the goal of intervention may be to enable a client to independently brush his or her teeth, or manage a checkbook, or become more alert to the body mechanics that help avoid injury on the job. Likewise, the goal of intervention may be to ensure that the client increases strength in the body part needed to perform a necessary task, or achieves better coordination for all activities, or becomes better able to enjoy life by developing a hobby, or participates more fully in life by developing social skills. The OT practitioner works with the client to identify those occupations that are meaningful and will improve his or her quality of life. Together, the OT practitioner and client focus intervention on maximizing occupational performance in these areas.

To understand the experience, the OT practitioner involves the client, family, and significant others in the OT process. The **client-centered approach** is central to OT practice since only the clients can determine his or her quality of life, and, consequently, they must help the practitioner understand their experience.

What Are the "Rules of Right Conduct"?

As discussed in Chapter 2, the profession of occupational therapy emerged from the era of Moral Treatment, which valued the humanitarian treatment of individuals who were mentally ill. Occupational therapy is still based on **humanism,** a belief that the client should be treated as a person, not an object.

Occupational Therapy Is Based on Humanism

From this humanistic perspective, values and attitudes central to the profession have evolved. In *Core Values and Attitudes of Occupational Therapy Practice,* AOTA identifies the concepts of altruism, equality, freedom, justice, dignity, truth, and prudence as the core values and attitudes of occupational therapy.[2]

Altruism is the unselfish concern for the welfare of others. OT practitioners demonstrate this commitment to the profession and to the client with caring, dedication, responsiveness, and understanding. **Equality** refers to treating all individuals equally with an attitude of fairness and impartiality and respecting each individual's beliefs, values, and lifestyles in the day-to-day interactions.[2]

The OT practitioner also values **freedom,** an individual's right to exercise choice and to "demonstrate independence, initiative, and self-direction."[2] Freedom is demonstrated through nurturing, which is very different from controlling or directing. OT practitioners nurture their clients by providing support and encouragement, enabling the client to develop his or her inherent potential. Nurturing encourages the development of independence in the client, rather than retaining all direction and control in the hands of the practitioner.

Justice is the need for all OT practitioners to abide by the laws that govern the practice and to respect the legal rights of the client. Through the value of **dignity,** the uniqueness of each individual is emphasized. OT practitioners demonstrate this value through empathy and respect for each person. **Truthfulness** is a value demonstrated through behavior that is accountable, honest, and accurate, and that maintains one's professional competence. **Prudence** is the ability to demonstrate sound judgment, care, and discretion.[2] These values and attitudes are reflected in the *Occupational Therapy Code of Ethics* (see Chapter 8) (see Appendix A).

Summary

This has been a *brief* introduction to the philosophy of occupational therapy and its role in shaping the knowledge base and practice of the profession. The philosophical base of a profession represents its core beliefs, values, and principles. The philosophy of the profession addresses questions concerning the nature of humankind, ethical practice, and rules of conduct.

OT practitioners work in a variety of settings with diverse clients. However, all practitioners abide by the philosophical principles of the profession which include valuing the following: a holistic and humanistic approach, occupation, purposeful activity, adaptation, and quality of life. The common bond between OT practitioners is the importance of occupation and the facilitation of occupational performance. From a holistic perspective, occupational therapy views humans as active beings. Occupation is seen as an essential part of human existence, and it refers to all of the daily activities in which people participate. The underlying goal of occupational therapy is to increase the individual's independence in any area of occupational performance; thus, the OT practitioner must recognize inhibitors of activity and be able to design client-centered intervention plans. Humans learn by doing and, through the process of adaptation, develop a mastery of self and competence. Improving a client's quality of life (particularly increasing a person's independence) is the focus of the services provided by OT practitioners. Occupational therapy facilitates the adaptive process by providing the client with opportunities to adapt and improve one's quality of life.

Learning Activities

1. Identify your values and beliefs. Do they relate to the values and beliefs of the occupational therapy profession?
2. Review Chapter 2 and research other historical occupational therapy resources to trace consistencies between the early and current philosophies of the profession.
3. From case study articles (i.e., *OT Practice*), gather examples of quality-of-life changes that result from occupational therapy intervention.
4. In your own words, write a description of occupational therapy.
5. In a small group, identify the various roles within which each person functions. Discuss how your different roles give individual meaning to the activities you perform.
6. List the core beliefs of OT. Interview a practitioner to identify how he or she has embodied the core beliefs and OT philosophy.

Review Questions

1. What is occupational therapy's view of humans?
2. What are the similarities and differences between occupation, activity, and tasks?
3. What is meant by the terms *occupation as a means* and *occupation as an end*?
4. What are the core concepts of occupational therapy practice? Provide examples of each of these.
5. What is the philosophical base of occupational therapy?

References

1. American Occupational Therapy Association: Occupational therapy practice framework: Domain and process, ed 2, *Am J Occup Ther* 62(6):625–683, 2008.
2. American Occupational Therapy Association: Core values and attitudes of occupational therapy practice, *Am J Occup Ther* 47:1085, 1993.
3. American Occupational Therapy Association: Position paper: Purposeful activity, *Am J Occup Ther* 47:1080, 1993.
4. American Occupational Therapy Association: The philosophical base of occupational therapy, *Am J Occup Ther* 49:1026, 1995. Reviewed by COE and COP in 2004.
5. Townsend EA, Polatajko HJ, Canadian Association of Occupational Therapists: *Enabling Occupation: An Occupational Therapy Perspective*, Ottawa, 2007, Canadian Association of Occupational Therapists.
6. Christiansen CH, Townsend EA, editors: *Introduction to Occupation: The Art and Science of Living*, Upper Saddle River, NJ, 2004, Prentice Hall.
7. Fidler GS: From crafts to competence, *Am J Occup Ther* 35:567, 1981.
8. Fidler GS, Fidler JW: Doing and becoming: Purposeful action and self actualization, *Am J Occup Ther* 32:305, 1978.
9. King LJ: Toward a science of adaptive responses, *Am J Occup Ther* 32:14, 1978.
10. Meyer A: The philosophy of occupation therapy, *Arch Occup Ther* 1:1, 1922. (Reprinted in *Am J Occup Ther* 31:10, 1977.)
11. Pierce D: Untangling occupation and activity, *Am J Occup Ther* 22:138–146, 2001.
12. Reed KL: The beginnings of occupational therapy. In Hopkins HL, Smith HD, editors: *Willard and Spackman's Occupational Therapy*, ed 8, Philadelphia, 1993, JB Lippincott.

13. Reed KL, Sanderson SN: *Concepts of Occupational Therapy*, ed 4, Philadelphia, 1999, Lippincott Williams & Wilkins.
14. Reilly M: Occupational therapy can be one of the great ideas of 20th century medicine, *Am J Occup Ther* 16:2, 1962.
15. Robeson HA: How can occupational therapists help the social service worker? *Occup Ther Rehabil* 5:279, 1926.
16. Shannon PD: Philosophy and core values in occupational therapy. In Sladyk K, Ryan SE, editors: *Ryan's Occupational Therapy Assistant: Principles, Practice Issues, and Techniques*, ed 4, Thorofare, NJ, 2005, Slack.
17. Slagle EC: Training aides for mental patients, *Arch Occup Ther* 1:13, 1922.
18. Trombly CA: Occupation: Purposefulness and meaningfulness as therapeutic mechanisms. The 1995 Eleanor Clark Slagle lecture, *Am J Occup Ther* 49:960–972, 1995.
19. Yerxa E: The philosophical base of occupational therapy. In *Occupational Therapy 2001 AD*, Bethesda, MD, 1979, American Occupational Therapy Association.
20. The Free On-line Dictionary of Computing. Philosophy (n.d.). Available at: http://dictionary.reference.com/browse/philosophy. Accessed August 12, 2011.

As I transitioned from being an occupational therapy assistant instructor to teaching GED, I realized how much occupational therapy is a part of who I am. We often hear about how transferable our skills are and how we can apply them to many situations. Knowledge of working with persons with learning disabilities, awareness of community resources, valuing the uniqueness of all people and not judging them, and, most of all, empathy have made my transition quite smooth. Working with a student who may need a safe place because his or her home life is in chaos or one who has had substance abuse problems and asks for a resource has provided me with intrinsic rewards that parallel working with a person with disabilities. Occupational therapy is much more than a profession; it is a way of life!

SUE BYERS-CONNON, MS, COTA/L, ROH
Former Instructor, Occupational Therapy Assistant Program
Instructor, GED Program
Mount Hood Community College
Gresham, Oregon

CHAPTER 4

Current Issues and Emerging Practice Areas

Key Terms

Aging in place
Assistive technology
Centennial vision
Driver rehabilitation specialists
Ergonomics
Evidence-based practice
Licensure laws
Participatory research
Vision

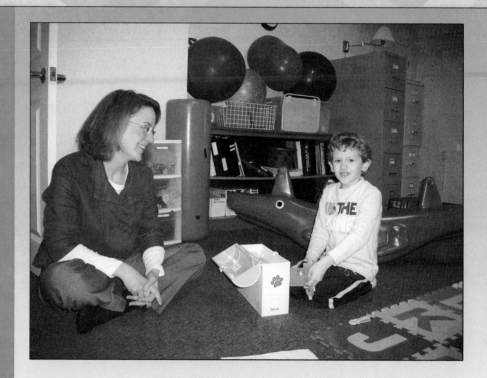

Objectives

After reading this chapter, the reader will be able to do the following:

- Identify current issues facing the occupational therapy profession
- Outline the centennial vision
- Describe emerging practice areas
- Discuss the value of evidence-based practice
- Discuss the influence of policy on practice

The role of the occupational therapy (OT) practitioner has developed significantly since its beginning work in positions such as reconstruction aide and working with injured veterans returning home. OT practitioners provide service to all ages (children to older adults) and diagnoses in such settings as hospitals, schools, rehabilitation clinics, private companies, and day treatment centers. With advances in science and technology, the OT practitioner today provides a wide range of technological and occupation-based service supported by research. The OT practitioner is skilled at problem-solving and clinical reasoning and adept at interpersonal interactions (e.g., therapeutic use of self). OT practitioners today

are consumers of research, and this enables them to provide quality evidence-based service to clients. They work in a variety of environments and thus must understand the legal implications of their services. They advocate for the rights of clients and participate in the political process to help generate policy to assist those in need. In general, today's OT practitioner is an informed, active professional whose interest in the client helps serve the public, the profession, and the individual. This chapter examines the latest trends in occupational therapy practice by providing an overview of the centennial vision and a description of emerging areas of practice.

Centennial Vision

A **vision** leads the future direction of a profession or organization. The vision is developed with the members and constituents over time, and it clarifies values, creates a future, and focuses the mission. Visioning helps organizations "stretch the horizon," develop a clear picture for the future,[11] and develop goals and objectives. Thus, a vision helps organizations move forward in a clear direction by encouraging all participants to work toward the same goals; 2017 will mark the centennial year of the occupational therapy profession. After much discussion and input from members, constituents, and consumers, AOTA adopted the centennial vision.[1]

AOTA's current vision statement is, "We envision that occupational therapy is a powerful, widely recognized, science-driven, and evidence-based profession with a globally connected and diverse workforce meeting society's occupational needs."[1] The vision for the occupational therapy profession emphasizes evidence-based practice and the value of the diversity of clients and practitioners. It highlights the work that OT practitioners do to meet society's needs and articulates the need for science to support practice.

Occupation

The centennial vision reflects the commitment to return to the roots of the profession: occupation (Box 4-1). Practitioners are encouraged to engage in occupation-based practice, focusing on helping clients re-engage in occupations, as opposed to focusing on specific component skills. The emphasis on occupation-based practice is prevalent in the occupational therapy literature, including the *Occupational Therapy Practice Framework*, standards for accreditation, conference programs, textbooks, and research publications. Educational programs have designed curricula around the uniqueness of occupation. Therefore, the trend to return to occupation remains a focus of research, education, and scholarly work.[1,2,9,13] OT practitioners embrace the uniqueness of the profession by helping persons do what they wish to do. Furthermore, research supports the premise that engagement in the actual occupation is beneficial and leads to increased physical, psychological, and social benefits.[2,6] Participation in occupations leads to increased motivation, generalization, and improved motor learning.[2,6,9]

Emerging Areas of Practice

As health care and society's needs change, opportunities and new areas of occupational therapy practice emerge. Events such as the aging of baby boomers (those persons born between 1946 and 1964), advancements in technology, and changes in health care policy provide OT practitioners with new opportunities. Former AOTA president Carolyn Baum identified six emerging areas of practice:

1. Aging in place
2. Driver assessments and training programs
3. Community health and wellness
4. Needs of children and youth
5. Ergonomics consulting
6. Technology and assistive-device developing and consulting[1,5]

These areas of practice illustrate the diversity of the profession and the breadth of services that OT practitioners provide. In addition to these areas of practice, OT practitioners continue to provide service in settings such as hospitals, skilled nursing facilities, community agencies, rehabilitation clinics, private clinics, schools, day care centers, and psychiatric facilities. OT practitioners provide services to underprivileged populations, including the homeless, migrant workers, and victims of disaster. Occupational therapy practitioners continue to work with returning veterans; they are examining the current issues these veterans face to better address their unique needs.

Priorities for 2011

The AOTA Board of Directors chose to focus activities on increasing the influence and recognition of the profession, ensuring that the profession is science driven and evidence based, and fostering the development of leaders. They outlined a series of activities to address these goals, including the development of the Coordinated Online Opportunities for Leadership (COOL) database, which allows members to volunteer for organization work in their area of expertise or desire more easily. Members identify their interests, areas of expertise, and preferences so that AOTA staff and committee chairpersons can find volunteers. Other priorities include developing a major image-building campaign and engaging in broad-based advocacy to ensure funding for OT in traditional and emerging areas. The priorities include building the research capacity of the profession and encouraging faculty to pursue doctoral degrees.

Aging in Place

With advances in medicine and health care, Americans are living longer, and more older adults wish to remain in their homes and live independently (or with minimal support).

Box 4-1

Definition of Occupation

"Activities . . . of everyday life, named, organized, and given value and meaning by individuals and a culture. Occupation is everything people do to occupy themselves, including looking after themselves . . . enjoying life . . . and contributing to the social and economic fabric of their communities."

From Law M, Polatajko H, Baptiste W, et al: Core concepts of occupational therapy. In Townsend E (ed): *Enabling Occupation: An Occupational Therapy Perspective*, p. 34, Ottawa, 1997, Canadian Association of Occupational Therapists.

This trend toward staying in the home is termed **aging in place.**[10] The OT practitioner offers a wide range of services to older individuals to allow them to remain at home and continue to be active in their community; these services include home modification, consultation, energy conservation, education, and remediation. Safety in the home includes the ability to manage medications, access emergency numbers, carry through with emergency procedures, show adequate judgment and cognition for daily living (e.g., cooking safety), demonstrate physical safety in the home, and the ability to safely protect oneself from strangers. Not only does the practitioner evaluate the client's skills, abilities, and safety in the home, but the OT practitioner also examines the support systems in place for the client (Box 4-2).

Socializing with others is important to the psychological well-being of individuals living at home. The OT practitioner may direct older persons to new social activities or help clients continue a previous activity with modifications or assistance. OT practitioners can be key players in developing creative programs to address the needs of the elderly. Clark et al. conducted a large, randomized control trial to examine the effectiveness of occupational therapy services on well older adults.[6] The results of this study support occupational therapy intervention as a cost-effective service to improve the health and quality of life of older adults.

Driver Assessments and Training Programs

Safe driving requires many factors (e.g., judgment, reaction time, sequencing, visual perceptual skills). OT practitioners determine a person's ability to drive after a trauma, illness, or decline in function by evaluating cognitive and physical abilities. Intervention is designed to remediate poor abilities or to make adaptations to accommodate dysfunctional skills. The OT practitioner and a team of providers are responsible for assessing whether the client is capable of driving safely; state laws provide driving licensure regulations. Clients may need special modifications to their vehicles in order to drive.

Box 4-2

Questions to Address for Staying in the Home

Is the client able to access emergency numbers?
How far away from emergency personnel does the client live?
How close are family members or support?
What is the disaster plan (e.g., hurricanes, flooding, snow)?
Can the client manage medications?
Is the client able to drive?
Who will be visiting the client on a regular basis?
Is the client able to access financial resources?
How will the client get around the community?
What are the social supports available to the client?
Is the home accessible to the client?
Can the client lock doors at night?

OT practitioners train individuals in the necessary foundation skills to ensure that drivers are safe. Because OT practitioners are trained to examine clients in a holistic manner, occupational therapists are well suited to succeed as **driver rehabilitation specialists.** Namely, the OT practitioner evaluates and intervenes in physical, social, cognitive, and psychosocial aspects of functioning that affect driving skills. OT practitioners may consult with technology specialists or mechanics on adapting vehicles to help clients with disabilities.

Community Health and Wellness

Because the goal of occupational therapy is to help individuals engage in activities of daily living, work, education, leisure, play, and social participation, OT practitioners may develop programs to keep communities healthy. Such programs focus on wellness and prevention of disability, and they help those with disabilities integrate into the community and contribute to society (e.g., vocational rehabilitation programs).

Advances in health care have enabled individuals to survive many conditions that interfere with functioning. Policy makers and consumers have begun to realize the benefits to helping individuals remain active in their community. OT practitioners facilitate health and wellness in communities through educational programs and services to individuals and groups. Providing services to the community promotes wellness and quality of life.

An individual's quality of life is based upon many things, including standard of living, finances, freedom, happiness, and access to goods and services. Therefore, helping older adults access health care, social groups, transportation, and daily living activities can increase their quality of life. For example, OTs may consult with a senior citizens' group about the benefits of physical activity, or speak to support groups on a variety of topics, including safety at home, driving tips, cooking modifications, and medication management.

The OT practitioner may design programs to increase wellness in the community or to address a specific concern, such as childhood obesity. They may work in the community to address the needs of the homeless, migrant workers, or victims of disaster. OT practitioners might also work with communities as consultants to assure accessibility for persons with disabilities (e.g., playgrounds, public buildings).

Needs of Children and Youth

The needs of children and youth continue to be a growing area for OT practitioners. Childhood obesity is a concern among this population. In fact, *Healthy People 2010* cited childhood obesity in America as one of the leading health issues.[8] Because there are many factors associated with childhood obesity, OT practitioners are becoming involved in developing programs for those children.

OT practitioners serve children in early intervention programs that begin as early as birth. Although federal law mandates these birth–to–3-year-old programs, states are responsible for the implementation of services. With limited funding and increased need for services, the OT practitioner working in early intervention may need to advocate for the children they serve. There continues to be a need for training and programming in this area.

When children with special needs transition to the public school system, an OT practitioner helps them function in the education environment. OT practitioners provide services within systems with limited funding, despite the vast needs. They may be involved in creating after school programs or evening social programs for children and youth. Creative solutions are needed to address the needs of children and youth.

Ergonomics Consulting

Ergonomics refers to the science of fitting jobs to people.[15] Ergonomics consulting involves providing recommendations to individuals and companies on work station set-up to promote safety, efficiency, and comfort to prevent work-related musculoskeletal injury. Examination of seating and positioning, lifting, and other physical requirements falls well within the OT practitioner's expertise. Proper ergonomics may prevent injury to the client, which may result in fewer missed work days and lower costs to the company and client.

Technology and Assistive-Device Developing and Consulting

Assistive technology, or adaptive technology, commonly refers to "products, devices or equipment, whether acquired commercially, modified, or customized, that are used to maintain, increase, or improve the functional capabilities of individuals with disabilities."[4] Assistive technology, which includes equipment to assist with communication, computer access, daily living, education and learning, hearing and listening, mobility and transportation, recreation and leisure, seating and position, vision and reading, and prosthetics and orthotics,[14] has improved life for those with disabilities. OT practitioners use technology to help clients function independently in many areas of performance. Because OT practitioners are skilled at analyzing activities, including the movement patterns required for success, many practitioners serve as consultants in the development of devices.

Frequently, the OT practitioner consults with the team on the type of assistive device and the physical, cognitive, or psychological skills the client possesses to use the device. The OT practitioner is an important member of the team because he or she determines whether the device helps the client perform in his or her daily occupations in a reasonable amount of time. The OT practitioner and client determine whether the device is practical and helpful to the client after careful analysis (Figure 4-1).

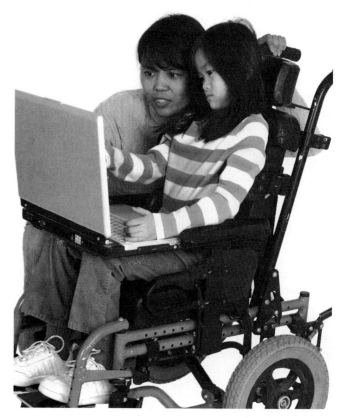

Figure 4-1 OT practitioners work with clients to help them use technology to engage in activity. This child works on a laptop computer for school and play. © iStockphoto.com

Educational Trends

Educators consistently evaluate how to teach OT and OTA students to succeed in clinical practice. Educators acknowledge that practitioners entering a diverse workplace with expanding areas of practice need to be lifelong learners and critical consumers of research. Practitioners must be able to support their decisions based upon available research. The need to justify intervention and examine evidence requires practitioners who are able to generate and critically analyze research. Basing practice on the best available research evidence is termed **evidence-based practice.** Insurance companies, consumers, and employers require professionals, including OT practitioners, to provide evidence for what they do. Given so many options for spending one's health care dollar, practitioners must show that therapy is beneficial and cost-effective.

This need to become critical consumers of research prompted the move to a Master's level degree as the entry-level requirement for therapists. This degree reflects the advanced critical analysis and synthesis required of today's practitioners, especially with regard to the ability to analyze research for practice. The associate's degree is still the educational requirement for OTAs.

The desire to prepare doctoral-trained faculty to teach, advance the research agenda of the profession, and generate evidence for interventions prompted the development of clinical doctorate programs. Many educational programs allow practitioners to focus on clinical work while pursuing an advanced degree. One technique to keep occupational therapy faculty in touch with clinical practice while fulfilling faculty commitments is **participatory research,** which helps close the gap between academia and practice. Participatory research involves the clinician, client, and faculty member in the research process, and it often results in relevant research while meeting a community or agency need.

Today's student is well versed in the use of technology, allowing educational programs to use distance education (including web-based courses and telecommunication courses) to reach practitioners who might otherwise not have educational opportunities. Educators use new teaching strategies to maximize learning with technology.

In summary, faculty strive to educate occupational therapy students who are critical and innovative thinkers—people who are able to interact therapeutically with clients and peers. Educators hope to bridge the clinical practice and theory gap so that students become practitioners who use current research and sound judgment to benefit their clients.

State Regulation

The practice of occupational therapy is regulated in most states through licensure laws that safeguard the public and protect the public from unethical, incompetent, or unauthorized practitioners. State **licensure laws,** also called practice acts, give a legal definition of occupational therapy and the domain of occupational therapy practice that differentiates it from other professions. These laws provide important guides for consumers, facilities, and providers, especially with regard to the minimum qualifications for practitioners.

OT practitioners need to keep up to date on the status of the licensure laws in their state and any proposed changes to the regulations. Government leaders and other professional organizations may oppose renewal of the licensure law, unless OT practitioners are actively involved in advocating for their profession. State licensure is discussed further in Chapter 8.

Policy and Reimbursement

OT practitioners must be aware of infringement from other professionals on their scope of practice and be proactive in such situations. Physical therapists, orthotists, and prosthetists have recently challenged the occupational therapy scope of practice. Typically, these challenges occur as other disciplines position themselves as a source for "one-stop shopping" in rehabilitation or for reimbursement purposes.[12] For example, the Federation of State Boards of Physical Therapy *Model Practice Act for Physical Therapy*[3] expands physical therapy's scope of practice to include "functional training in self-care and home management (including activities of daily living and instrumental activities

---

Box 4-3

Laws That Have Affected Occupational Therapy Services

1. *Section 504 of the Rehabilitation Act of 1973:* "No otherwise qualified handicapped individual in the United States . . . shall, solely by reason of . . . handicap, be excluded from participation in, be denied the benefits of, or be subjected to discrimination under any program or activity receiving federal financial assistance."[16] Section 504 provides rights and benefits to persons with disabilities and provides services to children in school systems who may not qualify for services under IDEA. This law requires that programs or activities receiving federal financial assistance provide reasonable accommodations so persons with disabilities may participate.

2. *The Americans with Disabilities Act (ADA) of 1990:* Provides protection from discrimination on the basis of disability. The ADA upholds and extends the standards for compliance set forth in Section 504 of the Rehabilitation Act of 1973 to employment practices, communication, and all policies, procedures, and practices that affect the treatment of students with disabilities.[16] ADA expanded services to include the workplace and public places. This law required that public places be accessible to those with disabilities. For example, occupational therapy professionals work with architects and employers to make work settings accessible to those with disabilities.

3. *Individuals with Disabilities Education Act (formerly PL 94-142 or the Education for All Handicapped Children Act of 1975):* Requires public schools to make available to all eligible children with disabilities a free appropriate public education in the least restrictive environment appropriate to their individual needs.[16] OT practitioners working in school systems work under this act. Thus, the role of the OT practitioner is to provide intervention that will allow the child to engage in education. Intervention takes place in the least restrictive environment and is appropriate to the child's needs.

4. *The Balanced Budget Act of 1997:* Set out to contain health care costs by placing caps on therapy services and resulted in a decrease in occupational therapy jobs. Many therapists changed settings during this time or moved on to private practice. Managed care pushed for productivity.[8]

5. *Medicare:* This health insurance program is for people 65 years of age or older and those with certain disabilities. It is a federally funded program that provides limits on spending and reimbursement for occupational therapy services.

of daily living)."[3] AOTA and state occupational therapy associations are concerned that this definition does not sufficiently speak to the limited scope of practice (i.e., functional skills related to physical movement and mobility) in which physical therapists address client needs in this area.[12] This definition infringes on what is traditionally the domain of occupational therapy and in which OT practitioners have extensive education and training.[12]

Policy affects health services, including occupational therapy. For example, the prospective payment system of 1983 resulted in shorter hospital stays, but OT practitioners continued to treat these clients in other settings (such as skilled nursing facilities and home health agencies).[7] Federal laws mandate services, but they require state legislation to determine how the laws will be carried out. OT practitioners must become familiar with policies while they are being developed and advocate for services for those with disabilities. Box 4-3 provides a partial listing of some of the laws that have affected occupational therapy services.

OT practitioners advocate for the profession by participating in policy making. Practitioners may advocate on local, regional, or national levels. The first step toward addressing these challenges is for OT practitioners to be familiar with the scope of practice and the foundations for it. Maintaining current on topics by reading professional journals, newsletters, and federal and state news can increase awareness of the issues that affect the profession. Practitioners can keep up to date on health care policy through active involvement in the state and national occupational therapy associations.

Summary

The centennial vision provides a message of growth and support for the profession.[1,5] Continued evidence supporting occupational therapy practice reinforces the work and ensures that the profession will thrive. The diversity of clients, as well as the diversity in practitioners, makes the profession exciting and valuable in a changing health care system. OT practitioners will need to continue to advocate for the profession and be involved in policy and reimbursement issues.

Learning Activities

1. Review five current *OT Practice* magazines and list the current issues. Present your findings to your classmates.
2. Review the AOTA national conference program to identify the current issues.
3. Pick one of the six emerging practice areas. Describe the role of the OT practitioner in the area and how you could develop future programs.
4. Develop a resource list around one of the six emerging practice areas.
5. Examine one health care policy, by discussing the history and intent of the policy. In small groups, describe how the policy has been implemented in practice.
6. Explore the licensure requirements in a state.

Review Questions

1. What are some current issues facing the occupational therapy profession?
2. What are the emerging practice areas?
3. What is evidence-based practice?
4. How has policy affected occupational therapy practice?
5. What are some current trends in occupational therapy education?

References

1. American Occupational Therapy Association: *AOTA's centennial vision: Shaping the future of occupational therapy*. Retrieved January 27, 2011, from http://www.aota.org/nonmembers/area16/index.asp.
2. American Occupational Therapy Association: Occupational therapy practice framework: Domain and process, *Am J Occup Ther* 56(6):609–639, 2002.
3. American Physical Therapy Association: *Guidelines: Physical Therapist Scope of Practice*, BOD G03-01-09-29, Board of Directors Standards, Positions, Guidelines, Policies and Procedures, Alexandria, VA, 2009, American Physical Therapy Association.
4. *Assistive Technology Act of 1998*. Retrieved January 27, 2011, from http://www.section508.gov/docs/AssistiveTechnologyActOf1998Full.pdf.
5. Brachtesende A: The turnaround is here! *OT Practice* 23(1):13–18, 2005.
6. Clark F, Azen SP, Zemke R, et al: Occupational therapy for independent-living older adults, A randomized controlled trial, *JAMA* 278(16):1321–1326, 1997.
7. Fisher G, Cooksey J: The occupational therapy workforce: Part I: Context and trends. In Brachtesende A, editor: *The turnaround is here! OT Practice*, vol 23(1), 2005, pp 13–18.
8. Office of Disease Prevention and Healthy Promotion (ODPHP): *Healthy People 2010*. Retrieved January 27, 2011, from www.healthypeople.gov.
9. Law M, Polatajko H, Baptiste W, et al: Core concepts of occupational therapy. In Townsend E, editor: *Enabling Occupation: An Occupational Therapy Perspective*, Ottawa, 1997, Canadian Association of Occupational Therapists, pp 29–56.
10. Pollak PB, DiGregorio DA: Aging in place, *J Extension* 26(4):1988. Retrieved January 27, 2011, from www.joe.org/joe/1998winter/a2.html.
11. Scott C, Jaffe D, Tobe G: *Organizational Vision, Values and Mission: Building the Organization of the Tomorrow*, Menlo Park, CA, 1993, Crisp Publishers.
12. Slater DY, Willmarth C: Understanding and asserting the occupational therapy scope of practice, *OT Practice* 10(19):CE-1–CE-8, 2005.
13. Clark F: The vision: What it is, Why it's right, 2011. Available at: http://www.aota.org/News/Centennial/Updates.aspx. Accessed August 12, 2011.
14. RehabTool LLC: *What's assistive technology?* Retrieved January 27, 2011, from http://www.rehabtool.com/at.html.
15. UCLA Ergonomics: *What is ergonomics and why is it important?* Retrieved January 27, 2011, from http://www.ergonomics.ucla.edu/what_and_why.html.
16. United States Department of Justice, Civil Rights Division, Disability Rights Section: *A guide to disability rights laws*, September 2005. Retrieved January 27, 2011, from http://www.ada.gov/cguide.pdf.

SECTION II

Occupational Therapy
The Practitioner

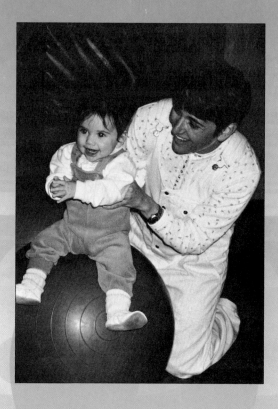

The most memorable aspects of my career in occupational therapy education were the wonderful students I had the privilege of knowing, and the opportunity I had to share with them my beliefs and philosophy about the health-giving value of occupation. My students taught me so much about life, teaching, and learning. It was a richly rewarding experience to facilitate and witness the evolution of the occupational therapy student to the professional occupational therapist.

LORRAINE WILLIAMS PEDRETTI, MS, OTR/RET.
Professor Emeritus
Department of Occupational Therapy
San José State University
San José, California

CHAPTER 5

From Student to Practitioner: Educational Preparation and Certification

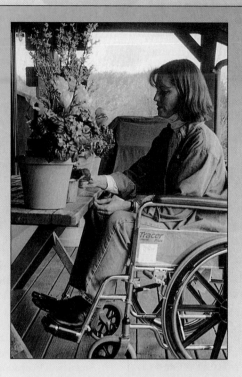

Objectives

After completing this chapter, the reader will be able to do the following:

- Describe the accreditation process for OT educational programs
- Identify the three categories of OT personnel
- Delineate the educational and professional requirements for each personnel category
- Describe the purpose of Level I and Level II fieldwork experiences
- Describe the Doctor of Occupational Therapy (OTD) and the Doctor of Philosophy (PhD)

The personnel who deliver occupational therapy services to consumers can be divided into three categories that vary in the type and amount of training they receive and the duties they perform. The most highly trained at the professional level is the **occupational therapist** (OT). The **occupational therapy assistant** (OTA) is trained at the technical level and works under the supervision of the OT. A third category of worker, the **occupational therapy aide,** does not receive specialized training before working in the field; rather, occupational therapy aides receive on-the-job training. In this chapter, the focus is on the educational preparation and certification process for the OT and the OTA.

Consistent with the terminology used by the American Occupational Therapy Association (AOTA), the term *occupational therapy personnel* is used when referring to *any* personnel (including OT students and aides) who deliver occupational therapy services. The term *occupational therapy practitioner* refers to any individual who is "initially certified to practice as either an OT or an OTA, or licensed or regulated by a state, district, commonwealth, or territory of the United States to practice as an OT or OTA and who has not had that certification, license, or regulation revoked due to disciplinary action."[5] When it is necessary to distinguish between the three categories of personnel, the respective titles are used.

Accreditation of Educational Programs

The **Accreditation Council for Occupational Therapy Education** (ACOTE) of the AOTA regulates entry-level education for both OT and OTA programs in the United States. Since 1935, AOTA sets standards for educational programs. The standards are reviewed and revised every 5 years by various constituency groups, educational program directors, and the public at large. The latest revision of the standards for occupational therapy Master's degree programs and OTA programs was completed in 2006. These standards are published in the *Standards for an Accredited Educational Program for the Occupational Therapist*[1] (Box 5-1) and in the *Standards for an Accredited Educational Program for the Occupational Therapy Assistant*[2] (Box 5-2).

ACOTE evaluates each educational program's compliance with the standards as part of the accreditation process. Each program must follow ACOTE procedures to

---

Box 5-1

OT Standards

(Effective 1/1/08)

Preamble

The rapidly changing and dynamic nature of contemporary health and human service delivery systems requires the entry-level occupational therapist to possess basic skills as a direct care provider, consultant, educator, manager, researcher, and advocate for the profession and the consumer.

A contemporary entry-level occupational therapist must:

- Have acquired, as a foundation for professional study, a breadth and depth of knowledge in the liberal arts and sciences and an understanding of issues related to diversity.
- Be educated as a generalist with a broad exposure to the delivery models and systems used in settings where occupational therapy is currently practiced and where it is emerging as a service.
- Have achieved entry-level competence through a combination of academic and fieldwork education.
- Be prepared to articulate and apply occupational therapy theory, evidence-based evaluations, and interventions to achieve expected outcomes as related to occupation.
- Be prepared to be a lifelong learner and keep current with evidence-based professional practice.
- Uphold the ethical standards, values, and attitudes of the occupational therapy profession.
- Understand the distinct roles and responsibilities of the OT and OTA in the supervisory process.
- Be prepared to advocate as a professional, for the occupational therapy services offered and for the recipients of those services.
- Be prepared to be an effective consumer of the latest research and knowledge bases that support practice and contribute to the growth and dissemination of research and knowledge.

Accreditation Council for Occupational Therapy Education of the American Occupational Therapy Association. Standards for a Master's degree educational program for the occupational therapist, *Am J Occup Ther* 61:652-661, 2007.

Box 5-2

OTA Standards

(Effective 1/1/08)

Preamble

The rapidly changing and dynamic nature of contemporary health and human service delivery systems requires the entry-level occupational therapy assistant to possess basic skills as a direct care provider, educator, and advocate for the profession and the consumer.

A contemporary entry-level occupational therapy assistant must:

- Have acquired an educational foundation in the liberal arts and sciences, including a focus on issues related to diversity.
- Be educated as a generalist, with a broad exposure to the delivery models and systems used in settings where occupational therapy is currently practiced and where it is emerging as a service.
- Have achieved entry-level competence through a combination of academic and fieldwork education.
- Be prepared to articulate and apply occupational therapy principles and intervention tools to achieve expected outcomes as related to occupation.
- Be prepared to be a lifelong learner and keep current with best practice.
- Uphold the ethical standards, values, and attitudes of the occupational therapy profession.
- Understand the distinct roles and responsibilities of the OT and OTA in the supervisory process.
- Be prepared to advocate as a professional, for the services offered, and for the recipients of those services.

Accreditation Council for Occupational Therapy Education of the American Occupational Therapy Association. Accreditation standards for an educational program for the occupational therapy assistant, *Am J Occup Ther* 61:62-671, 2007.

---

become accredited and to maintain accreditation. For example, institutions must inform ACOTE of their intention to begin a new program, and they must build a curriculum around the standards. Initial accreditation requires a review of the program design and an on-site inspection after at least 1 year of operation. After passing these requirements, the program becomes fully accredited and is then reviewed on a regular basis. To maintain accreditation, programs must complete a "Report of Self-Study" and undergo a site visit before the end of the period in which accreditation was awarded. The review board has the power to grant or withhold approval.

Accreditation of an occupational therapy educational program means that the minimal educational standards recommended by the profession have been met and the school has received formal approval by ACOTE. This approval ensures that graduates of an accredited program meet minimal entry-level standards and that they are qualified to take the national certification examination. As of 2010, there were 153 accredited occupational therapy programs and 160 accredited OTA programs in the United States and Puerto Rico.[3] A current listing of all programs can be found at AOTA's website, www.aota.org.

In selecting a school, prospective students are advised to seek information about the accreditation status, success of program graduates on the national certification examination, job placement rates, mission statement, and philosophy, as well as the emphasis of its educational program.

Entry-Level Educational Preparation

In practice, the roles of the OT and OTA are complementary and collaborative. Therefore, the curricula for the entry-level preparation of the OT and the OTA consist of a similar combination of classroom and clinical learning experiences that reflect current practice Table 5-1 summarizes the characteristics of the different levels of occupational therapy educational preparation. At both levels, students complete studies on anatomy, physiology, medical conditions, kinesiology, and general education courses that lead to a degree awarded by the respective college or university. Courses in the professional areas of the curricula are also similar in content. Students at both levels learn occupational therapy principles, practices, and processes. The difference in the education for the OT is the depth of theory provided in the core and professional curricula as well as a greater emphasis on evaluation and interpretation.

Each level of training requires practical experience, referred to as **fieldwork.** The purpose of fieldwork is to "provide ... students with the opportunity to apply the knowledge learned in the classroom to practice in the clinical setting."[6] Observation and participation in fieldwork are intended to enhance the academic coursework and to develop competent, entry-level practitioners. Frequently, OT and OTA students are scheduled to complete fieldwork at the same location. This provides students the opportunity to communicate and practice delegation of responsibilities with each other.

Students are expected to increase their technical and critical reasoning skills over time. Therefore, both OT and OTA educational programs require two levels of fieldwork. The initial level is referred to as **Level I fieldwork** and is completed concurrently with the academic coursework. The purpose of Level I fieldwork is to introduce the student to the profession and to the various applications of intervention. The amount of time required at this level varies by program.

Level II fieldwork experiences are designed to provide students with supervised, hands-on clinical training. OT students complete full-time fieldwork at a facility for a minimum of 24 weeks, whereas OTA students complete 16 weeks of full-time fieldwork. Students engaged in Level II fieldwork are immersed in occupational therapy practice, and, by the end of the experience, students are expected to be functioning as entry-level practitioners.

Educational Demographics of Occupational Therapy Practitioners

Demographic data are listed in Table 5-2, which shows that OT practitioners are primarily women; OTAs hold associate's degrees; and the majority of OTs have baccalaureate degrees. According to AOTA, 26% of OTs hold a Master's degree; this percentage is increasing as the Master's level is now the educational requirement for therapists (since 2007).[4]

Educational Preparation for the Occupational Therapist

Occupational therapists must complete a Master's degree to practice, as of 2007. Practitioners who obtained a bachelor of sciences or arts degree in occupational therapy prior to

Table 5-1 Characteristics of Levels of Preparation in Occupational Therapy

Degree	Distinctive Curricular Features	Average Program Length	Additional Requirements
Associate AA/ AS (required to practice as OTA)	Focus is on technical skills related to the methods and procedures used in occupational therapy.	2 years	16 weeks of Level II fieldwork
Entry-level master's MS/MA/MOT (required to practice as OT)	In-depth theory; greater emphasis on evaluation, interpretation, and intervention planning. Emphasis on critically analyzing research for practice. May have a baccalaureate degree in preoccupational therapy/health sciences or another field.	2 years post baccalaureate degree	24 weeks of Level II fieldwork; basic research project or thesis
Advanced master's MS or MA	Develop advanced research skills and specialization in practice area. Individual has a baccalaureate degree in occupational therapy.	1-3 years post baccalaureate degree	Master's thesis or advanced-level research project; may require additional fieldwork
PhD	Generate research and knowledge for the profession. Requires completion of Master's degree.	3-5 years	Dissertation
OTD	Advanced practice competencies; clinical leadership. Can be earned as entry-level degree or postgraduate.	3 years post baccalaureate	Clinical research project or practicum required

AA, Associate of Arts; *AS,* Associate of Science; *MA,* Master of Arts; *MOT,* Master of Occupational Therapy; *MS,* Master of Science; *OTD,* Doctor of Occupational Therapy; *PhD,* Doctor of Philosophy.

Table 5-2 Demographic Data on OT Practitioners

	OT	OTA
Men	6%	8%
Women	94%	92%
Associate's	N/A	81%
Baccalaureate	70%	11%
Certificate	2%	6%
Master's	26%	2%
Doctorate	1%	N/A

American Occupational Therapy Association. 2006 AOTA workforce and compensation survey: Occupational therapy salaries and job opportunities continue to improve [Electronic Version], OT *Practice* 11(17):10–12, 2006, from www.aota.org.

2007 are "grandfathered in" and may continue to practice. Some universities offer programs to help practitioners with baccalaureate degrees in occupational therapy progress to the advanced Master's level. Often, these courses are offered during evenings and weekends to accommodate the working therapist. Students who earned a baccalaureate degree in a related field (i.e., psychology, child development) may enter a basic Master's degree occupational therapy program. Students are encouraged to explore the educational options by communicating with local universities and colleges.

Doctor of Occupational Therapy and Postgraduate Education

Students may elect to obtain a **Doctor of Occupational Therapy** (OTD) degree. The OTD degree is a clinical or practice-based doctorate, also known as a professional doctorate. Pierce and Peyton described the OTD degree as one that focuses on the development of "sophisticated practice competencies rather than research or knowledge production."[8] With these competencies, the individual with the OTD degree is expected to contribute to outcomes research, program evaluation, and evidence-based practice. A person may earn an OTD as either an entry-level or as a postgraduate professional degree. For example, the individual may have a Bachelor of Art (BA)/Bachelor of Science (BS) or Master of Art (MA)/Master of Science (MS) in occupational therapy and return to school to earn an OTD degree.

The Doctor of Philosophy (PhD) is the traditional postgraduate degree and is a research-based degree. Doctorates such as the Doctorate of Education (EdD), Doctorate of Science (ScD), and Doctor of Public Health (DrPH) are also research-based degrees. Some academic institutes offer PhDs in occupational therapy, occupational science, and other related areas, such as psychology, which are appealing to professionals. An individual with a doctoral degree is trained to be an independent researcher, with importance placed on the discovery of knowledge.

Educational Preparation for the Occupational Therapy Assistant

In 1965, AOTA mandated that OTA programs be established in junior or community colleges. Gradually, OTA educational programs were lengthened from 9 to 12 months and then to 2 years. Beginning in 1977, OTA students were required to take the certification exam. Currently, OTA students must complete at least 2 years of postsecondary education in an accredited program, which may be obtained at a community college, junior college, or technical training school. The OTA student must successfully complete Level I and Level II fieldwork experiences. The type of associate's degree (science or arts) awarded depends on the institution. Students who have completed all of the educational requirements and Level II fieldwork are eligible to take the national certification examination for OTAs.

Box 5-2 shows the preamble of the *Standards for an Accredited Educational Program for the Occupational Therapy Assistant*, which describes the foundational requirements for an OTA.[2] Programs for the OTA typically focus less on theory and more on the "doing" aspects of the field, such as methods and procedures used in occupational therapy.[9]

OTA students may elect to further their education by seeking a baccalaureate degree in a related field and then obtain a basic Master's degree in occupational therapy. Some universities offer special arrangements so that the OTAs receive credit for the work they have completed toward advanced degrees. Nontraditional programs, such as weekend and online formats, are available to help OTAs advance their education. Those wishing to advance their education are urged to communicate with faculty and explore options.

Entry-Level Certification and State Licensure

Certification refers to the acknowledgment that an individual has the qualifications to be an entry-level practitioner, either a registered occupational therapist (OTR) or certified occupational therapy assistant (COTA). After completing the educational requirements and fieldwork, candidates at each educational level are eligible to sit for the national certification examination, administered by the **National Board for Certification in Occupational Therapy** (NBCOT). The certification exam is a 4-hour multiple-choice exam that covers evaluation and intervention planning for all areas of practice, ethics, delivery systems, and basic occupational therapy principles. Those candidates who pass the certification exam are entitled to use the appropriate professional designation after their names—OTR or COTA. Candidates residing in states that have licensure laws are eligible to apply for a state license to practice, once they have passed the exam. Candidates who do not pass the examination may retake the test. However, they must pay for each attempt. Typically, persons working under a temporary license who fail the examination may not continue working as an OT practitioner. They may work as aides until the test is passed.

History of Certification and Registration

Registration began in 1931 when AOTA listed OTs who had completed approved professional training and 1 year of subsequent work experience. Those individuals who qualified were granted the designation **registered occupational therapist.**[7] The first National Register, published in 1932, listed 318 OTs. In 1939, the standards for registration included the passage of a written essay examination. In 1947, the essay examination was converted to an objective multiple-choice examination, which is still in use today.

In the late 1950s, registration for OTAs was implemented for those individuals who graduated from an approved educational program. Initially, those individuals who had not graduated from an approved program but had worked a minimum of 2 years in one disability area were "grandfathered" in.[7] This plan was eliminated in 1963. The first OTA certification examination was administered in 1977.

In 1980, a category called "certified only" was created for practitioners who wanted to be certified without being a member of AOTA.[7] Additionally, during this time, state regulatory laws focused on competency in recertification.

The certification process underwent a major administrative change in 1986, when an autonomous certification board was created, separating AOTA membership and certification. This board was initially named the American Occupational Therapy Certification Board (AOTCB). In 1988, the AOTCB was incorporated as a separate entity from AOTA.[7] In 1996, AOTCB changed its name to the National Board for Certification in Occupational Therapy (NBCOT®). NBCOT consists of a 15-member board of directors composed of 8 OT practitioners and 7 public members. NBCOT functions independently in all aspects of initial certification. NBCOT has established procedures for and implemented a certification renewal program.

Summary

The OT and OTA are the two official levels of professionals in the field of occupational therapy, and each receives formal education in occupational therapy theory, philosophy, and process. The formal education of the OT and OTA is similar in content, but the OT receives more depth of theoretical knowledge and research. The OTA educational program typically takes 2 years to obtain an associate's degree; the OT degree requires a Master's degree (5-6 years of study). Students who complete the required coursework in an OT or OTA program are eligible to sit for the national certification exam and apply for state licensure (if required).

Learning Activities

1. Prepare a report on the logistics of the national certification examination.
2. Write a short paper on the history of occupational therapy education.
3. Interview an OT practitioner. Determine his or her motivation for entering the field. How did he or she learn about occupational therapy? Why did he or she decide to pursue the field? What is his or her educational background? Ask him or her to describe his or her fieldwork experiences.
4. Compare and contrast occupational therapy programs offered at two universities. Describe the levels of education and course and time requirements.
5. Examine the educational requirements for OT, OTA, OTD, and PhD programs.

Review Questions

1. What are the categories of OT personnel?
2. What are the educational requirements for each personnel category?
3. What are the professional requirements for each personnel category?
4. What is the Accreditation Council for Occupational Therapy Education?
5. What is the certification process for OT and OTA personnel?
6. What are the fieldwork requirements for OT and OTA personnel?

References

1. Accreditation Council for Occupational Therapy Education of the American Occupational Therapy Association: Standards for a master's degree educational program for the occupational therapist, *Am J Occup Ther* 61:652–661, 2007.
2. Accreditation Council for Occupational Therapy Education of the American Occupational Therapy Association: Accreditation standards for an educational program for the occupational therapy assistant, *Am J Occup Ther* 61:62–671, 2007.
3. American Occupational Therapy Association: *Academic programs annual data report: Annual year 2009–2010.* Retrieved February 2, 2011, from www.aota.org.
4. American Occupational Therapy Association: *Executive summary: September 2010. Membership Levels.* Retrieved January 27, 2011, from http://www.aota.org/Governance/ProceduralAdHoc/Minutes/Minutes9-10.aspx.
5. American Occupational Therapy Association: *The Reference Manual of the Official Documents of the American Occupational Therapy Association, Inc.,* ed 14, Bethesda, MD, 2009, American Occupational Therapy Association.
6. American Occupational Therapy Association: Occupational therapy fieldwork education: Value and purpose, *Am J Occup Ther* 63:393–394, 2009.
7. American Occupational Therapy Association: Chronology of certification issues dated through January 29, OT Week, 1997.
8. Pierce D, Peyton C: A historical cross-disciplinary perspective on the professional doctorate in occupational therapy, *Am J Occup Ther* 53(1):64–71, 1999.
9. Punwar AJ, Peloquin SM: *Occupational Therapy Principles and Practice,* ed 3, Baltimore, 2000, Lippincott Williams & Wilkins.

I stumbled upon the profession of occupational therapy quite serendipitously. I had originally intended to pursue a law degree in college but found myself drawn to courses in the sciences and arts. A university counselor recommended that I take a series of career tests, and the profession of occupational therapy appeared. Because I had never heard of this profession, the counselor provided me with information and names of individuals to contact regarding occupational therapy. I was amazed at the range of the profession and the creativity of the occupational therapists I encountered. This profession offered such variety!

As I reflect on over 25 years as an occupational therapist (I stopped counting after the quarter century mark!), I am so grateful to that counselor who opened my eyes to a profession that has provided me with such a tremendous opportunity for growth. This profession has allowed me to be a clinician, supervisor, educator, and researcher. Throughout the years, I have been so fortunate to learn from my clients, students, and colleagues in occupational therapy and other professions. They have taught me the true importance of occupation, whether playing a card game with friends, jumping rope on a playground, studying for an exam, or discussing the efficacy of various intervention methods. I have never ceased to be thankful that I found a profession as rewarding and fulfilling as occupational therapy.

WINIFRED SCHULTZ-KROHN, PhD, OTR/L, SWC, BCP, FAOTA
Associate Professor of Occupational Therapy
Department of Occupational Therapy
San José State University
San José, California

CHAPTER 6   Professional Organizations

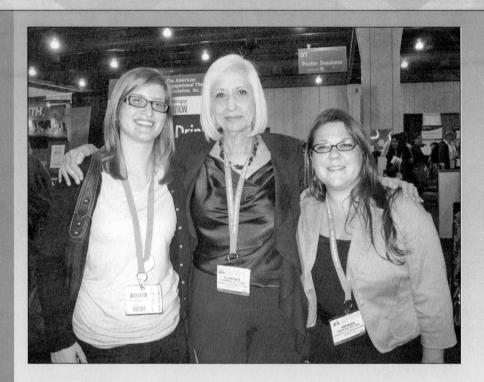

Objectives
After reading this chapter, the reader will be able to do the following:

- Describe the mission and major activities of the occupational therapy (OT) professional associations
- Describe the activities of the American Occupational Therapy Association, World Federation of Occupational Therapists, and state associations
- Describe how professional associations assure the delivery of quality occupational therapy services
- Identify ways professional organizations contribute to the professional development of their members

It is customary for professions to establish a professional association. The stronger and better supported the association is, the greater the benefits for the individual members. A **professional association** is organized and operated by its members for its members. It exists to protect and promote the profession it represents by (1) providing a communication network and channel for information, (2) regulating itself through the development and enforcement of standards of conduct and performance, and (3) guarding the interests of those within the profession.[1]

The professional organization for OT practitioners in the United States is the **American Occupational Therapy Association (AOTA).** Originally incorporated in 1917 as the National Society for the Promotion of Occupational Therapy, the association's name was changed to its present version in 1923. The **World Federation of Occupational**

Therapists (WFOT) was established in 1952 to help OT practitioners access international information, engage in international exchange, and promote organizations of occupational therapy in schools in countries where none exists.[3,5] Each state also has a professional organization for OT practitioners living in the state. Although there is frequent collaboration between AOTA and the individual state associations, the state associations are funded and operated independently from the national association. It is beneficial for OT practitioners to have a good understanding of the professional organizations and the services they provide. Because it would be impossible to discuss each state association in this text, this chapter describes the world and national associations. Readers are encouraged to join and support their professional associations at the world, national, state, and local levels. See Appendix D for the contact information for organizations.

American Occupational Therapy Association Mission

The mission of AOTA is "to advance the quality, availability, use and support of occupational therapy through standard-setting, advocacy, education, and research on behalf of its members and the public." In keeping with this mission statement, AOTA directs its efforts to (1) assure the quality of occupational therapy services, (2) improve consumer access to health care services, and (3) promote the professional development of its members.[1]

Membership

Three professional membership categories exist in AOTA: occupational therapist (OT), occupational therapy assistant (OTA), and occupational therapy student (OTS). Persons interested in the profession who are not OT professionals may join the organization as organizational or associate members. Membership categories determine the fees paid for membership and conferences, and who can attend special meetings, hold office, and vote. For example, organizational and associate members do not have voting privileges. Membership fees are higher for OTs. Membership fees for the OT student are lowest to encourage them to become involved in the organization and familiarize themselves with membership benefits.

Members at all levels are encouraged to become actively involved in AOTA by serving on committees, attending the annual conference, reviewing journal articles, presenting at conferences, and holding elected and volunteer positions. The COOL (Coordinated Online Opportunities for Leadership) database was developed to encourage membership participation at a variety of levels. Members complete a profile and indicate areas of expertise and interest. AOTA staff and committee chairpersons will use the database to find volunteers for a variety of organization and membership activities. Active membership helps OT practitioners become informed.[1]

Organizational Structure

AOTA is made up of a volunteer sector and paid national office staff. See Figure 6-1 for a description of the organizational structure of AOTA. The paid office staff is employed at the headquarters in Bethesda, Maryland, and performs the day-to-day operations under the management of the executive director. The national office staff is organized around four divisions: Business Operations Division (membership, marketing, corporate relations, and exhibits and advertising); Division of Public Affairs (federal affairs, reimbursement and regulatory policy, state affairs, and public/media relations); Professional Affairs Division (accreditation, education, practice, and professional development); and Finance, Information Technology, and Administration Division.

The volunteer sector consists of all of the members of the association and is represented by the executive board and the representative assembly. The executive board is charged with the administration and management of the association and includes elected officers. There are several standing committees of the executive board, including the representative assembly (RA), which is the legislative and policy-making body of the AOTA. The RA is composed of elected representatives from each recognized state, elected officers of the assembly and the association, a representative from the student committee, an occupational therapy assistant representative, the first delegate of the WFOT, and the chairpersons of the commissions. The standing commissions of the RA include the Commission on Education, Commission on Practice, Ethics Commission and Commission on Continuing Competence and Professional Development.[1]

Many occupational therapy educational programs have a club or organization for students. Student groups may participate in the **American Student Committee of the Occupational Therapy Association (ASCOTA),** a standing committee of the executive board of AOTA.

Assuring Quality of Occupational Therapy Services

The AOTA is responsible for ensuring the delivery of quality occupational therapy services. To this end, the association develops standards, produces official documents that identify the standards, and reviews the standards on a regular basis. Standards ensure that educational programs prepare students properly, that guidelines are in place articulating occupational therapy practice, and that a code of conduct is provided to clarify ethical issues. AOTA has developed standards of education, standards of practice, and ethical standards.

Standards for OT and OTA educational programs are developed and reviewed on a regular basis by the association's Accreditation Council for Occupational Therapy Education (ACOTE). Educational programs are accredited based on their compliance with these standards (see Chapter 5). These standards help ensure the delivery of quality educational programs in occupational therapy.

AOTA lends its support to states for the regulation of practice through licensure and other state laws. The *Occupational Therapy Scope of Practice*, developed by AOTA, is used by states as a model for their licensure laws.[6] As discussed in

THE AMERICAN OCCUPATIONAL THERAPY ASSOCIATION
2010 GOVERNANCE CHART

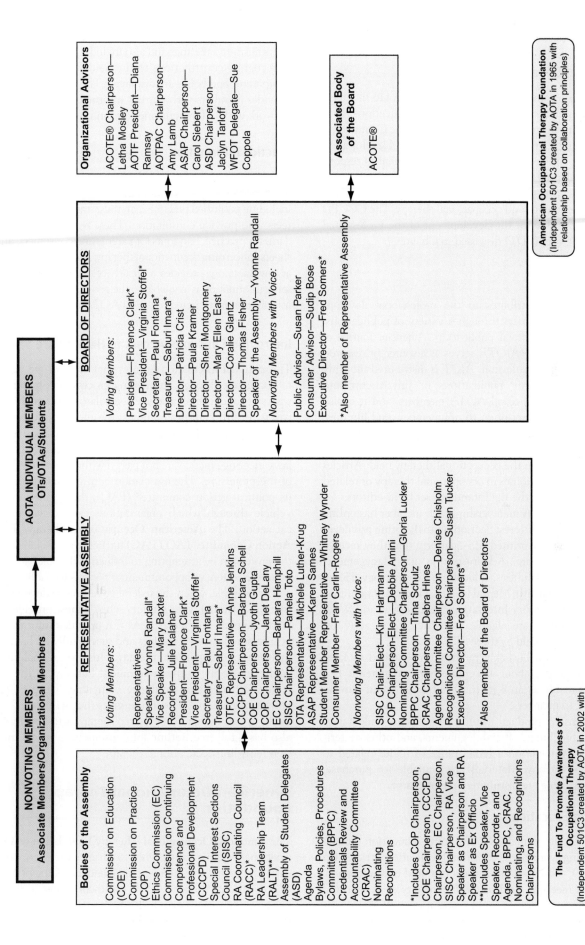

Figure 6-1 Organizational structure of the American Occupational Therapy Association. (Courtesy of the American Occupational Therapy Association, Bethesda, MD, www.aota.org/Governance/ProceduralAdHoc/Historical/Governance-Chart.aspx. Retrieved February 2, 2011.)

Chapter 8, state regulatory laws help ensure that practitioners meet specific competencies.

Professional Development of Members

AOTA promotes the professional development of its members through a number of activities, including publications, continuing education, and practice information. The Commission on Continuing Competence and Professional Development (CCCPD) is the designated body of the RA that is responsible for developing standards for continuing competency and for communicating to the various stakeholders' the issues surrounding competency and occupational therapy. The CCCPD was also responsible for the development of the Professional Development Tool (PDT) discussed in Chapter 7.

Publications

The association contributes to the professional development of OT practitioners through a variety of publications. The organization's official publication, *American Journal of Occupational Therapy (AJOT)*, serves as a source of research information for the profession. *AJOT* is distributed monthly (except for bimonthly publications in July/August and November/December) to all AOTA members, and it is also available through subscription to nonmembers and libraries. Subjects may include approaches to practice, programs and techniques, research, educational and professional trends, and areas of controversy in the occupational therapy field. Articles are written by professionals in occupational therapy or related fields and must meet the rigid standards set by its editors.

As a part of AOTA membership, each member has online access to 11 Special Interest Sections (SISs); voting privileges to three SISs, and 1 printed SIS quarterly that they receive by mail. The SISs are: Administration and Management, Developmental Disabilities, Education, Gerontology, Home and Community Health, Mental Health, Physical Disabilities, School System, Sensory Integration, Technology, and Work Programs. Members are eligible to participate in activities (such as meetings) held by three SISs.[1]

OT Practice is a biweekly publication designed to keep members informed about the profession in general. *OT Practice* (available as an e-journal) publishes useful clinical information to members.

An extensive product catalog lists books, videotapes, audiotapes, brochures, official documents, and other materials that are available on a broad range of topics related to occupational therapy. Materials are available for purchase, rent, or loan; some are distributed free of charge.

Continuing Education

AOTA sponsors numerous continuing education activities, including workshops, continuing education articles (in *OT Practice*), self-paced clinical courses, and online courses. The annual meeting, held in a different city each year and hosted by the area's local or state association, provides a variety of continuing education opportunities. All members are encouraged to attend. The conference hosts presentations ranging from poster sessions, panel discussions, and workshops, to formal presentations. The national conference conducts business meetings and also includes an awards ceremony to recognize contributions to the field. The latest materials, equipment, and books are displayed. The national conference provides members with current information and a chance to network with OT practitioners around the country.

Practice Information

In addition to all of the publications mentioned, AOTA has developed resources for information on all of the practice areas, including published practice materials, staff experts, and volunteers who provide consultation. These resources include standards for practice, handouts for parents and consumers, and fact sheets concerning occupational therapy. AOTA's official website at www.aota.org provides a wealth of information. Although some information is available to the general public, much of the information is restricted to use by AOTA members.

Improving Consumer Access to Health Care Services

The national association ensures that services are accessible to consumers through an ongoing process of communication with state and federal lawmakers, regulatory bodies, third-party payers, health care professionals, the media, and the public. For example, AOTA keeps abreast of proposed legislation and special committees within the government, ensuring that new laws affecting practice are not passed without hearing the voice of the profession. The association is in communication with its political action committee (PAC), the legally sanctioned vehicle through which organizations can engage in political action. The **American Occupational Therapy Political Action Committee (AOTPAC)** furthers the legislative aims of the profession by attempting to influence the selection, nomination, election, or appointment of persons to public office.[2]

For example, when the federal government developed legislation outlining what services schools must provide for the Handicapped Children Act, AOTA provided information on occupational therapy services and successfully lobbied for the inclusion of occupational therapy. This professional vigilance applies not only to the government but also to the private sector. When major insurance companies write or rewrite policies regarding the health services they will cover, AOTA works to ensure that occupational therapy is included. AOTA also has a toll-free hotline for consumers to access information regarding occupational therapy.

American Occupational Therapy Foundation

The **American Occupational Therapy Foundation (AOTF)** is a national organization designed to advance the science of occupational therapy and increase public understanding of the value of occupational therapy. AOTF was incorporated as a separate not-for-profit organization in 1965.[4] It is a vehicle for providing resources to programs and individuals for the purpose of carrying out occupational therapy education and research. AOTF also operates a library that contains books and journals related to occupational therapy. AOTF provides grant opportunities, scholarships, and research support.[4] Donations and bequests from AOTA members, corporations, and private foundations are collected and managed by AOTF to support these programs.

Since 1980, AOTF has published the *Occupational Therapy Journal of Research (OTJR)*, now named *OTJR: Occupation, Participation and Health*, to address the need for more publication opportunities. This journal is published quarterly and is available for a subscription fee.

World Federation of Occupational Therapists

The World Federation of Occupation Therapists (WFOT) was developed in 1952 with the objectives to promote and advocate for occupational therapy and establish minimum educational standards for member countries.[5] WFOT also serves as a vehicle for international information exchange among occupational therapy associations, practitioners, and other allied health personnel. The organization is responsible for many publications, including the WFOT journal. WFOT is organized into five program areas, which include standards and quality, education and research, promotion and development, international cooperation, and executive programs.[5] An international conference is sponsored by WFOT every 4 years. As the worldwide practice of occupational therapy continues to grow and develop, WFOT is a valuable mechanism for exchange of information with OT practitioners in other countries.

Summary

AOTA is the national organization representing OT practitioners. Its major activities include assuring the delivery of quality occupational therapy services, improving consumer access to health care, and promoting the professional development of its members.

AOTA ensures the delivery of quality services through the development and enforcement of standards, accreditation of educational programs, research, and support for regulation. To encourage the professional development of its members, AOTA conducts continuing education programs, publishes materials, and provides practice information. AOTA distributes information to federal and state lawmakers, insurance providers, media, public, and other health care providers.

At the international level, WFOT provides an information exchange and advances the practice and standards of occupational therapy around the world. OT practitioners are encouraged to participate in professional organizations at the international, national, state, and local levels.

See Appendix D for a list of professional organizations.

Learning Activities

1. Go to AOTA's website (www.aota.org), and retrieve information on an aspect of AOTA that is of special interest to you; write a brief paper on your findings.

2. Gather information on the next AOTA conference (e.g., when, where, cost, theme), and prepare a bulletin board display or poster.

3. Hold a class brainstorming session to compile a list of topics appropriate for a 15-minute conference short paper.

4. Gather information on your state occupational therapy association; prepare an informational handout for your class.

5. Prepare an overview of a topic from the WFOT conference. Discuss the current issues and topics with classmates.

6. The following is a recommended series of exploratory *American Journal of Occupational Therapy* investigations. Each stage is a bit more demanding and thus builds an increasing familiarity with both the publication and research techniques. These can become a series of projects over a period of time. Each class member is to do the following:
   - Locate the place and manner in which *American Journal of Occupational Therapy* is housed (current and past volumes).
   - Read an article of interest from *American Journal of Occupational Therapy*; give a 5-minute oral report on the topic, the source information, and the point of interest.
   - Research an article on an assigned topic; give a 5-minute oral report. (Further research may be required to gain information on the topic before the article search.)
   - Read an article from any occupational therapy source; write a half-page summary of the topic.
   - Gather information on an intervention technique by summarizing and critiquing at least three research articles.

Review Questions

1. What are the purposes of a professional organization?
2. List five benefits to membership in AOTA, WFOT, and state organizations.
3. How can members participate in professional organizations?
4. What resources are available to OT practitioners through the professional organizations?
5. What is your local occupational therapy association? Describe the activities of this association.

References

1. American Occupational Therapy Association: *About AOTA*. Retrieved January 30, 2011, from www.aota.org/About.aspx.
2. American Occupational Therapy Association: *AOTPAC fact sheet*. Retrieved January 30, 2011, from http://www.aota.org/Practitioners/Advocacy/AOTPAC/About/36338.aspx.
3. American Occupational Therapy Association: *Frequently asked questions about the World Federation of Occupational Therapists (WFOT)*. Retrieved January 30, 2011, from http://www.aota.org/Practitioners/Resources/Intl/WFOT/40549.aspx.
4. American Occupational Therapy Foundation: *Did you know? Facts about the American Occupational Therapy Foundation*. Retrieved January 30, 2011, from http://www.aotf.org/aboutaotf.aspx.
5. World Federation of Occupational Therapy: *WFOT information*. Retrieved January 30, 2011, from www.wfot.org.au/inside.asp.
6. American Occupational Therapy Association: Scope of practice, *Am J Occup Ther* 58:673–677, 2004.

I like helping people.

Okay, so maybe that sounds a little simplistic, but it is true. I like solving problems, connecting people with resources, working with an individual eye to eye, and setting and meeting goals. I like looking at not only the "forest," but also the "trees," and seeing each "tree" for the individual that he or she is and recognizing the unique and special characteristics that each person has to offer. I like treating a person with respect and dignity, and through the knowledge and skills that I possess as an occupational therapist, helping that person to achieve a life that is purposeful and meaningful to him or her, not by my definitions, but by what he or she defines as important. I like looking at the whole person, not just a body part or specific function, but as a precious asset to society, complex and dynamic. I like the look on someone's face when he or she realizes that he or she can accomplish far more than he or she ever thought he or she would be able to do before working with an occupational therapist. I like when "can't" becomes "can" and "doesn't" becomes "done."

I like helping people; I love being an OT.

JILL J. PAGE, OTR/L
Industrial Rehabilitation Consultant
ErgoScience, Inc.
Birmingham, Alabama

CHAPTER 7

The Occupational Therapy Practitioner: Roles, Responsibilities, and Relationships

Key Terms

Activity director
Advanced-level practitioner
Board certification
Career development
Client-related tasks
Close supervision
Continuing competence
Direct supervision
Entry-level practitioner
General supervision
Interdisciplinary team
Intermediate-level practitioner
Multidisciplinary team
Non–client-related tasks
Professional development
Relationship
Roles
Routine supervision
Service competency
Specialty certification
Supervision
Transdisciplinary team

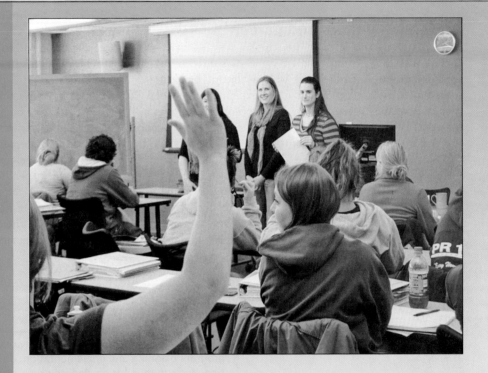

Objectives

After completing this chapter, the reader will be able to do the following:

- Identify the different roles an occupational therapy (OT) practitioner may assume
- Describe the three levels of performance for OT practitioners
- Explain the role of activity director
- Discuss the minimum responsibilities of the occupational therapist (OT) and the occupational therapy assistant (OTA) in service delivery as described in the *Standards of Practice*
- Understand the levels of supervision and parameters that affect these levels
- Identify the practices that contribute to successful supervisory relationships
- Describe service competency
- Describe the different types of teams in health care and recognize the importance of interdisciplinary teams
- Understand the importance of lifelong learning and professional development
- Describe tools that can be used to maintain and document continuing competency

When a student graduates from an accredited educational program and passes the National Board for Certification in Occupational Therapy (NBCOT®) exam, there is a basic level of competence that is assumed, and a state license (in states that have licensure) is granted. At this point, the practitioner is considered to be an entry-level practitioner. This is an exciting point in time for OT and OTA students, with many career opportunities and experiences for learning. In this chapter, we first discuss the various roles in which an OT practitioner may function. The responsibilities of the entry-level OT practitioner in service delivery are outlined, along with guidelines for supervision. Next, we describe relationships found in service delivery and how the OT practitioner can work effectively within those relationships. Finally, we discuss how the entry-level practitioner develops knowledge and skills to maintain competency and advance in the profession. By understanding the available roles and responsibilities and their requirements, the entry-level OT practitioner can control the direction of his or her career.

Professional Roles and Career Development

It is important to understand what is meant by professional roles and relationships. Crist explained that **roles** specify positions or sets of stipulated job-related responsibilities.[13] Each role carries with it specific expectations for job performance and responsibilities. An individual's ability to function in a role is based on educational preparation, professional boundaries and responsibilities, and prior experience in the role.[13] As in life, most people working in organizations have multiple roles. The connection of different roles to one another is a **relationship.** Working organizations are made up of many relationships. The combination

of roles and relationships defines expectations in the organization and clarifies interactions.[13]

Direct client care is the role most commonly assumed by the OT practitioner who is just entering the field. However, there are an additional 10 roles identified by the profession that can potentially be held by OTs and OTAs. These include consumer educator, fieldwork educator in a practice setting, supervisor, administrator in a practice setting, consultant, academic fieldwork coordinator, faculty, academic program director, researcher/scholar, and entrepreneur. Each of these roles and a description of its major functions are shown in Table 7-1. Often, OT practitioners function in more than one role—at times within the same job. For example, an OT may provide direct client services and perform the functions of an administrator; an OTA may hold positions as both a faculty member and clinician.

As the career of an OT practitioner progresses, he or she may wish to advance within the service delivery path or transition into a role outside of service delivery. This is referred to as **career development.** How the individual develops in a career will depend upon previous choices about roles and relationships.[13]

There are three ways in which career development occurs in occupational therapy: vertical movement within a setting, lateral movement across settings, and maturation within

Table 7-1 Occupational Therapy Roles

Role	Major Function
Practitioner—OT	Provides quality occupational therapy services, including evaluation, intervention, program planning and implementation, discharge planning–related documentation, and communication. Service provision may include direct, monitored, and consultative approaches.
Practitioner—OTA	Provides quality occupational therapy services to assigned individuals under the supervision of an OT.
Educator (consumer, peer)	Develops and provides educational offering or training related to occupational therapy to consumer, peer, and community individuals or groups.
Fieldwork Educator (practice setting)	Manages Level I or II fieldwork in a practice setting. Provides OT students with opportunities to practice and carry out practitioner competencies.
Supervisor	Manages the overall daily operation of occupational therapy services in defined practice area(s).
Administrator (practice setting)	Manages department, program, services, or agency providing occupational therapy services.
Consultant	Provides occupational therapy consultation to individuals, groups, or organizations.
Academic Fieldwork Coordinator	Manages student fieldwork program within the academic setting.
Faculty	Provides formal academic education for OT or OTA students.
Academic Program Director	Manages the educational program for OT or OTA students.
Researcher/Scholar	Performs scholarly work of the profession, including examining, developing, refining, and evaluating the profession's body of knowledge, theoretical base, and philosophical foundations.
Entrepreneur	Entrepreneurs are partially or fully self-employed individuals who provide occupational therapy services.

Adapted from American Occupational Therapy Association: Career exploration and development: A companion guide to the occupational therapy roles document. In COTA *Information Packet: A Guide for Supervision,* Bethesda, MD, 1995, AOTA.
Note: Many jobs involve more than one role, and job titles vary by setting.

a role.[13] In vertical movement within a setting, the practitioner moves up in the organization to progressively higher positions. For example, a practitioner may move to the role of fieldwork educator, then department supervisor, and eventually manager of a rehabilitation clinic. A lateral movement across settings might involve an expert clinician transitioning to the role of a clinical instructor in a university setting. The third means of career development is the maturation of the individual within a specific role from entry level, to intermediate level, to an advanced level, for example, from entry-level clinician to advanced clinical specialist.

Levels of Performance

OT practitioners perform at one of three levels: entry, intermediate, or advanced. An individual's level of performance is not based on years of experience in the field because this is not a valid indicator of performance. Instead, the practitioner's level of performance is based on attaining a higher skill level through work experience, education, and professional socialization.[9]

Table 7-2 describes the levels of performance and demonstrates how a practitioner's career may develop as knowledge and skill increase. The **entry-level practitioner** is expected to be responsible for and accountable in professional activities related to the role. In states with licensure laws, entry-level practice is defined by the licensure law and supporting regulations. The **intermediate-level practitioner** has increased responsibility and typically pursues specialization in a particular area of practice. The **advanced-level practitioner** is considered an expert, or a resource, in the respective role.

Each individual progresses along this continuum at a different pace. Some individuals never progress past the entry level in a particular role, or a person may transition to a new role, wherein his or her level of performance is classified at entry level. For example, an individual who has worked as an OT at the advanced level may transfer into an administrative role at the entry level. An OTA at the intermediate level may transition to the role of an entry-level faculty member. Even at the entry level, individuals in both situations may need to acquire additional knowledge and skill to satisfactorily perform the new job functions. It is also possible for an individual to function in two roles at different levels. For example, an OTA intermediate-level practitioner may assume new responsibilities as a fieldwork educator. In the new role, this OTA would initially perform the job function at the entry level.

For any type of role advancement or transition, the OT practitioner must be aware of what the expectations are for the new role and prepare accordingly. Methods to achieve role advancement or transition are discussed later, in the section on professional development.

Specialized Roles

There are specialized roles in which OT practitioners can function; however, these roles are typically outside of the profession. These include roles such as case manager, supervisor of other allied health care professionals, consultant, and activity director. These roles are advanced-level positions for OT practitioners. We discuss the role of activity director in the following section because it is a role that the OTA can function in without supervision.

Activity Director

The role of **activity director** is one for which the OTA is well qualified and can function independently.[21] Activity directors are typically employed in group homes, institutions for people with mental retardation, assisted living facilities, and long-term care facilities for older persons. In these types of facilities, residents may withdraw and become isolated. The activity director is responsible for planning, implementing, and documenting an ongoing program of activities that meet

Table 7-2 **Levels of Performance**

Role	Major Focuses
Entry	• Development of skills • Socialization in the expectations related to the organization, peer, and profession *Acceptance of responsibilities and accountability for role-relevant professional activities is expected.*
Intermediate	• Increased independence • Mastery of basic role functions • Ability to respond to situations based on previous experience • Participation in the education of personnel *Specialization is frequently initiated, along with increased responsibility for collaboration with other disciplines and related organizations. Participation in role-relevant professional activities is increased.*
Advanced	• Refinement of specialized skills • Understanding of complex issues affecting role functions *Contribution to the knowledge base and growth of the profession results in being considered an expert, resource person, or consultant within a role. This expertise is recognized by others inside and outside of the profession through leadership, mentoring, research, education, and volunteerism.*

Adapted from American Occupational Therapy Association: Occupational therapy roles, *Am J Occup Ther* 47:1087, 1993.

the needs of the residents. The activity director needs to be aware of and adhere to regulations for activity programs and personnel that have been set forth by Medicare, state health departments, and licensing agencies.

The *Standards of Practice*[18] for the National Association of Activity Professionals classifies activities that are provided to the client as supportive, providing maintenance, or empowering. Supportive activities are commonly provided to individuals who do not have the cognitive or physical ability to participate in a group program. The purpose of these activities is to promote a comfortable environment and to provide stimulation to those individuals. Examples include placing meaningful objects in the person's room and providing background music. Maintenance activities are those that provide opportunities for the individual to maintain physical, cognitive, social, emotional, and spiritual health. Examples of maintenance activities are exercise groups, games such as shuffleboard, creative writing, and choir. Empowering activities are geared toward promoting self-respect, and they offer opportunities for self-expression, personal responsibility, and

social responsibility. Writing a facility newsletter or forming a council dedicated to resolving residents' issues are examples of empowering activities.[18] Detailed information on the role of the OTA as an activity director can be found in *Ryan's Occupational Therapy Assistant*.[21]

Roles and Responsibilities During Service Delivery

The Standards of Practice for Occupational Therapy[6] defines the minimum requirements for OT practitioners working in service delivery. The standards are delineated into four areas: (1) professional standing and responsibility; (2) screening, evaluation, and reevaluation; (3) intervention; and (4) outcomes. These standards are summarized in Table 7-3 and printed in full in Appendix B.

It is important to remember that these standards are guidelines developed by the American Occupational Therapy Association (AOTA) that support the *Scope of Practice for*

Table 7-3 Responsibilities of the Occupational Therapist and Occupational Therapy Assistant During the Delivery of Occupational Therapy Services

Service	Occupational Therapist	Occupational Therapy Assistant
Evaluation	Directing the evaluation process. Directing all aspects of the initial contact during the evaluation, including need for service, defining the problems within the domain of occupational therapy, determining client goals and priorities, establishing intervention priorities, determining further assessment needs, and determining assessment tasks that can be delegated to the OTA. Initiating and directing the evaluation, interpreting the data, and developing the intervention plan.	Contributing to the evaluation process by implementing delegated assessments. Providing verbal and written reports of observations and client capacities to the OT.
Intervention planning	Overall development of the occupational therapy intervention plan. Collaborating with the client to develop the plan.	Collaborating with the client to develop the plan. Being knowledgeable about evaluation results and for providing input into the intervention plan, based on client needs and priorities.
Intervention implementation	The overall implementation of the intervention. Providing appropriate supervision when delegating aspects of intervention to the OTA.	Being knowledgeable about the client's occupational therapy goals. Selecting, implementing, and modifying therapeutic activities and interventions that are consistent with demonstrated competency levels, client goals, and the requirements of the practice setting.
Intervention review	Determining the need for continuing, modifying, or discontinuing occupational therapy services.	Contributing to this process by exchanging information with and providing documentation to the OT about the client's responses to and communications during intervention.
Outcome evaluation	Selecting, measuring, and interpreting outcomes that are related to the client's ability to engage in occupations.	Being knowledgeable about the client's targeted occupational therapy outcomes and providing information and documentation related to outcome achievement. Implementing outcome measurements and providing needed client discharge resources.

Adapted from American Occupational Therapy Association: Standards of practice for occupational therapy, *Am J Occup Ther* 64(6):415–420, 2010.

Occupational Therapy.[8] They are often used by states in the formation of licensure laws and supporting regulations for occupational therapy practice. State licensure laws provide a legal definition of practice for that state and may delineate specific responsibilities for the OT and OTA related to role delineation, supervision, documentation, and advanced practice (see Chapter 5). The OT practitioner must provide services in accordance with the laws or regulations of the state in which he or she practices. Other regulatory agencies, such as the Centers for Medicare and Medicaid Services (CMS), also have regulations that supersede these guidelines.

The first standard delineates requirements related to professional standing and responsibility for all OT practitioners. Key points related to Standard I are that the OT practitioner: (1) deliver services that reflect the philosophical base of occupational therapy; (2) be knowledgeable about and deliver services in accordance with AOTA standards, policies, and guidelines, and state and federal regulations; (3) maintain current licensure, registration, or certification as required; (4) abide by the AOTA *Occupational Therapy Code of Ethics*,[4] and *Standards for Continuing Competence*;[5] (5) maintain current knowledge of legislative, political, social, cultural, and reimbursement issues; and (6) be knowledgeable about evidence-based research.[6]

The second standard outlines the practitioner's responsibilities during screening, evaluation, and reevaluation. An OT accepts and responds to referrals and initiates the screening, evaluation, and reevaluation process. The OT is responsible for analyzing and interpreting the evaluation data. The OTA contributes to the process by performing assessments that have been delegated by the OT. The OTA communicates verbally or in writing to the OT his or her observations of the assessment and the client's abilities. The OT then completes and documents the evaluation results. The OTA contributes to the documentation of the evaluation results. The OT recommends additional consultations or refers clients to appropriate sources as needed.[6]

Practitioner responsibilities during the intervention stage of service delivery are described in Standard III. The OT has the overall responsibility for documentation and implementation of the intervention, based on the evaluation, client goals, current best evidence, and clinical reasoning. The OTA can select, implement, and modify therapeutic activities (consistent with his or her demonstrated competency, delegated responsibilities, and intervention plan). The OT, with contributions from the OTA, modifies the intervention plan throughout the process and documents the client's responses and any changes to treatment.[6]

Requirements and responsibilities related to outcomes are delineated in Standard IV. The OT selects, measures, documents, and interprets outcomes that are related to the client's ability to engage in occupations. The OT is responsible for documenting changes in the client's performance and for discontinuing services. A discontinuation plan or transition plan is prepared by the OT, with contributions from the OTA regarding the client's needs, goals, performance, and follow-up services. Either practitioner facilitates the transition process in collaboration with the client, family members, and significant others. The OT evaluates the safety and effectiveness of the occupational therapy processes and interventions; the OTA contributes to this evaluation of safety and effectiveness.[6]

Supervision

After initial certification and applicable state licensure, the entry-level practitioner functions independently in delivering occupational therapy services. It is recommended that he or she seek supervision and mentoring from a more experienced OT to grow professionally and to develop best approaches to practice. OTAs require supervision from an OT to deliver occupational therapy services. The OT is ultimately responsible for all aspects of the services provided by the OTA, the occupational therapy aide, and the OT student.

The document *Guidelines for Supervision, Roles, and Responsibilities During the Delivery of Occupational Therapy Services*[7] provides a definition of supervision and parameters for supervision. However, it is important for the OT practitioner to adhere to state and federal regulations, the *Occupational Therapy Code of Ethics*[4] (see Chapter 5), and the policies of the workplace. The regulations that delineate the specific responsibilities and supervisory requirements for the OT and OTA vary considerably from state to state. Each OT practitioner needs to be responsible for familiarizing him or herself with the appropriate state regulations. The AOTA website (www.aota.org) provides a summary of the supervision requirements for each state. Outside accreditation bodies and third-party payers also have specific requirements related to supervision. For example, CMS specifies requirements regarding provision of services by students. Any facility that is reimbursed by Medicare needs to abide by these requirements.

Supervision is defined by AOTA as a "cooperative process in which two or more people participate in a joint effort to establish, maintain, and/or elevate a level of competence and performance."[7] The supervisor is an individual "who has some official responsibility to direct, guide, and monitor the supervisee's practice."[12] It is important that the OT and OTA work collaboratively to develop and implement a plan for supervision that ensures safe and effective service delivery and promotes professional competence and development.[7]

Levels of Supervision and Parameters That Affect Supervision Levels

Supervision can be quantified by the number of hours and the level or intensity of supervision that is provided. State and federal regulations specify requirements for levels of supervision. The OT student needs to be aware of terminology that may be used to describe the different levels of supervision.

It is helpful for the student to conceptualize supervision along a continuum as shown in Figure 7-1.[2,11] Supervision ranges from a level of being in direct contact at all times with

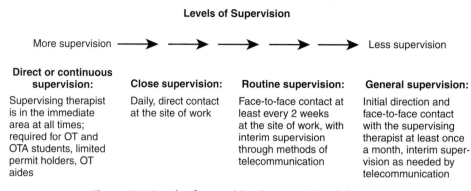

Figure 7-1 Levels of supervision in occupational therapy.

the supervisee to a level wherein face-to-face contact occurs on a monthly basis. At the high end of the continuum is **direct supervision** (or continuous supervision), wherein the supervising OT is on site and available to provide immediate assistance to the client or supervisee if needed. **Close supervision** is the need for direct, daily contact. **Routine supervision** involves direct contact at least every 2 weeks, with interim supervision as needed. **General supervision** is described as at least monthly face-to-face contact.[9]

Contact between a supervisor and supervisee can be face-to-face or via telecommunication. Some state regulations are very specific about the amount of face-to-face contact that is to take place at the different levels. For example, descriptors such as "daily," "once every seventh treatment," "one hour per 40 occupational therapy work hours," or "every 21 calendar days" may be used by states to regulate the amount of face-to-face contact. Many state regulations specify that when the OT is not providing direct supervision, he or she must be available via methods of telecommunication at all times while the OTA is treating clients. These methods include the use of cell phones, voice mail, and laptops with the capability of sharing client data and e-mailing each other.

Elaine is an OTA with over 10 years of experience in home health. She works under the supervision of an OT but only sees her face-to-face once a month. She takes a cell phone and a laptop with her to every home visit. After her first visit of the day is complete, she checks her e-mail using her laptop computer. She has an e-mail message from her supervising OT that there is a new client whose evaluation has recently been completed, and the client needs to be scheduled for therapy. Elaine then goes into the agency database on her laptop and searches for the new client. In the client's electronic file, Elaine finds and reads the OT's evaluation report and intervention plan. Elaine locates the client's phone number and schedules an appointment for later that afternoon.

Most state regulations specify the number of OTAs whom an OT can supervise at any one time. For example, current regulations in California stipulate that an OT may supervise up to two OTAs; in Delaware, the maximum number of OTAs

who can be supervised is three.[2] In some cases, states also stipulate how many years of experience the supervising OT needs to have before he or she can supervise an OTA.

Supervision is an ongoing process that changes with the setting and the individuals involved. The frequency, method, and content of supervision depends on several parameters. First, it is important to determine the regulatory requirements and requirements of the practice setting that pertain to supervision. The supervisor and supervisee also need to understand each other's level of competence, experience, education, and credentials. After these parameters have been established, supervision is based on the following:

- The complexity of client needs
- The number and diversity of clients
- The skills of the OT and OTA
- The type of practice setting

A level of supervision that is *more frequent* than the minimum level required by the practice setting and regulatory agencies may be required if (1) the needs of the client and the occupational therapy process are complex and fluctuating; (2) a large number of clients with diverse needs are served by occupational therapy in the practice setting; and (3) it is determined by the OT and OTA that additional supervision is necessary for the delivery of safe and effective occupational therapy services.[7] Based on all of these factors, the OT working with the OTA determines how much and what type of supervision is appropriate. Collaboratively, they develop and document a plan for supervision.

Supervisory contacts should be documented, including the frequency of supervisory contact, the methods(s) or types(s) of supervision, content areas addressed during the contact, evidence to support areas and levels of competency, and signatures and credentials of the individuals participating in the supervisory process.[7] Keeping such records will meet regulatory requirements and also allow both the supervisor and supervisee to observe the progress made, to adjust job expectations as needed, and to provide evidence of professional development activities for both individuals.[11]

The supervising OT may co-sign treatment notes completed by the supervisee as another way of documenting that supervision has taken place. As a rule of thumb, documentation by either an OT or OTA student needs to be signed by the supervisor. Individuals (OTs and OTAs) holding a temporary license or limited permit must also have a co-signature on documentation until the permanent license is received. OTAs do not necessarily need their documentation co-signed. However, state and federal regulations, third-party reimbursement policies, and the policies of the practice setting may request it. The supervisory process is an interactive one; it requires more than paper review and a co-signature on documentation.

Service Competency

Because the OT is responsible for the performance level of the OTA, he or she must have confidence that the OTA will obtain the same results when providing occupational therapy services. **Service competency** is a useful mechanism to ensure that services are provided with the same high level of confidence. Service competency is defined as "the determination, made by various methods, that two people performing the same or equivalent procedures will obtain the same or equivalent results. In test development, this is known as interrater reliability. The same concept can be applied to professionals working together in the service provision process. It stems from the assumption that the practitioners employ currently acceptable practices."[10]

The methods and standards to establish service competency vary, depending on the task or procedure involved. Methods such as independent scoring of standardized tests, observation, videotaping, and co-treatment can be used. Service competency is more easily established for frequently used procedures. It may take longer to establish competency for uncommon procedures. Service competency is established for a particular procedure, when the practitioners meet the acceptable standard of performance on three successive occasions.[10] It is important that service competency be established for each procedure.

Supervision of the Occupational Therapy Aide

An occupational therapy aide is an individual who supports the OT and OTA by performing specifically delegated tasks.[7] Occupational therapy aides may also be referred to as restorative aides, service extenders, or rehabilitation aides/technicians. Depending on state law, either an OT or an OTA may supervise the occupational therapy aide; however, the OT remains the individual ultimately responsible for the actions of the aide. He or she directs the development, documentation, and implementation of a supervisory plan. The person working as an aide is not required to have any special training; typically, he or she receives on-the-job training from the OT practitioners. Because the level of training is limited, it is important that supervision remain close.

The aide is assigned to perform delegated, selected, client-related and non–client-related tasks for which the aide has demonstrated competency.[7] **Non–client-related tasks** include the preparation of the work area and equipment, clerical tasks, and maintenance activities. Examples of these types of tasks include setting up for a group activity in an outpatient

mental health setting, making the daily schedule in an inpatient rehabilitation setting, and cleaning equipment in an outpatient hand clinic. The aide may provide routine **client-related tasks** where the aide may interact with the client but not as the primary service provider of occupational therapy.[7] These tasks must have (1) a predictable outcome; (2) a situation in which the client and environment are stable and that does not require the aide to make judgments, interpretations, or adaptations; (3) a client who has demonstrated prior ability to perform the task; and (4) a clearly established task routine and process.[7] The supervisor ensures that the aide is competent in carrying out selected tasks and in using related equipment. The aide must be instructed in how to perform the task with the specific client and be aware of precautions, signs, or symptoms the client may demonstrate that indicate that assistance is needed.[7] The practitioner documents the supervision of the aide.

Occupational Therapist–Occupational Therapy Assistant Partnership: Strategies for a Successful Supervisory Relationship

Beyond the practical need to determine appropriate duties and supervision, each OT practitioner needs to be aware that the roles of the OT and OTA are intentionally interrelated. The relationship is a partnership. For that partnership to be effective, there needs to be mutual respect and trust.

There are many factors that contribute to a successful supervisory relationship. The supervisor should have a solid knowledge base related to the practice of occupational therapy and guidelines for supervision. It is also important that the supervisor have an understanding of the different ways in which individuals learn and an awareness of his or her own learning style as well as that of the supervisee. Communication is a key element in successful supervisory relationships. Both parties must listen actively, give and receive constructive feedback, be assertive and tactful, and resolve conflicts.[11] Instead of providing quick and easy answers to concerns brought up by the supervisee, the supervisor provides resources and direction that facilitate problem solving and clinical reasoning.

Berger identifies some helpful practices to increase the likelihood for success in the supervisory process.[11] Setting a designated and prioritized time for supervision meetings will save time and make it more likely that the process will take place. Having a written agenda so that both the supervisor and supervisee know the issues and the priority in which they will be discussed ensures that the time allotted is used most efficiently. As supervisory topics come up during the course of a week, it is helpful to jot these down on a running list of topics for supervisory meetings. Active participation by both supervisor and supervisee is critical to the success of the supervision process. Both parties should be involved in actively evaluating and discussing levels of competency, seeking feedback on performance, setting goals for the future, and maintaining records of professional development.[11]

Health Care Teams and Teamwork

Practitioners also need to navigate relationships within the health care team. Box 7-1 lists some common disciplines that may be on a team with the OT practitioner. In health care today, working as a member of an interdisciplinary team is the norm. Entry-level practitioners need to first establish a solid identity in their own profession and its uniqueness.[14] The OT practitioner needs to have knowledge of the roles and responsibilities of other health professionals and good interpersonal, communication, and team-building skills.[20] Once this foundation is established, the practitioner is capable of building productive relationships with members of other disciplines.[14] An experienced OT practitioner may in time have the responsibility for coordinating the interdisciplinary treatment team and supervising team members. Responsibilities of this role include organizing and leading team meetings, managing client data, and communicating results to doctors and administrators.

There are three different types of teams: multidisciplinary, interdisciplinary, and transdisciplinary. In a **multidisciplinary team,** there are a variety of disciplines that work together in a common setting. However, the relationship between the team members is not interactive. At the other extreme is the **transdisciplinary team,** in which members cross over professional boundaries and share roles and functions.[12] In this approach, there is a blurring of traditional practitioner roles. The **interdisciplinary team** is commonly found in health care today. Members of an interdisciplinary team maintain their own professional roles while using a cooperative approach that is interactive and centered on a common problem to solve.

In the interdisciplinary team approach, various disciplines meet and plan the overall care of the client, maintaining an awareness of his or her needs, responses, and goals. Team members become mutual sources of information and support in treatment. It is not uncommon for team members using this approach to co-treat (treatment provided by each team member at the same time) a client. For example, the team OT and speech-language pathologist may both treat a client with a swallowing disorder at mealtime. The OT will focus treatment on the client's skill of bringing the food to his mouth and chewing it, whereas the speech-language pathologist may be focused on producing an effective swallow. In this case, the common problem the therapists are working to remediate is the client's swallowing disorder. Each member focuses on what he or she does best and supports the other during the intervention.

There are many similarities between the working partnership of the OT and the OTA and interdisciplinary teams of professionals who work in health care. Similarities include the need to have an understanding about the roles of team members, knowledge of professional boundaries, knowledge of the group process (see Chapter 16), and good communication skills. Teams whose members are open minded, willing to hear and try new things, and tolerant of change are the most effective.[14]

Lifelong Learning and Professional Development

The focus of this chapter has been on the roles and responsibilities of the entry-level practitioner who has a minimum skill base. But what about the OT practitioner who has been in practice 5, 10, or 15 years? In health care, changes in technology, research evidence, best practices, delivery mechanisms, and regulations occur constantly. A practitioner who does not keep up with these changes is opening himself or herself up to consequences ranging from self-dissatisfaction with one's performance to employer or client dissatisfaction and potential client harm.[16] How do the employer, third-party payers, and consumer know that the practitioner has kept abreast of these changes and continues to be competent to practice? Who is responsible for making certain that a practitioner remains competent?

To keep pace with these changes, the OT practitioner needs to continually acquire new knowledge, skills, and other assets. The Code of Ethics states that the OT practitioner is responsible for achieving and maintaining competence in order to practice.[4] Thus, OT practitioners are obligated by the profession's Code of Ethics to commit to lifelong learning to ensure that they are competent to practice. Organizing and personally managing a cumulative series of work experiences to add to one's knowledge, motivation, perspectives, skills, and job performance is referred to as career development or **professional development.**[20]

Box 7-1

Professionals Who Team with Occupational Therapy Practitioners

Adapted physical educator
Audiologist
Biomedical/rehabilitation engineer
Case manager
Dietician
Durable medical equipment provider
Nurse
Orthotist and prosthetist
Physical therapist
Physicians (primary care provider, physiatrist, neurologist, psychiatrist, ophthalmologist, orthopedist, cardiologist)
Psychologist
Rehabilitation counselor
Respiratory therapist
Recreation therapist
Social worker
Special educator
Speech-language pathologist
Vocational counselor

Adapted from Cohn ES: Interdisciplinary communication and supervision of personnel. In Crepeau EB, Cohn ES, Schell BAB (eds): *Willard and Spackman's Occupational Therapy,* ed 11, Philadelphia, 2009, Lippincott Williams & Wilkins.

An element of lifelong learning and professional development is continuing competence.[16] **Continuing competence** is defined as "a dynamic, multidimensional process in which the professional develops and maintains the knowledge, performance skills, interpersonal abilities, critical reasoning skills, and ethical reasoning skills necessary to perform his or her professional responsibilities."[15] The Standards for Continuing Competence establishes criteria in each of these areas useful to practitioners when examining their own competence (Table 7-4). The practitioner uses these standards as a guide for assessing the current level of competence, developing capacity for the future, and documenting continuing competence.[5] The standards also serve as a foundational element in the development of AOTA's board certifications and specialty certifications.

Table 7-4 **Standards of Continuing Competence**

Standard	Description
Standard 1: Knowledge	OTs and OTAs shall demonstrate understanding and comprehension of the information required for the multiple roles and responsibilities they assume. The individual must demonstrate the following: • Mastery of the core of occupational therapy as it is applied in the multiple responsibilities assumed • Expertise associated with primary responsibilities • Integration of relevant evidence, literature, and epidemiological data related to primary responsibilities and to the consumer population(s) served • Integration of current Association documents and legislative, legal, and regulatory issues into practice
Standard 2: Critical reasoning	OTs and OTAs shall employ reasoning processes to make sound judgments and decisions. The individual must demonstrate the following: • Deductive and inductive reasoning in making decisions specific to roles and responsibilities • Problem-solving skills necessary to carry out responsibilities • The ability to analyze occupational performance as influenced by environmental factors • The ability to reflect on one's own practice • Management and synthesis of information from a variety of sources in support of making decisions • Application of evidence, research findings, and outcome data in making decisions
Standard 3: Interpersonal abilities	OTs and OTAs shall develop and maintain their professional relationships with others within the context of their roles and responsibilities. The individual must demonstrate the following: • Use of effective communication methods that match the abilities, personal factors, learning styles, and therapeutic needs of consumers and others • Effective interaction with people from diverse backgrounds • Use of feedback from consumers, families, supervisors, and colleagues to modify one's professional behavior • Collaboration with consumers, families, and professionals to attain optimal consumer outcomes • The ability to develop and sustain team relationships to meet identified outcomes
Standard 4: Performance skills	OTs and OTAs shall demonstrate the expertise, aptitudes, proficiencies, and abilities to competently fulfill their roles and responsibilities. The individual must demonstrate expertise in the following: • Practice grounded in the core of occupational therapy • Therapeutic use of self, the therapeutic use of occupations and activities, the consultation process, and the education process to bring about change • Integration of current practice techniques and technologies • Updating performance, based on current research and literature • Quality improvement processes that prevent practice error and maximize client outcomes
Standard 5: Ethical reasoning	OTs and OTAs shall identify, analyze, and clarify ethical issues or dilemmas to make responsible decisions within the changing context of their roles and responsibilities. The individual must demonstrate the following: • Understanding and adherence to the profession's Code of Ethics, other relevant codes of ethics, and applicable laws and regulations • The use of ethical principles and the profession's core values to understand complex situations • The integrity to make and defend decisions based on ethical reasoning

Adapted from American Occupational Therapy Association: Standards for continuing competence, *Am J Occup Ther* 64(6):411–413, 2010.

The mission of AOTA, the National Board for Certification in Occupational Therapy (NBCOT®) and state regulatory boards is to protect the public and ensure quality services. Therefore, they have a vested interest in the continuing competency of OT practitioners. Many states require continuing competence in order for the individual to renew his or her license. The OT practitioner demonstrates continuing competence through participation in various continuing education activities. The practitioner earns a certain number of contact hours or continuing education units. The number of contact hours required is specified in each state's licensure regulations. There are many avenues and resources available to practitioners for professional development. It is the practitioner's responsibility to determine what to do and which resources to use.

Strategies for Professional Development and Continuing Competence

Each OT practitioner needs to accept personal ownership of his or her career and manage his or her own process for professional development and continuing competency. The key is for the OT practitioner to develop an idea of the direction he or she wants his or her career to take and set goals and activities to get there. Many activities are available for professional development and continuing competency. For example, the individual can participate in professional development activities at work, at conferences, at universities, or online. Practitioners are advised to develop a habit of reading a wide range of literature and attend state, regional, and national occupational therapy conferences.[14] Attending conferences allows one to network with other practitioners and learn about the latest practice and research influencing the profession. A summary of typical professional development activities is listed in Box 7-2.

Tools, such as the Professional Development Tool (PDT), assist practitioners in the professional development process. The PDT, developed by AOTA, is available on the AOTA website. The objectives for the use of the PDT are the following[1]:

- Assess learning needs and organized professional growth activities toward self-identified professional or career outcomes
- Identify and pursue professional development opportunities that will improve practice and career opportunities
- Promote quality in the profession and contribute to the growth of the profession
- Fulfill one's responsibility for continuing competence

Using the PDT, the practitioner completes steps to identify personal and professional development interests and needs, create a professional plan, and document completion of activities in a professional development portfolio. There are other resources that can assist practitioners in developing a professional portfolio.[17] Many students learn about professional portfolios and start the development of a portfolio during their educational process.

Box 7-2

Examples of Professional Development Unit Activities

These are examples of professional development activities that qualify for PDUs by NBCOT®. Professional development activity requirements for state licensing boards may be different.

- Attend outside workshops, seminars, lectures, professional conferences
- Complete self-assessment and professional development plan
- Develop instructional materials such as training manual
- Complete external self-study series or telecommunication course
- Find fellowship training in specific area
- Teach academic courses in occupational therapy or occupational therapy assistant program as a guest lecturer
- Complete independent learning/study with and without assessment component (e.g., continuing education article, video, audio, and/or online courses)
- Present at state, national, or international workshops, seminars, and conferences
- Make presentations for local organizations/associations
- Make peer presentations on specific treatment approaches or case studies
- Become a primary investigator in scholarly research
- Review a professional manuscript for journals or textbooks
- Join a professional study group/online study group
- Provide professional in-service training
- Publish an occupational therapy article in non–peer-reviewed publication (e.g., *OT Practice, SIS Quarterly, Advance, Community Newsletters*)
- Publish chapter(s) in occupational therapy or related professional textbook
- Do reflective OT practice in collaboration with an advanced-certified OT colleague
- Volunteer services to organizations, populations, or individuals

Refer to the NBCOT website for complete and updated information: www.nbcot.org.
NBCOT, National Board for Certification in Occupational Therapy; PDU, personal development unit.

Certification renewal with NBCOT is another mechanism that can be used to facilitate the process of professional development and continuing competency. When a practitioner is initially certified with NBCOT, he or she can use the credential Registered Occupational Therapist® (OTR®) or Certified Occupational Therapy Assistant® (COTA®). This initial certification is in effect for 3 years. Every 3 years, the practitioner must complete NBCOT requirements for certification renewal to continue to use the OTR or COTA credential. Renewal of certification with NBCOT is voluntary, yet may be required by employers or for state licensure. To renew, practitioners submit proof of having completed a minimum of 36 professional development units (PDUs) within each 3-year certification renewal cycle. At least 50% of those units must be directly related to the delivery of occupational therapy services.[19] PDUs can be earned through a number of methods. Box 7-2 lists professional development activities that may apply to NBCOT renewal.

Obtaining an advanced practice credential or specialty certification is another avenue for pursuing and documenting competency. Many OT practitioners gain advanced knowledge, skill, and experience in a specialized area of practice. The OT practitioner who completes the requirements for an advanced practice credential or specialized certification can represent himself or herself to employers, payers, and consumers as having a certain level of expertise and the qualifications to practice in the specialized area. Table 7-5 shows examples of credentials for advanced practice or specialty certification that OT practitioners may obtain.

AOTA currently provides **specialty certification** for both OTs and OTAs in driving and community mobility; environmental modification; feeding, eating, and swallowing; and low vision.[3] Competencies unique to each of these areas of practice have been defined. Practitioners must document a minimum of 2000 hours of experience as an OT or OTA and 600 hours of delivering occupational therapy services in the certification area to clients over the last 3 calendar years. After these requirements are met, the applicant submits an application, verification of employment, and a reflective portfolio demonstrating achievement of defined competencies.

AOTA offers **board certification,** which incorporates more generalized areas of practice that have an established knowledge base in occupational therapy. Board certification is targeted specifically for OTs and is offered in gerontology, mental health, pediatrics, and physical rehabilitation.[3] Certification is based on the completion and peer review of a portfolio, a professional development plan, and a rigorous

self-assessment that is grounded in the Standards for Continuing Competence[5] instead of an exam. To apply for board certification, the practitioner needs to have a minimum of 5000 hours of experience as an OT in the certification area in the last 7 calendar years and a minimum of 500 hours of experience delivering occupational therapy services (paid or voluntary) in the certification area to clients in the last 5 calendar years.

Several other organizations offer voluntary certification based on the passage of an examination, evidence of experience, or both (see Table 7-5). Sensory Integration International offers a specialty certification in sensory integration (SI). The American Society of Hand Therapists certifies individuals in hand therapy, and those who pass the examination are allowed to use the designation of certified hand therapist (CHT) after their names. The Rehabilitation Engineering and Assistive Technology Society of North America (RESNA) offers a specialty certification in assistive technology. Those who submit verification of a certain amount of work experience and pass the examination are allowed to use the designation of assistive technology provider (ATP) after their name. These are just a few examples of the many specialty certifications currently available.

Summary

The primary role for the entry-level OT practitioner is in service delivery. Once a practitioner increases his or her level of expertise and knowledge, he or she can assume or transition to various other roles within and outside of occupational therapy. The *Standards of Practice* delineates the responsibilities of OT practitioners in service delivery. The OT and OTA

Table 7-5 **Specialty Certification/Advanced Practice Credentials**

Examples of Advanced Practice and Specialty Certification Credentials	Credential Awarded	Granting Organization*
Advanced Practitioner (for OTAs)	AP	AOTA
Board Certified in Pediatrics (for OTs)	BCP	AOTA
Board Certified in Mental Health (for OTs)	BCMH	AOTA
Board Certified in Gerontology (for OTs)	BCG	AOTA
Board Certified in Rehabilitation (for OTs)	BCR	AOTA
Assistive Technology Practitioner	ATP	RESNA
Certified Case Manager	CCM	CCMC
Certified Driving Rehabilitation Practitioner	CDRS	ADED
Certified Hand Therapist	CHT	ASHT
Certified Professional Ergonomist	CPE	BCPE
Certified Vocational Evaluation Specialist	CVE	CCWAVES
Trained in Neuro-developmental Therapy	NDT	NDTA
Certified to administer the Sensory Integration and Praxis Tests	SIPT	WSP/USC; SII

Adapted from Schell BAB, Crepeau EB, Cohn ES: Professional development. In Crepeau EB, Cohn ES, Schell BAB (eds): *Willard and Spackman's Occupational Therapy*, ed 10, Philadelphia, 2003, Lippincott Williams & Wilkins.
*ADED, Association for Driver Rehabilitation Specialists; AOTA, American Occupational Therapy Association; ASHT, American Society of Hand Therapists; BCPE, Board of Certification in Professional Ergonomics; CCMC, Commission for Case Manager Certification; CCWAVES, Commission on Certification of Work Adjustment and Vocational Evaluation Specialist; NDTA, Neuro-developmental Training Association; RESNA, Rehabilitation Engineering and Assistive Technology Society of North America; SII, Sensory Integration International; WSP/USC, Western Psychological Service/University of Southern California.

have a collaborative partnership in which they plan, implement, and document frequency and methods of supervision. For health care professionals, involvement in lifelong learning and professional development is important to maintain competency for practice.

Learning Activities

1. Develop a career plan based on your education. In what role(s) and at what level of performance do you want to be functioning in 5 years? 10 years? 15 years?
2. AOTA has published papers that describe the specialized knowledge and skills needed to practice in specific areas. Find these documents online or in your library, and identify the areas of practice that have developed special knowledge base and skills. Why have these been developed? How are these different from the minimum standards of practice?
3. Some states' licensure laws delineate advanced areas of practice in which the OT practitioner is required to have specialized knowledge and skills. Research the regulations for the state in which you live, and identify any areas requiring advanced knowledge and skills.
4. Box 7-1 lists a number of professionals with whom OT practitioners may team. Are you familiar with the roles of each of these professionals? Research professional roles that are not familiar to you, and write down their primary functions.
5. Interview an OT practitioner. Write a paper describing his or her job, requirements, supervision, and role within the team. Provide examples of the level of performance the practitioner functions.
6. Observe an OT and OTA working together. Describe the relationship and the type of supervision the OTA receives from the OT. Interview each practitioner to gain insight on how this relationship works or could be improved. Write a summary of your findings, and present it to the class.
7. Compare and contrast in a short paper the role of the OT practitioner when working in a multidisciplinary, transdisciplinary, or interdisciplinary team.
8. Develop a presentation on professional development opportunities in your state. Complete the AOTA Professional Development Tool.[1] Provide a summary of your findings.

Review Questions

1. Describe the three levels of performance that OT practitioners progress through as they obtain experience.
2. What are the minimum requirements (hint: standards) for OTs and OTAs working in service delivery?
3. What is meant by service competency, and how may it be achieved?
4. Describe the OT/OTA relationship.
5. Describe the OT practitioner's role in multidisciplinary, transdisciplinary, and interdisciplinary teams.

References

1. American Occupational Therapy Association: *Professional Development Tool*, Bethesda, MD, 2003, AOTA. Retrieved January 30, 2011, from http://www.aota.org/Practitioners/ProfDev/PDT.aspx.
2. American Occupational Therapy Association: *Occupational therapy assistant supervision requirements*, June 2006. Retrieved January 30, 2011, from http://www.aota.org/Practitioners/Licensure/StateRegs/Supervision/36455.aspx.
3. American Occupational Therapy Association: *AOTA board and specialty certification programs*. Retrieved January 30, 2011, from http://www.aota.org/Practitioners/ProfDev/Certification.aspx.
4. American Occupational Therapy Association: Occupational therapy code of ethics and ethics standards, *Am J Occup Ther* 64(6):151–160, 2010.
5. American Occupational Therapy Association: Standards for continuing competence, *Am J Occup Ther* 64(6):411–413, 2010.
6. American Occupational Therapy Association: Standards of practice for occupational therapy, *Am J Occup Ther* 64(6):415–420, 2010.
7. American Occupational Therapy Association: Guidelines for supervision, roles, and responsibilities, *Am J Occup Ther* 63(6):797–803, 2009.
8. American Occupational Therapy Association: Scope of practice, *Am J Occup Ther* 64(6):389–396, 2010.
9. American Occupational Therapy Association: Occupational therapy roles, *Am J Occup Ther* 47:1087, 1993.
10. American Occupational Therapy Association: Entry-level role delineation for registered occupational therapists (OTRs) and certified occupational therapists (COTAs), *Am J Occup Ther* 44:1091, 1990.
11. Berger S: Personnel considerations and supervision. In Solomon A, Jacobs K, editors: *Management Skills for the Occupational Therapy Assistant*, Thorofare, NJ, 2003, Slack Inc.
12. Cohn ES: Interdisciplinary communication and supervision of personnel. In Crepeau EB, Cohn ES, Schell BAB, editors: *Willard and Spackman's Occupational Therapy*, ed 11, Philadelphia, 2009, Lippincott Williams & Wilkins.
13. Crist P: Roles, relationships, and career development. In Johnson M, editor: *The Occupational Therapy Manager*, rev ed, Bethesda, MD, 1996, American Occupational Therapy Association.
14. Gilkeson GE: *Occupational Therapy Leadership: Marketing Yourself, Your Profession, and Your Organization*, Philadelphia, 1997, FA Davis.
15. Hinojosa J, Bowen R, Case-Smith J, et al: Standards for continuing competence for occupational therapy practitioners, *OT Practice* 5(20):CE-1–CE-7, 2000.
16. Moyers PA, Hinojosa J: Continuing competence. In McCormack GL, Jaffe EG, Goodman-Lavey M, editors: *The Occupational Therapy Manager*, ed 4, Baltimore, 2003, American Occupational Therapy Association Press.
17. Nagayda J, Schindehette S, Richardson J: *The Professional Portfolio in Occupational Therapy: Career Development and Continuing Competence*, Thorofare, NJ, 2005, Slack Inc.
18. National Association of Activity Professionals: *Standards of Practice: Section A—Standards of Care*, Washington, DC, 1991, National Association of Activity Professionals.
19. National Board for Certification in Occupational Therapy: *PDU activities chart*. Retrieved January 30, 2011, from http://www.nbcot.org/pdf/renewal/pdu_chart.pdf.

20. Punwar AJ: Roles and functions of the occupational therapist and occupational therapy assistant. In Punwar AJ, Peloquin SM, editors: *Occupational Therapy: Principles and Practice*, Baltimore, 2000, Lippincott Williams & Wilkins.

21. Ryan SE, Sladyk K: The occupational therapy assistant as activity director. In Sladyk K, Ryan SE, editors: *Ryan's Occupational Therapy Assistant: Principles, Practice Issues and Techniques*, Thorofare, NJ, 2005, Slack Inc.

I chose the field of occupational therapy because the profession seemed limited only by the individual professional. As an occupational therapist, I have had numerous choices of work settings and ages of clients with whom I have interacted. I have worked in acute care hospitals, comprehensive outpatient and adult day care settings, public school settings, regular day care settings, preschool settings for children with special needs, as well as home environments. I have had the pleasure of working with clients of all ages from diverse cultural backgrounds. I taught for many years at a community college. Our typical OTA student was nontraditional in age and historical background. Now I am providing services to children throughout the school district.

I am rewarded on a regular basis as my clients progress, gaining more active interaction with others and control of themselves and their environment. I believe I have been able to significantly impact the quality of life of my clients. In essence, it is not how long we live (quantity) but rather how we live (quality). Occupational therapists are in a unique position to assist in improving the quality of life of the persons whom we serve.

JEAN W. SOLOMON, MHS, OTR/L
Berkeley County School District
Charleston, South Carolina

CHAPTER 8

Practicing Legally and Ethically

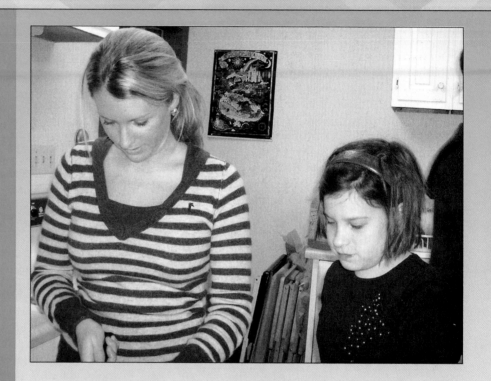

Objectives

After reading this chapter, the reader will be able to do the following:

- Understand the purpose of a code of ethics
- Identify the seven principles in the *Occupational Therapy Code of Ethics*
- Describe the function of the Ethics Commission
- Outline the steps to ethical decision-making
- Distinguish between ethical and legal behavior
- Explain the purpose and implementation of state laws regulating occupational therapy (OT)
- Describe the disciplinary processes developed by state regulatory boards and the professional association
- Discuss the similarities and differences of morals, ethics, and laws and their connection to the practice of occupational therapy

Health care today is very complicated, and systems often place the practitioner in a position to deal with ethical dilemmas. The need for increased productivity, managed care policies, and an increase in consumer activism have placed extra burden on practitioners for decision-making. Occupational therapy practitioners are confronted daily with situations that require decisions. Morals, ethics, and laws have the potential to affect the clinician's decision-making in practice.

Morals are related to character and behavior from the point of view of right and wrong. Morals develop as a result of background, values, religious beliefs, and the society in which a person lives. Thus, OT practitioners bring their individual morals to situations and those morals may or may not be in agreement with the client's morals. Professional decisions may or may not agree with the practitioner's morals; rather, decisions are based upon ethics. Practitioners are required to comply with professional ethics and legal mandates.[13]

Ethics is the study and philosophy of human conduct. Ethics is "a systematic reflection on and an analysis of morals."[12] Ethics guide how a person behaves and makes decisions so that the best or "right" conduct is carried out. **Law** is defined as "a binding custom or practice of a community: a rule of conduct or action prescribed or formally recognized as binding or enforced by a controlling authority."[11] Laws are established by an act of the federal or state legislature. Laws are intended to protect citizens from unsafe practice, whereas ethics compel the professional to provide the highest level of care.

Ethics and laws are closely intertwined. However, ethics differ from laws and rules in that ethical standards are more general, and their intent is to give positive guidance rather than impose binding and negative limits to specific situations. However, because ethics are blended with laws to form professional standards, ethical misconduct may also constitute a violation of the law.[13]

In this chapter, the *Occupational Therapy Code of Ethics* and an approach to ethical decision-making are described. State licensure laws and regulations of the profession are also discussed, including potential sanctions when a practitioner violates the regulations.

Practicing Ethically

Frequently, OT practitioners encounter situations in which they must weigh alternatives and make decisions about a course of action. Some situations are easy to resolve, whereas others may challenge one's decision-making abilities. Clinicians frequently rely on their own values and morals when deciding a course of action. However, professional decision-making relies on a systematic ethical problem-solving process.

Clinical reasoning involves understanding the client's diagnoses, strengths, weaknesses, prognosis, and goals. Practitioners use clinical reasoning to develop and provide intervention to address goals and make necessary adaptations. Clinical reasoning requires problem-solving and professional judgment; therefore, it improves with experience, reflection, and critical analysis. Practitioners use clinical reasoning along with morals and ethics when making professional decisions.

A professional **code of ethics** provides direction to members of a profession for mandatory behavior and protects the rights of clients, subjects, their significant others, and the general public.[13] For example, the code of ethics dictating that OT practitioners treat each client equitably describes a basic principle of the occupational therapy profession. Ethical codes provide guidelines for making correct or proper choices and decisions of health care practice in the field.[4,12] These guidelines are usually stated in the form of principles.

American Occupational Therapy Association Code of Ethics

The American Occupational Therapy Association (AOTA) *Occupational Therapy Code of Ethics*[4] was initially adopted by AOTA's Representative Assembly in April 1977 (see Appendix A). This code provides guidelines to practitioners to help them recognize and resolve ethical dilemmas, to practice at the expected standard using guiding principles, and to educate the public (see Appendix A). The *Code of Ethics* is meant to inspire professional conduct for quality and empathetic occupational therapy while respecting the diversity of clients. The *Code of Ethics* is based upon the core values of the profession.[9]

The *Occupational Therapy Code of Ethics* consists of seven principles, each addressing a different aspect of professional behavior.[4] Following is a brief description of each principle and an example to illustrate professional application.

Principle 1: Beneficence

In general terms, the principle of **beneficence** means that the OT practitioner will contribute to the good health and welfare of the client. Principle 1 of the *Occupational Therapy Code of Ethics* has four parts, each of which is related to the well-being of the recipient of services. This principle highlights the need for OT practitioners to (1) treat each client fairly and equitably, (2) advocate for recipients to obtain needed services, (3) promote public health and safety and well-being, and (4) charge fees that are reasonable and commensurate with the services provided.[4]

Mr. Parker can no longer pay for occupational therapy services. His occupational therapist (OT), Karen, started a daily self-feeding program for Mr. Parker prior to his funds running out. Karen visits Mr. Parker at mealtime and explains the proper use of the adaptive equipment to the aide. She discusses how to work on independence and what assistance may still be needed upon discharge. The therapist does not bill for this instructive visit, knowing that Mr. Parker will receive better care after she has personally addressed the issues.

This example illustrates the principle of beneficence in that the OT practitioner shows concern for the client by ensuring that the aide is properly trained in feeding techniques. The OT practitioner advocates that the client receive the services he needs.

When serving as a consultant to a residence facility for individuals who have severe intellectual disability, Judy, the OT, becomes aware that another therapist, Sam, is billing for one-half-hour individual intervention sessions. In reality, Sam only passes through the unit and briefly talks with the clients and does not provide treatment. After observing the pattern for several weeks, Judy speaks with Sam, who brushes off the inquiry, "Look, we all have plans on file, but these kids aren't going to progress no matter what we do." Judy documents the situation and brings the matter to the attention of the administrator.

In this case, Judy must address the breech of ethical conduct by Sam. Sam is financially exploiting the client by charging for intervention services that do not take place.

Principle 2: Nonmaleficence

The principle of **nonmaleficence** means that the practitioner should not inflict harm on the client. This principle ensures that OT practitioners maintain therapeutic relationships that do not exploit clients physically, emotionally, psychologically, socially, sexually, or financially. Furthermore, the OT practitioner is obligated to identify and address problems that may impact professional duties and bring concerns regarding professional skills of colleagues to the appropriate authority.[4] In that OT practitioners work with a variety of clients, it is the practitioner's responsibility to address concerns and foresee possible harmful situations so that harm can be avoided. The principle of nonmaleficence requires practitioners avoid any relationships, activities, or undue influences that may interfere with services.[4]

Tonya, a 15-year-old teen attending an outpatient group for eating disorders, becomes exceptionally attached to the OT practitioner, Mark. The teen calls Mark at home to discuss her intervention plan, telling Mark she got his phone number from her cousin, whom Mark knows from school. Mark limits the call and speaks to Tonya the next day at group, explaining to Tonya that it is inappropriate to call him at home and reiterating the professional nature of their relationship. Tonya is upset, but agrees that she will not call him. Mark asks a colleague to work with Tonya. He does not completely stop working with Tonya because he does not want her to feel rejected, but rather reinforces professional boundaries.

This example illustrates nonmaleficence (i.e., do no harm). Mark believes the relationship between himself and the teen may be harmful to the teen's intervention plan. Tonya has become too attached and is unsure of the boundaries. Mark is truthful with the teen and brings the situation up with the team so that no emotional harm will come to Tonya. The team supports him in continuing to serve on the team so that

he does not completely reject Tonya. The team fears that complete rejection may harm Tonya emotionally and result in slower progress or regression in her treatment.

Principle 3: Autonomy and Confidentiality

Principle 3 protects the client's right of **autonomy** and **confidentiality**. Autonomy is the freedom to decide and the freedom to act.[11] Confidentiality refers to the expectation that information shared by the client with the OT practitioner, either directly or through written or electronic forms, will be kept private and shared only with those directly involved with the intervention (under conditions expected by the client).[2,12] Confidentiality also stipulates that the client will determine how and to whom information may be shared. This principle requires OT practitioners to respect a client's right to refuse treatment, and it protects all privileged communication.[12]

According to Principle 3, the OT practitioner (1) collaborates with clients and caregivers to determine goals; (2) informs clients of the nature, possible risks, and outcomes of services; (3) receives informed consent for services; (4) respects a client's decision to refuse treatment; and (5) maintains confidentiality concerning information.[4]

Informed consent refers to the "knowledgeable and voluntary agreement by which a client undergoes intervention that is in accord with the patient's values and preferences."[12] Thus, clients have the right to refuse intervention and the right to be made aware of the risks, benefits, and cost of occupational therapy intervention.

Mrs. Jones, who is indigent and lives in a nursing home, resists going to occupational therapy but rather constantly asks to return to her room. The therapist, Andrea, learns that Mrs. Jones is afraid someone will steal her things. Andrea deals with the issue by making an intervention plan to address Mrs. Jones's fear that she will lose her hairbrush, an old mirrored compact, a brocade change purse, a bottle of toilet water, and a pair of underpants. Mrs. Jones does not want to tell anyone, but with her consent Andrea obtains a wheelchair carrier. Part of Mrs. Jones's intervention plan is the use of a checklist to pack her carrier with these treasured belongings each morning and to unpack it at the end of each day. The staff is informed that using a daily checklist is part of her occupational therapy program. Now Mrs. Jones goes to activities and therapy without protest.

This example illustrates a respect for the rights of both autonomy and confidentiality. The therapist allowed Mrs. Jones the freedom to choose to keep her treasures with her. This autonomy gave Mrs. Jones the assurance and comfort to participate in occupational therapy activities. The therapist respected her confidences by being careful to only discuss the contents of the carrier with Mrs. Jones, but informing the team of the intervention plan. The therapist respected Mrs. Jones's right to decide if and how she will participate in therapy and allowed her to contribute to the intervention planning process. The practitioner respected Mrs. Jones's right to confidentiality by not discussing with others the reasons she refused to go to therapy.

Principle 4: Social Justice

Principle 4 stipulates that OT practitioners provide services in a fair and equitable manner to all. Accordingly, individuals and groups should receive fair treatment and be afforded the same opportunities. Therefore, OT practitioners must advocate for their clients and provide opportunities for their clients to participate equally in occupations. This principle suggests that practitioners advocate for clients, promote activities for all patients, provide services to all (regardless of race, socioeconomic status, religion, or culture), and take responsibility to educating the public and society about the value of occupational therapy services.

> Brie is an OT working in private practice. The recent economic crisis has made it difficult for Brie's clients to continue coming to occupational therapy weekly. She is concerned for her clients and at the same time, she has to keep her business afloat. She meets with her employees and they decide to offer rates on a sliding scale so that the clients continue to receive therapy. She also contacts a local university to inquire if the OT students could conduct home visits as a classroom project. She is aware that some of her clients need home adaptations.

In this example, the therapist is seeking services for her clients in a fair and equitable manner. She is making adjustments to provide fair and equitable services for all clients. By using the university resources, Brie is able to provide additional services to her clients while maintaining her practice.

Principle 5: Procedural Justice

OT practitioners are obligated to comply with the laws and regulations that guide the profession. The OT practitioner must be aware of and follow federal, state, and local laws, as well as institutional policies. The practitioner may also need to inform employers, employees, and colleagues about these laws and policies. OT practitioners must accurately report and document information related to professional activities.[4]

> Before Kaitlin, an occupational therapy assistant (OTA), moves to a new state, she requests a copy of the licensure law and notes that the new state limits some treatment modalities. Once employed, she reads the employer's policies and procedures manual regarding facility records and acquaints herself with the department's style of record-keeping. The facility uses a specific style for documenting intervention. Although not familiar with the style of charting, Kaitlin refreshes her understanding with the format and implements it in her documentation.

The OT practitioner in this example is in compliance with state laws related to intervention procedures and with the documentation policies delineated by the facility where she works.

Principle 6: Veracity

Veracity refers to the duty of the health care professional to tell the truth. OT practitioners must accurately represent their qualifications, education, training, and competence.[2,4] Practitioners may not use any form of false advertising or exaggerated claims. The OT practitioner must disclose instances that pose actual or potential conflicts of interest. Furthermore, the OT practitioner must accept responsibility for actions that reduce the public's trust in occupational therapy services.

> Kevin, a therapist who is opening a private practice, makes certain that the advertising circulars promoting his private practice center do not the make any exaggerated claims about the center's ability to "cure" or make unrealistic promises of creating a "new life."

This example illustrates the principle of veracity because the clinician assures that advertisements for his private practice are truthful while promoting its services.

Principle 7: Fidelity

Fidelity, or faithfulness, in professional relationships describes the interactions between an OT practitioner and his or her colleagues and other professionals. Such aspects as the importance of maintaining confidentiality in matters related to colleagues and staff; accurately representing qualifications, views, and findings of colleagues; and reporting any misconduct to the appropriate entity are considered part of fidelity.[4] This principle includes statements concerning taking measures to discourage, prevent, expose, or correct any breeches of the code.[4]

> Lindsay, an OT student, just completed her thesis for her Master's degree, and her faculty advisor wants to present the results at a national conference. The faculty advisor asks Lindsay for permission to submit a conference proposal describing the results of her thesis with the understanding that Lindsay will be listed as the principal author. Lindsay is also encouraged to present the paper with the faculty advisor, if the proposal is accepted.

In this example, the professor demonstrates the principle of fidelity to her student colleague. By ensuring that both the faculty advisor's name and the student's name are on the paper, she is accurately reporting who has been involved in both gathering the data and reporting the findings.

Solving Ethical Problems

Ethical problems may be divided into three categories: ethical distress, ethical dilemma, or locus of authority problems. **Ethical distress** situations challenge how a practitioner maintains his or her integrity or the integrity of the profession.[12] An **ethical dilemma** is a situation in which two or more ethical principles collide with one another, making it difficult to determine the best action. Problems with **locus of authority** require decisions about who should be the primary decision-maker.[12] These situations rely on the ethical decision-making process.

Generally, six steps are used to resolve an ethical problem[11,12]:

1. Gather all of the relevant facts about the situation. Describe the clinical, contextual, individual, and personal preferences concerning the situation.
2. Identify the type of ethical problem (e.g., distress, dilemma, locus of authority). Determine the ethical principles involved (e.g., beneficence, nonmaleficence, justice, veracity, autonomy, confidentiality, fidelity).
3. Clarify professional duties in this situation that may be outlined in the *Code of Ethics* (e.g., do no harm, tell the truth, keep promises, and be faithful to colleagues). What is the conduct required of each professional (including yourself)?
4. Explore alternatives, including the desired outcome and consequences of actions.
   a. Describe features that are pertinent to this situation, including facts, laws, wishes of others, resources, risks, *Code of Ethics*, degree of certainty of the facts on which a decision is based, predominant values of the others involved.[3,12]
   b. Who are the other people involved? What are the consequences of the actions for the interested parties?
5. Complete the action.
6. Evaluate the process and the outcome.

The ability to decide which action to take may be developed by understanding the steps and discussing situations in which there are conflicting elements. Examining ethical distress, dilemmas, and locus of authority problems provides the opportunity to base professional decisions on ethical reasoning. Examining situations systematically benefits clients, professionals, and the employer.

The case application in Box 8-1 provides an example of the ethical decision-making process.

Box 8-1

Dave: A Case Application of the Ethical Decision-Making Process

Dave, a 13-year-old boy, has reached his occupational therapy goals. He was injured in an automobile accident wherein the driver had excellent insurance coverage, so the insurance is still available. Reportedly, his home situation is not good; both parents are alcoholics and have difficulty staying employed; there is concern for his welfare. Dave enjoys the attention he receives in therapy and works hard on his goals. In the time the OT practitioner has worked with him, his whole attitude has improved.

He wants to keep coming to occupational therapy, but he has achieved occupational therapy goals. The OT practitioner is meeting with the team and must make a recommendation as to whether or not to continue intervention. The practitioner enjoys working with Dave and has established a meaningful and positive therapeutic relationship.

Following is a description of how to work through this case using the ethical decision-making process.

Steps in the Ethical Decision-Making Process	Consideration and Analysis of the Steps
1. Gather all of the relevant facts about the situation. Describe the clinical, contextual, individual, and personal preferences concerning the situation.	• *Dave will be returning home to a less than optimal situation.* • *Dave's parents are both alcoholics who have difficulty keeping employment.* • *Dave has moved frequently.* • *Dave's parents are inconsistent in visiting him.* • *Dave loves the attention he gets during occupational therapy intervention.* • *Dave is well liked by his older peers in the rehabilitation setting.* • *If Dave continues to come to occupational therapy services, he may become dependent upon a support structure that is not readily available to him upon eventual discharge. The team is concerned for the welfare of the child; social workers are involved in the case.* • *Dave has a tutor, who will make home visits upon discharge. The teacher, school psychologist, and family physician are all important members of the team.*

Continued

Box 8-1—Cont'd

2. Identify the type of ethical problem (e.g., distress, dilemma, locus of authority). Determine the ethical principles involved (e.g., beneficence, nonmaleficence, justice, veracity, autonomy, confidentiality, fidelity).

- *Ethical distress is illustrated as the OT practitioner examines whether Dave should continue to receive occupational therapy services after meeting his goals. The OT practitioner, experiencing ethical distress, wonders if her integrity would be compromised by providing services to a child who may not require them.*
- *The ethical dilemma can be defined as discharging Dave now that he has reached his goals or continuing occupational therapy services, which may require new goals.*
- *Locus of authority problem is depicted in that the child (a minor) wants to continue with therapy, yet his parents (who have substance abuse issues) may not serve his best interest. The OT practitioner must decide if she will rely on the wishes of the parents, the child, or the institution (which supports continued treatment due to financial income) to determine intervention.*
- *The OT practitioner may hypothesize that occupational therapy services could still help the child and that returning home to an unsupportive environment may do more harm. Thus, the principle of beneficence (do well) is being challenged. Furthermore, the the professional issue of providing services to a child who has reached his goals may challenge the principle of veracity (truthfulness). The OT practitioner may have to be less than truthful in saying the child requires occupational therapy services. Fidelity is challenged by not trusting other colleagues to serve the child.*

3. Clarify professional duties in this situation that may be outlined in the *Code of Ethics* (e.g., do no harm, tell the truth, keep promises, and be faithful to colleagues).

- *The OT practitioner is responsible for helping Dave return to the occupations that he desires, including school, community activities, and activities of daily living. Although the child has reached the physical and social goals, as per his intervention plan, the practitioner believes Dave may require some modifications to be successful in school. The OT practitioner also remains concerned that Dave's support system (e.g., his parents) may not adequately assist him. After careful consideration, the practitioner acknowledges that other professionals, such as the social worker and school psychologist, may be able to address these issues.*

4. Explore alternatives, including the desired outcome and consequences of actions.

- *The OT practitioner could develop new goals for occupational therapy intervention. This way Dave would stay in the current system. He may become attached to the center and have difficulty transitioning to home, school, or the community.*
- *Dave could be discharged from occupational therapy services and attend a new program for children with learning issues (due to head injuries), which takes place close to his community. The social worker may be able to secure transportation. However, the child may still be in a chaotic home environment and benefit from outside support. The school psychologist recommends a Big Brother/Big Sister program and a parent support group for the parents (who may be willing, with encouragement from the team).*

5. Complete the action.

- *The team meets to discuss the courses of action and the consequences for each. After a thorough analysis, the OT practitioner feels informed and prepared to discuss the options that are in Dave's best interest. Although the initial reaction of the practitioner was to continue Dave's occupational therapy by reworking several goals, the practitioner realizes that the other alternatives might benefit him. In this case, the team works together to address the issues and discharges the client to a successful situation. Dave will attend a support program in his local area for teens. This program will address his emotional needs and help him transition to the school. The OT practitioner will consult with the director and staff members concerning Dave's physical and social needs. The OT practitioner agrees to attend a session with Dave so that he feels some continuity of care.*

6. Evaluate the action.

- *The OT practitioner felt supported by the team. The careful analysis of the alternative plans provided a solution that maintained the integrity of the profession and supported the child. Dave benefited from the work of all members and saw the team as advocates. The school and community support provided the child with the independence to engage in activities with his peers.*

Practicing Legally

At both the state and federal levels, there are different types of laws that govern certain aspects of occupational therapy practice. The U.S. Constitution and state constitutions are the primary sources of legal authority. After the federal and state constitutions, statutory law is the next source of legal authority.[13] **Statutes** are laws that are enacted by the legislative branch of a government. There are federal and state statutes. The federal Congress or state legislature votes to pass a law, which then is assigned to an agency. The agency itself, or a designated board, follows up with the development of regulations to implement and enforce the law. The **regulations** describe in specific terms how the intent of the law will be carried out. In this section, we discuss both statutes and regulations that affect the practice of occupational therapy. More information on state and federal laws and regulations can be found on the Internet.

Federal Statutes

Federal statutes, which are passed by Congress in Washington, DC, pertain to all 50 states. Federal statutes can be enforced through the federal court systems. Violating a federal statute may result in fines, injunctions, or prison time. Examples of some of the important federal statutes that affect the practice of occupational therapy include the following:

- The Health Insurance Portability and Accountability Act (HIPAA) established national standards for electronic health care transactions and addressed the security and privacy of health care data.[10]
- The Individuals with Disabilities Education Act (IDEA) requires public schools to make available to all eligible children with disabilities a free, appropriate public education in the least restrictive environment appropriate to their individual needs. OT practitioners working in school systems practice under this act. Thus, the role of the OT practitioner is to provide intervention that will allow the child to engage in education.
- The Americans with Disabilities Act (ADA) provides protection from discrimination on the basis of disability. The ADA upholds and extends the standards for compliance set forth in Section 504 or the Rehabilitation Act of 1973 to employment practices, communication, and all policies, procedures, and practices that impact the treatment of students with disabilities.[17]
- The Social Security Amendments of 1965 established, among other provisions, the foundation for the Medicare and Medicaid programs. Medicare is a federally subsidized health insurance program for individuals 65 and older. Medicaid is a joint federal- and state-funded program that provides health care services to the poor. Occupational therapy services are covered under both of these programs.

State Statutes

State statutes are passed by state legislatures. Accordingly, regulations will vary from state to state. Most state statutes are organized by subject matter and published in books referred to as codes. Typically, a state has a family or civil code, a criminal code, a welfare code, and a probate code, in addition to many other codes dealing with a wide variety of topics.

States are permitted by the federal constitution to regulate areas such as education, insurance (private and public), and licensing. Consequently, state statutes may affect the practice of occupational therapy through regulation of the insurance industry, including health maintenance organizations, workers' compensation insurance programs, and health care services for the indigent. Child abuse and elder abuse laws are also within the state purview. All states have passed some form of law requiring **mandatory reporting** of suspected child abuse and neglect. Mandatory reporting is the requirement that certain professionals, including health care providers, report suspected child abuse. A health care provider who fails to report suspected abuse may be criminally liable.[15]

One of the most significant statutes affecting occupational therapy practice is the state occupational therapy practice act. With the recognition that laws and regulations will vary from state to state, the next section focuses on general principles of state regulation of occupational therapy.

State Regulation of Occupational Therapy

State regulation of occupational therapy practice has been in place since the 1970s and includes licensure, statutory certification laws, registration, and trademark laws. Occupational therapy is regulated through one of these forms in all 50 states, the District of Columbia, Puerto Rico, and Guam.[1] Table 8-1 shows the breakdown of state regulation as of 2006. The primary purpose of regulation is to protect the consumer from practitioners who are unqualified or unscrupulous.

Under statutory certification and registration, a person may not use the title of or proclaim to be *certified* or *registered* unless he or she has met specific entry-level requirements. State trademark laws (also called *title control*) are similar to statutory certification in that they prevent non–OT

Table 8-1 **State Regulation of Occupational Therapy**		
	Occupational Therapists	Occupational Therapy Assistants
Licensure	46 states, District of Columbia, Guam, Puerto Rico	43 states, District of Columbia, Guam, Puerto Rico
Certification	1 (Indiana)	2 (California and Indiana)
Registration	2 (Hawaii and Michigan)	1 (Michigan)
Trademark	1 (Colorado)	0
No regulation	0	4 (Virginia, New York, Hawaii, and Colorado)

From American Occupational Therapy Association: State licensure requirements, July 24, 2006. Retrieved August 17, 2006, from www.aota .org/members/area4/links/links03.http://www.aota.org/Practitioners/ Licensure/StateRegs.aspx.

practitioners from representing and charging for occupational therapy services. Neither statutory certification nor trademark laws define the scope of practice of the profession.

Licensure, the most stringent form of regulation, is "the process by which an agency of government grants permission to an individual to engage in a given occupation upon finding that the applicant has attained the minimal degree of competence required to ensure that the public health, safety, and welfare will be reasonably protected."[16] State licensure is one way to ensure the public that the person delivering services has obtained a degree of competency required by the profession and has permission to engage in that service. In the states with licensure laws, it is illegal to offer occupational therapy services without a license.

In addition to listing the qualifications needed for a person to practice, licensure laws also define the scope of practice of a profession and, therefore, are often referred to as practice acts. The scope of practice defined in the licensure law is a legal definition of occupational therapy's domain of practice. This is another step toward ensuring consumer protection. The scope of practice also defends occupational therapy from challenges of other professions that may question the qualifications of practitioners to provide particular services or that may infringe upon occupational therapy's scope of practice.[14] Most states use the *Definition of Occupational Therapy Practice for the AOTA Model Practice Act*[6] and the *Scope of Practice*[8] as model language for state licensure laws and regulations. These documents are not statutes and do not have the force of the law, but they are intended to support state laws and regulations that govern the practice of occupational therapy.

OTs are legally responsible for services provided by OTAs or aides under their supervision. The roles and supervision of OTAs and aides are also delineated in state regulations. Two AOTA documents provide guidelines that are used by states to develop these regulations. *The Standards of Practice for Occupational Therapy*, which was last revised in 2005, describes the minimum standards of practice for professional standing and responsibility, screening, evaluation, re-evaluation, intervention, and outcomes.[5] *The Guidelines for Supervision, Roles, and Responsibilities During the Delivery of Occupational Therapy Services*[7] outlines parameters of supervision for OT personnel (see Appendix B).

An appointed state regulatory board carries out the tasks involved in implementing the licensure law and regulations. These licensure boards vary in structure from an advisory board to an autonomous body. Licensure boards are responsible for writing the regulations that govern the license, collecting fees and issuing licenses, investigating complaints, and delineating requirements for continuing competency. Licensure boards cannot change the scope of practice enacted through state legislation. They may advise the legislature or make suggested amendments. In some states, OT practitioners are appointed to serve on the board. OT practitioners can provide input into the regulatory process through their state association or by attending hearings, which are typically announced ahead of time and open to the public.

To be licensed in a state generally requires that the practitioner provide proof that he or she has completed the academic and fieldwork requirements of an Accreditation Council for Occupational Therapy Education (ACOTE)–accredited occupational therapy or occupational therapy assistant program and has passed the National Board of Certification for Occupational Therapy (NBCOT®) certification exam. An application is completed, fingerprints are submitted for a background check, and a fee is paid. Upon satisfying all legal requirements, the practitioner is issued a license to practice in that state. Each state requires its own licensing, and it is not permissible to practice in a state requiring licensure without a license. A practitioner may become licensed in as many states as he or she wishes.

States require practitioners to renew their license at specific intervals, usually every 1 to 2 years. Many state regulations require that practitioners complete a number of continuing education hours or continuing competence requirements to renew licensure. It is the responsibility of the practitioner to keep his or her knowledge up to date with current practice. Again, requirements vary from state to state, and each practitioner needs to be aware of the particular continuing competence requirements for his or her state. Strategies for professional development and continuing competence are discussed in Chapter 7.

Disciplinary Processes

Law and professional ethics are often intertwined. This blending may be related to the highly legalistic nature of today's society in which "one in seven Americans may be embroiled in civil litigation at any given time." Another reason is the fact that consumers of health care services have become more aware of their rights and more willing to assert those rights, which might mean using the legal system.[13] With this blending of law and professional ethics comes the potential to process violations in a number of different ways. In Box 8-2, we present a case study that exemplifies the blending of ethics and law.

The *Occupational Therapy Code of Ethics* applies to individuals who are or were members of AOTA.[4] Therefore, AOTA has jurisdiction over complaints against members who are suspected of unethical conduct. The Ethics Commission (EC) of AOTA ensures compliance with the *Code of Ethics*, and it establishes and maintains enforcement procedures. Any individual, group, or entity within or outside of AOTA may file a formal, written complaint against a member of AOTA for unethical conduct.[3] The EC conducts a preliminary assessment and determines if there is sufficient ground to carry the complaint forward to a full investigation. If the member is found to have committed an ethical violation, one of the following disciplinary sanctions is imposed: reprimand, censure, probation of membership subject to terms, membership suspension, or revocation of membership in AOTA (see Box 8-3).[3] It is the policy of AOTA to communicate with NBCOT® and state regulatory

Box 8-2

Case Study: Blending of Ethics and Law

An OT student is completing her Level II fieldwork in a mental health setting. Her clinical supervisor, Kent, repeatedly asks her if she would like to join him in activities outside of work hours. She makes up excuses or manages to avoid the question. After a group session, he makes a comment to her about her breasts. The student is afraid to say anything to her supervisor or the department manager for fear that it will affect how she is evaluated on her fieldwork. The student keeps quiet about the situation until the end of her fieldwork, when she reports the situation to the academic fieldwork coordinator. Preceding her statement to the coordinator, she asks that the information she is about to divulge remain confidential.

* Is this a legal issue? An ethical issue? Or both?
* What actions should the academic fieldwork coordinator take at this time?
* Should the student pursue any further actions? If so, what?

Box 8-3

Possible Sanctions Imposed by the American Occupational Therapy Association

Reprimand: A formal expression of disapproval of conduct communicated privately by letter from the Chairperson of the Ethics Committee that is nondisclosable and noncommunicative to other bodies
Censure: A formal expression of disapproval that is public
Probation: Failure to meet terms will subject a member to any of the disciplinary actions or sanctions
Suspension: Removal of membership for a specified period of time
Revocation: Permanent denial of membership

From American Occupational Therapy Association: Enforcement procedures for occupational therapy code of ethics, *Am J Occup Ther* 64(6):137–148, 2010.

boards when disciplinary actions have been taken against an OT practitioner.

It is the responsibility of the licensure board to protect the public from direct or potential harm that may be caused by unqualified or incompetent practitioners. The regulatory board follows established disciplinary processes and guidelines that are clearly spelled out in each state's regulations. In cases in which there is not direct or potential harm to the public (e.g., practicing without a current and active license, failing to disclose a conviction or convictions in the application process), the licensure board may assess a fine, which would vary depending upon the gravity of the situation. An abatement, or order of correction, is also usually given to the practitioner and must be completed in a designated amount of time. In situations in which there is clear evidence of direct or potential harm to the public, the consequences for the practitioner are more severe. Disciplinary actions that could be taken against the practitioner include public censure, suspension, or revocation of licensure or practice privileges. Each state has jurisdiction only over practitioners licensed in the state.

Summary

The *Occupational Therapy Code of Ethics* provides standards of conduct for OT practitioners. The Ethics Commission enforces the principles of the *Code of Ethics*. The seven principles include beneficence, nonmaleficence, autonomy and confidentiality, social justice, procedural justice, veracity, and fidelity. Using ethical decision-making guidelines helps practitioners make professionally sound decisions.

Standards of practice provide guidelines for the delivery of quality occupational therapy services to the consumer. State licensure is the legal means of regulating occupational therapy practice. Both the *Code of Ethics* and state licensure laws have procedures for processing disciplinary actions. OT practitioners are responsible for understanding and following the ethical and legal standards of practice.

Ethics, laws, and regulations serve primarily to protect the public from unqualified or unscrupulous practitioners. Laws and regulations in particular establish a legal scope of practice for the profession and differentiate it from other professions. OT practitioners obtain rights and protection as a result of these laws and regulations, but they must also assume the responsibilities and limits imposed by regulation.

Learning Activities

1. Obtain a series of ethical situations, including suggested solutions, from faculty members or practicing therapists. In small groups, discuss the scenarios; and, using the ethical decision-making guidelines, develop a solution. Discuss each scenario, and use the suggested solutions to provide alternatives.
2. Compare and contrast the *Occupational Therapy Code of Ethics* to those of two other allied health professions.
3. View a film such as *The Kevorkian Files*, *The Tuskegee Study*, or the *Life of David Gale* to promote discussion on ethical decision-making. Ask students to identify one or two ethical issues from the film, define them, and discuss the stakeholders and alternatives.
4. Ask students to bring in an ethical issue from current news. Using the ethical decision-making process, discuss this issue and possible solutions.
5. Research the licensure laws from three states. Compare and contrast the occupational therapy practice guidelines for each of these states.

Review Questions

1. What is a code of ethics?
2. Provide an example of ethical distress, ethical dilemma, and locus of authority problems.
3. List and describe the seven principles in the *Occupational Therapy Code of Ethics*.
4. List the six steps to ethical decision-making.

References

1. American Occupational Therapy Association: *State licensure requirements*. Retrieved January 30, 2011, from http://www.aota.org/Practitioners/Licensure/StateRegs.aspx.
2. American Occupational Therapy Association: Guidelines to the occupational therapy code of ethics, *Am J Occup Ther* 60:652–658, 2006.
3. American Occupational Therapy Association: Enforcement procedures for occupational therapy code of ethics, *Am J Occup Ther* 64(6):137–148, 2010.
4. American Occupational Therapy Association: Occupational therapy code of ethics, *Am J Occup Ther* 64(6):151–160, 2010.
5. American Occupational Therapy Association: Standards of practice for occupational therapy, *Am J Occup Ther* 64(6):415–420, 2010.
6. American Occupational Therapy Association: *Definition of Occupational Therapy Practice for the AOTA Model Practice Act*, Bethesda, MD, 2007, American Occupational Therapy Association.
7. American Occupational Therapy Association: Guidelines for supervision, roles, and responsibilities, *Am J Occup Ther* 63(6):797–803, 2009.
8. American Occupational Therapy Association: Scope of practice, *Am J Occup Ther* 64(6):389–396, 2010.
9. American Occupational Therapy Association: Core values and attitudes of occupational therapy practice, *Am J Occup Ther* 47:1085–1086, 1993.
10. Centers for Medicare and Medicaid Services: *HIPPA—General information*, 2010. Retrieved January 30, 2011, from httphttp://www.cms.gov/HIPAAGenInfo/.
11. Davis CM: *Patient Practitioner Interaction: An Experiential Manual for Developing the Art of Health Care*, ed 4, Thorofare, NJ, 2006, Slack.
12. Purtilo R, Doherty R: *Ethical Dimensions in the Health Professions*, ed 5, Philadelphia, 2010, WB Saunders.
13. Scott R: *Professional Ethics: A Guide for Rehabilitation Professionals*, St. Louis, 1998, Mosby.
14. Slater DY, Willmarth C: Understanding and asserting the occupational therapy scope of practice, *OT Practice* 10(October 17), 2005. Presentation retrieved August 12, 2011 from: http://www.aota.org/Practitioners/Advocacy/Tools/Presentations/41786.aspx.
15. Smith SK: *Mandatory Reporting of Child Abuse and Neglect*, Hartford & Avon, CT, July 12, 2009. Retrieved January, 30, 2011, from http://www.smith-lawfirm.com/mandatory_reporting.htm.
16. United States Department of Health, Education, and Welfare, Public Health Service: *Credentialing Health Manpower*, [Publication No. (OS) 77-50057], Bethesda, MD, 1977, United States Department of Health, Education, and Welfare, Public Health Service.
17. United States Department of Justice: *Civil Rights Division, Disability Rights Section: A Guide to Disability Rights Laws*, September 2005. Retrieved January 30, 2011, from http://www.ada.gov/cguide.pdf.

SECTION III

The Practice of Occupational Therapy

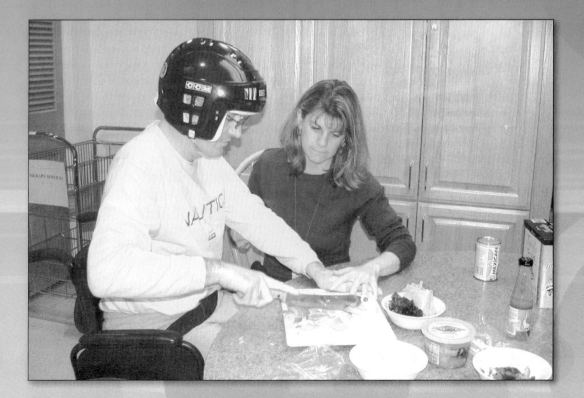

My entrance into the profession was influenced and sustained by the efforts and examples of some very remarkable mentors. My mother, a registered nurse, regaled my sisters and me with tales of her nursing experiences in the Army Nurse Corps during World War II. I read every Cherry Ames book (nurse/detective à la Nancy Drew), and I loved my stint as a candy striper at the local hospital, but somehow I knew that nursing wasn't quite what I was looking for in my career future. I remember first hearing about occupational therapy from Dr. Marian Diamond, the esteemed professor of anatomy and physiology at the University of California at Berkeley and my instructor. Based upon my high regard for her and her suggestion that I would be a perfect OT (whatever that was), I followed suit and met with Doris Cutting, the chair of the OT department at San José State University, who made me want to be a part of whatever it was she was. Armed with my bachelor's in humanities from Berkeley, I smiled as I picked up my OT class schedule and saw neuroanatomy, psychology, and weaving on my list—now this was a program that was meant for me!

OT school was a dream—each of the assignments a step closer to my newly chosen profession. Professors Amy Killingsworth, Lorraine Pedretti, and many others further nourished my enthusiasm for OT through their obvious passion for the profession, conveyed through stories of their caring and creative interactions with clients. I was privileged to begin my career at Rancho Los Amigos Medical Center with incomparable role models of superb OT practice, including Dottie Wilson, Lois Barber, Doris Heredia, Sarah Kelly, and numerous others who mentored their colleagues, facilitating and celebrating each other's successes. I remember driving to work with a smile on my face and eagerly looking forward to each day and the new stories I would be developing with my clients—a wish I have for every budding OT.

All of these mentors, through their example, inspired pursuit of further learning and scholarship as a commitment to furthering excellence in client care as well as advancing the knowledge base of the profession. In response, I chose to study at the graduate level and subsequently seek an academic position—both environments where I was again treated to the supportive mentoring climate I have come to know throughout my occupational therapy experience. Elizabeth Yerxa, Florence Clark, Lela Llorens, Ruth Zemke—among many others in academia—exemplified for me the importance of nurturing and celebrating the accomplishments of others to strengthen and enrich the profession we love so well. In tribute to these generous and amazing mentors, I encourage my OT colleagues and strive myself to reach out, encourage, and support developing occupational therapists.

HEIDI MCHUGH PENDLETON, PhD, OTR/L, FAOTA
Professor
Department of Occupational Therapy
San José State University
San José, California

CHAPTER 9

Occupational Therapy Practice Framework: Domain and Process

Key Terms

Activities of daily living
Activity demands
Client-centered approach
Client factors
Client satisfaction
Consultation
Context
Education
Evaluation
Health
Instrumental activities of daily living
Occupational performance
Occupation-based activity
Performance patterns
Performance skills
Preparatory methods
Purposeful activity
Quality of life
Role competence
Therapeutic use of occupations and activities
Wellness

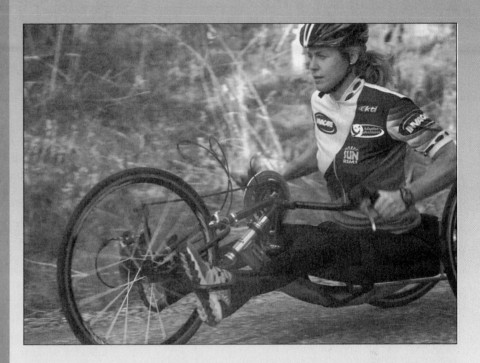

Objectives

After reading this chapter, the reader will be able to do the following:

- Define the domains of occupational therapy (OT) practice
- Outline the occupational therapy process
- Analyze activities in terms of areas of performance, performance skills, performance patterns, and client factors
- Provide examples of how contexts influence occupations
- Describe intervention approaches

The American Occupational Therapy Association developed the *Occupational Therapy Practice Framework (OTPF)* as a revision to *Uniform Terminology for Occupational Therapy*, which provided a unified language for the profession.[3] Although *Uniform Terminology* helped practitioners "speak the same language," this document did not provide information on the process of providing occupation-based intervention. The *OTPF* was developed to help practitioners use the language and constructs of occupation to serve clients and educate consumers.[1]

The *OTPF* clearly and concisely describes the occupational therapy profession, including the process and terminology, for students, clinicians, and consumers. The emphasis is on occupation, client-centered care, and the dynamic nature of the therapy process. This chapter provides readers with an overview of the *OTPF*. See Appendix C-OTPF for a description of the terms and concepts in the *OTPF*.

Areas of Occupation

The goal of occupational therapy is to help clients engage in occupation.[1,6,8,9] Occupations are the everyday things that people do and that are essential to one's identity.[1,5,9]

The areas of occupation include activities of daily living (ADL), instrumental activities of daily living (IADL), rest and sleep, education, work, play, leisure, and social participation.[1] The following paragraphs provide descriptions of the areas of occupation along with clinical examples.

Activities of Daily Living

Activities of daily living refer to activities involved in taking care of one's own body and include such things as dressing, bathing/showering, personal hygiene and grooming, bowel and bladder management, functional mobility, eating, feeding, personal device care, toileting, sexual activity, and sleep/rest.[1]

> Craig is a 2-year-old boy, small for his age, whose mother is concerned that he does not like many foods. Upon evaluation, the occupational therapist (OT) determines that Craig exhibits oral motor control issues (e.g., tongue thrusting) and oral hypersensitivity that interfere with his eating. The OT develops an intervention plan to address this ADL.

Instrumental Activities of Daily Living

Instrumental activities of daily living refer to activities that may be considered optional and involve the environment. IADLs include care of others, care of pets, child rearing, communication device use, community mobility, health management, financial management, home establishment and management, meal preparation and clean up, safety and emergency procedures, religious observance, and shopping.[1]

> Raiser is a 19-year-old man with mild intellectual deficits. He recently graduated from a group home and will be living alone in the next few months. The OT practitioner works with Raiser on living independently by practicing how to purchase, use, and maintain household equipment (e.g., toaster, microwave). In another session, the practitioner works with Raiser on using the telephone to call the landlord for assistance with the household. These skills are part of home management.

Rest and Sleep

Rest and sleep are restorative activities that support healthy participation in occupations.[1] These activities include all of those tasks to get ready for sleep, such as grooming, undressing, and establishing sleep patterns.

> Tom is a 5-year-old boy who is having difficulty sleeping through the night. His parents report that he sleeps only 2-3 hours a night. During the day, Tom takes frequent naps. The OT practitioner works with Tom and his family on establishing healthy routines for sleep and rest.

Education

Education is an area of occupation that includes formal (e.g., school, university, coursework) and informal (e.g., obtaining topic-related information or skills, instruction/training in areas of interest) learning.

> David is a 7-year-old second grader who is experiencing difficulty with handwriting. His teacher is concerned that David is falling behind others in his class and makes a referral to occupational therapy. The OT practitioner evaluates David's handwriting skills and begins intervention to improve strength and coordination for handwriting. Because children spend approximately 30% of the school day writing,[11] this is a necessary ability for his education.

Work

Work refers to paid or volunteer activities and includes the entire range of employment activities such as interests, pursuits, job seeking, and job performance, to retirement preparation and adjustment, as well as volunteer exploration and participation.[1]

> Kylie is experiencing difficulty returning to her job as a legal secretary because of her motor vehicle accident, which resulted in a traumatic brain injury. The OT practitioner emphasizes work habits such as getting to work on time, organizing her work space, limiting conversation with others, and completing her work. The OT practitioner arranges a meeting with Kylie and her supervisor to review the firm's standards and the necessary job skills. The supervisor agrees to provide the OT practitioner with a description of Kylie's "typical day" so the OT practitioner may prepare her more adequately.

Play

Play refers to "any spontaneous or organized activity that provides enjoyment, entertainment, amusement, or diversion."[1,13] OT practitioners work with clients on play exploration and participation.

Karl is a 12-year-old boy who does not engage in play activities with his peers at school or at home. His teachers and parents are concerned that Karl does not find any enjoyment in his childhood. The OT practitioner works with Karl to identify play activities and invites two friends to a session in which they engage in a variety of outdoor games as a means of exploring the types of play that Karl may enjoy.

Gloria is a 52-year-old woman with a diagnosis of schizophrenia. She has difficulty in many social settings. The OT practitioner begins intervention by helping Gloria succeed in community settings by reviewing basic social manners, including dress, language, and how close she stands to others. As part of the intervention, Gloria attends several outings in the community, including the art museum, library, and a coffee shop. Standards of behavior vary with the type of social participation activity.

Leisure

Leisure refers to nonobligatory activity. This area of occupation includes planning as well as participating in the activity. Exploring areas of interest is considered part of leisure occupations.

Jana is a 66-year-old woman who is dealing with the loss of her husband. She and her husband retired to a new state just prior to his death, and Jana therefore has few friends. Upon evaluation, the OT discovers that Jana participates in few enjoyable activities. In fact, Jana cannot articulate any leisure interests. The OT invites Jana to several community outings that she thinks Jana may enjoy. The practitioner watches for any nonverbal or verbal indication of enjoyment so that she may elaborate or expand on areas of interest for Jana. Exploring one's options is often the first step in developing leisure occupations.

Social Participation

Social participation refers to activities involving interactions with others, including family, community, and peers/friends.[1] OT practitioners examining social participation analyze the behaviors and standards for given social situations.

As shown in the above examples, performance in areas of occupation varies greatly, depending upon the client's age, motivation, interests, culture, and abilities. Further analysis of occupations is necessary to fully understand how to provide meaningful intervention.

Analysis of Occupational Performance

The *OTPF* supports a top-down approach in that the OT practitioner evaluates the areas of performance and occupations in which the client hopes to engage first, followed by an analysis of the performance skills or client factors interfering with performance. This approach differs from reductionistic approaches that analyze components first and subsequently design intervention based upon deficits. The *OTPF* encourages practitioners to keep occupation central to practice. See Figure 9-1 for an overview of the domain of occupational therapy.

Once the practitioner has identified the occupations in which the client would like to engage, the practitioner analyzes **performance skills**—including motor, process, communication/interaction skills, emotional regulation, sensory, perceptual, and cognitive skills—required to complete the occupation. Performance skills are small units of performance. When an OT practitioner examines performance, he or she identifies performance skills that are effective or ineffective.[1] For example, the practitioner may decide that the client's poor fine-motor skills are interfering with the ability

AREAS OF OCCUPATION	CLIENT FACTORS	PERFORMANCE SKILLS	PERFORMANCE PATTERNS	CONTEXT AND ENVIRONMENT	ACTIVITY DEMANDS
Activities of Daily Living (ADL)*	Values, Beliefs, and Spirituality	Sensory Perceptual Skills	Habits	Cultural	Objects Used and Their Properties
Instrumental Activities of Daily Living (IADL)	Body Functions	Motor and Praxis Skills	Routines	Personal	Space Demands
Rest and Sleep	Body Structures	Emotional Regulation Skills	Roles	Physical	Social Demands
Education		Cognitive Skills	Rituals	Social	Sequencing and Timing
Work		Communication and Social Skills		Temporal	Required Actions
Play				Virtual	Required Body Functions
Leisure					Required Body Structures
Social Participation					
*Also referred to as *basic activities of daily living (BADL)* or *personal activities of daily living (PADL)*.					

Figure 9-1 Domain of occupational therapy. (From American Occupational Therapy Association: Occupational therapy practice framework: Domain and process, ed 2, *Am J Occup Ther* 62:625–683, 2008.)

to get dressed in the morning. The client may have difficulty problem-solving how to make breakfast or be unable to make eye contact with peers. These types of performance skills may need to be addressed before the client can engage in desired occupations. Performance skills are dependent upon client factors, activity demands, and context.[1]

Client factors are even more specific components of performance that may need to be addressed for clients to be successful. Client factors include values, beliefs, spirituality, body functions, and body structures. Client factors include such things as range of motion, strength, endurance, posture, visual acuity, and tactile functions. OT practitioners analyze occupational performance at the basic level so that they can help clients fine-tune their skills and obtain the standards they wish.

Patterns of performance are another component of occupational performance analyzed by the OT practitioner. **Performance patterns** refer to the client's habits, routines, roles, and rituals.[1] Three types of habits are described in the *OTPF*: useful habits support occupations, impoverished habits do not support occupations, and dominating habits interfere with occupations. Examining performance patterns helps the OT practitioner understand how the occupation is actually accomplished for the individual client. An example of a client with an impoverished habit is one who has difficulty consistently getting up on time and performing morning self-care in a timely manner. As a result of this, the client will have a poorly established or ineffective routine and experience difficulty carrying out his or her desired roles.

When choosing an activity to help a client reach his or her goals, OT practitioners also examine the **activity demands,** which include the objects used and their properties, space demands, social demands, sequencing and timing, required actions, required body functions, and required body structures.[1] For example, Mrs. Salazar is a client in occupational therapy who finds the occupation of baking for her family very meaningful. Due to her recent stroke, she has difficulty sequencing the steps for baking a cake. The OT practitioner modifies the demands of the activity by writing each step out very clearly on a sign that is placed in front of Mrs. Salazar while she bakes a cake. Evaluating activity demands allows the OT practitioner to match appropriate activities to the client's needs and to determine how to modify, adapt, or delete aspects of the activity so the client can be successful.

The activity demands change as a result of the **context** or setting in which the occupation occurs. Context changes the requirements and performance skills, patterns, and demands of the activity. For example, cooking a meal at home for one is much different than having five friends over for a holiday dinner. According to the *OTPF*, contexts include aspects related to the cultural, personal, physical, social, temporal, and virtual areas.[1] See Table 9-1 for definitions of each. Each context must be examined in terms of the demands placed on the occupation.

Case Application

The following case provides an overall view of how the *OTPF* is used in clinical practice.

An OT working at a home health agency evaluates 2-year-old David, who has developmental delays, and finds out the following:

- The parents are concerned because David does not "play like other children."
- David does not sleep through the night, does not eat a variety of foods, and is small for his age.
- David drools and is difficult to understand. He talks using one-word sentences. He still sucks his thumb.
- David reaches with and uses a palmar grasp to hold objects. He walks with a wide-based gait.
- David smiles on approach and makes brief eye contact.
- David lives at home with three siblings (ages 7, 5, and newborn).

Using the *OTPF* as a guide, the OT decides to focus intervention on play and feeding issues. Play and activities of daily living are areas of occupation within the domain of occupational therapy. After considering areas of performance and patterns of performance, the OT practitioner examines David's motor, processing, and communication/interaction skills (performance skills). The practitioner explores the contexts in which the activities will occur. Specifically, the clinician finds out that David will play with his 7- and 5-year-old sisters, who enjoy playing musical games and pretend. The family has a safe and well-stocked playroom. David will get plenty of practice if the sisters participate in the sessions.

Contextually, the practitioner identifies that meal times may be very stressful, as Dad has an inconsistent work schedule, leaving meal times to Mom (with four small children). Thus, the practitioner decides to focus feeding intervention strategies to snack times and subsequently provides adaptations (e.g., finger foods) to compensate for poor skills to ensure successful independent meal times. The activity demands of the feeding intervention are changed by modifying the types of food served to David, for example, by having him eat finger foods instead of foods that require a utensil. Furthermore, David is gaining weight and not experiencing any malnutrition. The OT practitioner examined body functions and structures to determine how they may be influencing David's performance.

This example provides an overall look at how to use the *OTPF* to guide intervention. Much more detail can be uncovered by examining each aspect of the framework. Furthermore, many occupational therapy models of practice also provide comprehensive guidelines that are congruent with the framework (see Chapter 14).

Occupational Therapy Process

The *OTPF* provides a description of the process involved in occupational therapy. Specifically, OT practitioners are involved in evaluation, intervention, and outcome of

Table 9-1 **Context or Contexts**

Context	Definition	Example
Cultural	Customs, beliefs, activity patterns, behavior standards, and expectations accepted by the society of which the individual is a member. Includes political, such as laws that affect access to resources and affirm personal rights. Also includes opportunities for education, employment, and economic support.	Ethnicity, family, attitude, beliefs, values
Physical	Nonhuman aspects of contexts. Includes the accessibility to and performance within environments having natural terrain, plants, animals, buildings, furniture, objects, tools, or devices.	Objects, built environment, natural environment, geographic terrain, sensory qualities of environment
Social	Availability and expectations of significant individuals, such as spouse, friends, and caregivers. Also includes larger social groups that are influential in establishing norms, role expectations, and social routines.	Relationships with individuals, groups, or organizations; relationships with systems (political, economic, institutional)
Personal	"[F]eatures of the individual that are not part of a health condition or health status." Personal context includes age, gender, socioeconomic status, and educational status.	25-year-old unemployed man with a high school diploma
Temporal	"Location of occupational performance in time."[12]	Stages of life, time of day, time of year, duration
Virtual	Environment in which communication occurs by means of airways or computers and an absence of physical contact.	Realistic simulation of an environment, chat rooms, radio transmissions

From American Occupational Therapy Association: Occupational therapy practice framework: Domain and process, ed 2, *Am J Occup Ther* 62: 625–683, 2008.

services.[1] The OT is primarily responsible for the evaluation and interpretation of assessments. However, the occupational therapy assistant (OTA) may assist the OT, and he or she contributes to the evaluation by providing data, after service competency has been determined. Service competency refers to verifying that the OTA is able to produce similar consistent results as the OT. The OTA is not responsible for the interpretation of the results. The OT is responsible for developing the intervention plan.[2,4] The key points of the occupational therapy process emphasized by the *OTPF* are listed in Box 9-1.

The **evaluation** includes an occupational profile and analysis of occupational performance. An occupational profile provides background information on the client's goals, habits,

occupations, and history.[1] Generally, the occupational profile is obtained through an interview. However, the OT practitioner may also administer assessments to obtain the information. Box 9-2 presents the information collected for an occupational profile.

Box 9-1

Key Points of the Occupational Therapy Process

1. The process outlined is dynamic and interactive in nature.
2. Context is an overarching, underlying, and embedded influence on the process of service delivery.
3. The term *client* is used to name the entity who receives occupational therapy services.
4. A client-centered approach is used throughout the Framework.
5. "Engagement in occupation" is viewed as the overarching outcome of the occupational therapy process.

From American Occupational Therapy Association: Occupational therapy practice framework: Domain and process, ed 2, *Am J Occup Ther* 62:625–683, 2008.

Box 9-2

Occupational Profile

1. Who is the client (individual, caregiver, group, population)?
2. Why is the client seeking service, and what are the client's current concerns relative to engaging in occupations and in daily life activities?
3. What contexts support engagement in desired occupations, and what contexts are inhibiting engagement?
4. What is the client's occupational history (i.e., life experiences, values, interests, and previous patterns of engagement in occupations and in daily life activities; the meanings associated with them)?
5. What are the client's priorities and desired targeted outcomes?
   - Occupational performance
   - Client satisfaction
   - Role competence
   - Adaptation
   - Health and wellness
   - Prevention
   - Quality of life

From American Occupational Therapy Association: Occupational therapy practice framework: Domain and process, ed 2, *Am J Occup Ther* 62:625–683, 2008.

The evaluation process involves a **client-centered approach**; the OT practitioner is interested in the client's viewpoint, narrative, and desires. Because the aim of therapy is to help the client re-engage in occupations, the practitioner determines from the client, if possible, the occupations of interest. A client-centered approach involves working collaboratively with clients and is considered a foundational component of occupational therapy practice.[1,9]

During the evaluation, the OT analyzes the client's performance skills and client factors to determine strengths and limitations for the client. The OT may choose to use formal assessments, including standardized tests or protocols, when evaluating clients. The OTA may assist in the process, once he or she has demonstrated competency in administering the assessment or protocol. However, the OT is responsible for the interpretation of the data.

Intervention Plan

An intervention plan is developed once the evaluation is completed and the OT determines the client's strengths and weaknesses, and analyzes the areas of performance and contexts in which the occupations are performed. The intervention plan is developed with the client to address those areas important to him or her.[1,9] See Table 9-1 for a definition of the contexts.

The intervention plan includes a description of the goals and objectives of intervention. Although the OT develops the plan, the OTA may also contribute to its development (upon establishment of service competency). Goals are designed to be meaningful, relevant to the client, measurable, and occupation-based.

Once the goals and objectives have been established, the intervention approach is developed. The *OTPF* identifies five general approaches to intervention: create, establish, maintain, modify, and prevent. The following paragraphs describe each approach and provide a clinical example.

Create/Promote (Health Promotion)

This approach provides opportunities for people with and without disabilities. The OT practitioner sets up a program or activity in the hope that all those who participate will benefit by enhanced performance.

Mary, the OT for a local school, developed an after-school handwriting program to help third through fifth graders. The program provided fun strengthening and coordination activities, along with games to do at home. Mary created this program as a service to the children. Occupational therapy students from the local university helped run the groups.

Establish/Restore (Remediate)

The OT practitioner uses strategies and techniques to change client factors to establish skills that have not yet developed or to restore those that have been lost.[1,7]

Brian, the OT practitioner in a local rehabilitation hospital, worked with Jasmine, a 54-year-old woman who lost use of her right side after a cerebral vascular accident. The goal of the therapy sessions included increasing the use of her right hand and arm so she could prepare meals for her children again. Brian helped Jasmine improve right arm range of motion, strength, motor control, and eye–hand coordination. Remediation of these client factors ensures that Jasmine is able to meet her goals and cook for her family.

Maintain

This intervention approach provides support to allow the client to continue to perform in the manner in which he or she is accustomed. OT practitioners using this approach help clients keep the same level of performance and not decline in functioning.

Harry is an 89-year-old man who still lives on his own in a small first-floor apartment. Harry experienced a mild heart condition, which resulted in a brief hospitalization. The physician requested an occupational therapy evaluation to determine how to help Harry. Harry informed the OT practitioner that he wants to remain living alone; his family is close by for support. The OT practitioner conducted a home evaluation and made some changes in the environment to ensure safety (e.g., removed some scatter rugs, installed grab bars). These changes allowed Harry to maintain his current living situation, despite his decreased endurance and other natural effects of the aging process.

Modify (Compensation, Adaptation)

Sometimes activities are changed so that clients may continue to perform them despite poor skill level. Compensation refers to changing the demands of the activity or the way the client performs the activity.[1] This is useful when client factors are not changeable in a practical amount of time and the client wishes to engage in the activity.

Gerard, a 10-year-old diagnosed with developmental coordination disorder (DCD),* is extremely disorganized and has difficulty writing quickly. The OT practitioner provides Gerard with a simple day planner (as opposed to a large complicated system) and requests that the teacher provide a list for the child's homework. These compensations allow Gerard to be successful in a regular classroom until his handwriting skills are adequately developed.

---

*Developmental coordination disorder is characterized by marked motor coordination deficits that interfere with activities of daily living that are not due to physical, sensory, or neurological impairments.

Prevent

OT practitioners are interested in keeping clients well, and as such they may help clients engage in activities to prevent or slow down disease, trauma, or poor health.

Conrad is the OT practitioner in a rural community with a high percentage of families with obesity. Conrad and his colleagues develop a program for children to engage in physical activity and to educate families about nutrition. The OT practitioner adapts the physical activity as necessary and provides group activities to enhance self-esteem, self-concept, and healthy choices. This program is designed to prevent childhood obesity and the complications that arise from obesity.

The previously mentioned intervention approaches show the range of possibilities for servicing clients. OT practitioners use clinical judgment, experience, and research to determine which type of approach works for the specific client within the particular setting. The OT practitioner considers the context(s), client factors, performance skills, performance patterns, and activity demands when determining the intervention approach. Once the approach is identified, the practitioner develops the intervention plan for therapeutic use of occupations. The following section describes the types of occupational therapy interventions.

Types of Occupational Therapy Interventions

The *OTPF* lists therapeutic use of self (see Chapter 16), therapeutic use of occupations and activities, consultation, and education as the types of occupational therapy intervention.[1] The evaluation process helps the OT practitioner determine what type of intervention strategy he or she will use. Furthermore, the OT practitioner bases these decisions on models of practice (ways to organize one's thoughts[10,14]) and frames of reference (ways to implement therapy). Upon determining the client's goal for therapy, the OT practitioner decides the best strategy for meeting the goals.

Therapeutic use of occupations and activities refers to selecting activities and occupations that will meet the therapeutic goals.[1] OT practitioners may use **preparatory methods** or activities designed to get the client ready to engage in occupations.[1,8] Preparatory activities may include such methods as

stretching, range of motion, exercise, and applying heat or ice; and they are designed to get the client ready for purposeful or occupation-based activity. Preparatory activities should be conducted as one part of the intervention session rather than making up the entire session.[8]

Purposeful activities involve choice, are goal-oriented, and do not assume meaning for the person. **Purposeful activity** leads to occupation and may be a part of the occupation. For example, practicing folding towels is considered purposeful activity for the occupation of household maintenance.

The goal of occupational therapy is for clients to engage in occupations that they find meaningful. Therefore, **occupation-based activity** refers to participation in the actual occupation, which has been found to be motivating and which results in better motor responses and improved generalization. Occupation-based activity requires that the activity be completed in the actual context in which it occurs.

Consultation involves "a type of intervention in which practitioners use their knowledge and expertise to collaborate with the client. The collaborative process involves identifying the problem, creating possible solutions, and altering them as necessary for greater effectiveness. When providing consultation, the practitioner is not responsible for the outcome of the intervention."[1,6] **Education** involves imparting knowledge to the client.[1] This intervention type involves providing clients information about the occupation, but it may not result in actual performance of the occupation. For example, an OT practitioner who is treating a young child for a feeding problem may be at the house on one visit when it would be inappropriate to have the child eat. The practitioner can educate the mother by using pictures of the proper way to position the child during feeding.

Outcomes

Occupational therapy intervention is designed to help clients engage in occupations. It is important for OT practitioners to measure the outcome of their intervention and to determine whether the overarching goal of engagement in occupations has been met. This is a very broad end result, and OT practitioners use the following more specific outcomes to measure the results of intervention.

The OT practitioner can measure improvement or enhancement of the client's ability to carry out activities of daily living, or what is called **occupational performance.** For example, a client at admission to a skilled nursing facility following hip replacement may not have been able to dress himself due to decreased endurance and prescribed precautions because of the surgery. The client receives occupational therapy intervention to improve his activities of daily living and upon discharge is independent in dressing with the use of assistive devices. The outcome in this case is his ability to independently function in the activity of dressing. Occupational performance outcomes are the most commonly used outcomes in occupational therapy.

As clients improve skills and perform occupations, they show improved **role competence,** that is, the ability to meet the demand of roles.[1] Furthermore, clients become more able to adapt or change to varying situations. Another outcome that can be measured following occupational therapy intervention is **client satisfaction.** This is a measure of the client's perception of the process and the benefits received from occupational therapy services. Because occupational therapy is a client-centered approach, one hopes that the clients are pleased with the outcomes and the process.

Engagement in occupations and activities influences a client's **health** and **wellness.** Health refers to the state of physical, mental, and social well-being, whereas wellness refers to the condition of being in good health.[1]

Because clients often become active in their lives again after occupational therapy intervention, **quality of life** may improve and thus is considered a desired outcome of intervention. Quality of life measures determine the client's appraisal of his or her satisfaction with life at that given time. Finally, another goal of occupational therapy intervention is prevention of further disease and the promotion of a healthy lifestyle. Whether or not further disease has been prevented and the person is following a healthier lifestyle are also outcomes of occupational therapy that can be measured. The type of outcomes used will depend upon the practice setting.

Outcomes are identified from the very beginning of the occupational therapy process, during the evaluation. Practitioners select the types of outcomes and measures they will use to determine success. They focus intervention on meeting the desired outcomes and reevaluate the client's progress toward the desired goal(s) throughout. Modifications to intervention and decisions (i.e., continue intervention, discontinue intervention) about further intervention are based on the client's needs and performance.

Summary

The *OTPF* provides a description of the occupational therapy domain and process for OT practitioners, students, and consumers. The framework is comprehensive and emphasizes occupation-based intervention. This framework may be used with a variety of models of practice and frames of reference. Together, the OT and OTA (upon reaching service competency) develop intervention goals by collaborating with the client. Once an intervention plan has been developed, the OT and OTA provide intervention that may include therapeutic use of self, therapeutic use of occupation or activity, preparatory methods, consultation, or education. The outcomes of occupational therapy include improving occupational performance, role competence, and quality of life. Occupational therapy intervention may promote client satisfaction, health and wellness, adaptation, and prevention.

Learning Activities

1. Match a list of activities with the area of performance under which they fall.
2. Select an occupation that is important to you. Analyze the performance skills, client factors, and performance patterns required to engage in the occupation. Describe the context(s) in which you most frequently engage in this occupation.
3. Provide a clinical example for each of the five general approaches to intervention. Present these to your classmates.
4. Review research articles exploring occupational therapy intervention. Present to the class a review of how the current literature describes therapeutic use of occupation and activities. Write a three-page paper describing therapeutic use of occupations. Include a short PowerPoint slide show presentation.

Review Questions

1. What are the differences between areas of performance, performance skills, and client factors?
2. How is the occupational therapy process described according to the *OTPF?*
3. What are the types of occupational therapy intervention?
4. What are the five general approaches to intervention?

References

1. American Occupational Therapy Association: Occupational therapy practice framework: Domain and process, ed 2, *Am J Occup Ther* 62:625–683, 2008.
2. American Occupational Therapy Association: Guide for supervision of occupational therapy personnel, *Am J Occup Ther* 48:1045, 1994.
3. American Occupational Therapy Association: Uniform terminology for occupational therapy, ed 3, *Am J Occup Ther* 48:1047, 1994.
4. American Occupational Therapy Association: Entry-level role delineation for registered occupational therapists (OTRs) and certified occupational therapy assistants (COTAs), *Am J Occup Ther* 44:1091, 1990.
5. Christiansen CH, Baum CM, editors: *Occupational Therapy: Enabling Function and Well-Being,* Thorofare, NJ, 1996, Slack Inc.
6. Dunn W: *Best Practice in Occupational Therapy in Community Service with Children and Families,* Thorofare, NJ, 2000, Slack Inc.
7. Dunn W, McClain LH, Brown C, et al: The ecology of human performance. In Neidstadt ME, Crepeau EB, editors: *Willard and Spackman's Occupational Therapy,* ed 9, Philadelphia, 1998, Lippincott Williams & Wilkins, pp 525–535.
8. Fisher AG: Uniting practice and theory in an occupational framework, *Am J Occup Ther* 52(7):509–519, 1998.
9. Law M, Cooper B, Stewart D, et al: The person-environment-occupation model: A transactive approach to occupational performance, *Can J Occup Ther* 63(1):9–23, 1996.
10. MacRae N: *Unpublished lecture notes. OT 301 foundations of occupational therapy,* 2001, University of New England.

11. McHale K, Cermak SA: Fine motor activities in elementary school: Preliminary findings and provisional implications for children with fine motor problems, *Am J Occup Ther* 46:898–903, 1992.

12. Neidstadt ME, Crepeau EB, editors: *Willard and Spackman's Occupational Therapy*, ed 9, Philadelphia, 1998, Lippincott Williams & Wilkins.

13. Parham LD, Fazio LS, editors: *Play in Occupational Therapy for Children*, St. Louis, 1997, Mosby.

14. Solomon J, O'Brien J: Scope of practice. In Solomon J, O'Brien J, editors: *Pediatric Skills for Occupational Therapy Assistants*, ed 3, St. Louis, 2010, Mosby.

I remember my first months in practice as an occupational therapist. I simply could not believe that anyone would pay me for doing what was pure fun and enjoyment. Today, some 23 years later, I no longer mind being paid for my services as a pediatric therapist. However, I continue to love the practice of occupational therapy with children and marvel that something as fun as therapy is considered to be a "job." Perhaps we should keep it a secret!

Why does occupational therapy with children continue to be personally exciting and stimulating? First, it forces me to critically analyze and solve problems. Simultaneously, I must be concerned about (1) the child's behavior and performance; (2) the parents' perceptions, desires, and concerns; (3) the conditions in the environment that seem to relate to my first two concerns; and (4) the interests and concerns of other adults invested in the child (e.g., physical therapist, teacher, speech therapist). While analyzing all of the variables that influence the child's functional performance and behavior, I must select interaction styles, therapeutic activities, and recommendations that will optimally benefit the child and promote development. What a challenge! Understanding the child–family–environment interaction, solving problems related to the child's function and behavior, and implementing the steps that will lead to a mutually agreed-upon vision for the child is just the right challenge for me.

JANE CASE-SMITH, EdD, OTR/L, FAOTA
Professor
Division of Occupational Therapy
Ohio State University
Columbus, Ohio

CHAPTER 10

Occupational Therapy Across the Life Span

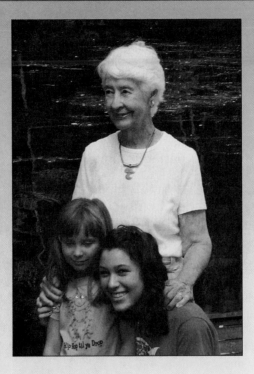

Objectives

After reading this chapter, the reader will be able to do the following:

- Understand the changes in occupation across the life span
- Understand the developmental tasks throughout the life span
- Understand client factors across the life span
- Describe the types of clients with whom occupational therapy (OT) practitioners work
- Understand the unique services provided by occupational therapy at each developmental stage

Evan is a premature infant weighing 4 pounds, 5 ounces, at birth. The OT practitioner works with him in the neonatal intensive care unit (NICU) to help facilitate feeding, sleep/wake cycles, and regulation. The practitioner considers the medical context of Evan's intervention sessions along with the parent and family needs. Evan's family travels far to see him each day, and the toll of the long drive to the hospital begins to show on his parents' faces. The OT practitioner carefully negotiates suggestions so as to support the family and help the client.

Meanwhile, an OT practitioner works with Grace, a 98-year-old woman who hopes to remain at home despite a recent fall. Grace has lived alone since her husband died 25 years ago. She maintains a small house and entertains family on occasion. Grace walks to the post office for her mail daily. She has lived in the small rural town all her life. The occupational therapist (OT) evaluates the safety of her home and makes simple suggestions to Grace and the family so that Grace may remain at home.

These examples illustrate the varied approaches an OT practitioner may take with clients who range in age and ability. Because OT practitioners work with clients of all ages, practitioners need to understand the developmental tasks throughout the life span. The following paragraphs provide descriptions of the developmental tasks expected of typical age groupings. Not all persons fit exactly into these groupings. Thus, practitioners must view each person individually while being aware of developmental progressions.

Infancy

How big was your child at birth? At what age did your child roll, sit, crawl, walk, talk, or feed himself or herself? When did your baby sleep through the night? What are your child's favorite playthings? With whom does your child like to play? Is your child a picky eater? How would you describe your child's temperament?

OT practitioners ask these questions to learn about infants. Frequently, parents of infants wonder if their child is developing "typically." Because a wide range of "typical" behavior exists, OT practitioners must understand the normal range of development to provide parents with answers for promoting infant development and to provide effective intervention.

Developmental Tasks of Infancy

Infancy represents the period of birth through 1 year. (Figure 10-1). During this period, infants grow rapidly and achieve motor, social, and cognitive skills (Box 10-1). Gross and fine motor skills develop as infants begin to voluntarily reach, grasp objects, roll, sit, crawl, and eventually walk. Notably, infants grow in size, height, and weight. Frequently, pediatricians chart the infant's growth pattern as a sign of early development. Pediatricians also test an infant's reflexes. Primitive reflexes are present at birth or soon after, which is an indication of the infant's neurological development.[1] Reflexes are motor responses to sensory stimuli, such as moving one's foot when the sole of the foot is stroked or quickly

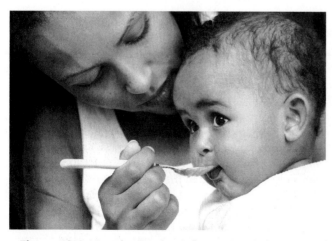

Figure 10-1 Mom feeding her infant. © iStockphoto.com

Box 10-1
Developmental Tasks of Infancy (0-1 Year of Age)
Exploration phase: child explores self and environment Motor milestones: integration of primitive reflexes, rolling, prone-on-elbows, sitting, crawling, walking Oral motor control: learning to eat different textures and types of food Social trust develops, including smiling and interactions with others Regulates sleep/wake cycle Fine motor development: holding and releasing objects, picking up objects Engages in solitary play and sensory movements

Adapted from Llorens L: *Application of a Developmental Theory for Health and Rehabilitation*, Rockville, MD, 1982, American Occupational Therapy Association.

putting one's hands in front to avoid falling. Infants possess a variety of reflexes. For example, the sucking reflex, which promotes nutrition, is present.[1] Over the course of the first year, the primitive reflexes typically disappear. Thus, the practitioner evaluates for the presence or absence of reflexes as an indicator of development. An infant who continues to have reflexes past the "typical" age may have sustained neurological trauma.[1]

Typically developing infants establish a sleep/wake cycle, and they experience periods of playfulness and express discomfort through crying.[2] They can be consoled and stop crying once their needs are met. Infants who are not consolable may have sensory regulation disorder. These children may benefit from occupational therapy to help regulate their behaviors.

Socially, infants interact by smiling and expressing emotions to family members. Infants play pat-a-cake, make eye contact, and smile. Between 8 and 10 months, infants develop stranger anxiety and may cry when approached or held by strangers. Social language begins in infancy with sounds, vocalizations such as cooing, listening, speaking words, and learning to respond to simple verbal directions.[5] Infants begin to reciprocate by taking turns vocalizing or smiling, which is observed when they play "peek-a-boo."

Activities of daily living develop as infants learn to recognize food sources and begin to hold utensils. They may allow caregivers to dress them, and they may enjoy bath time. Infants may begin to pick up food and put it in their mouth. However, infants are dependent on adults to maintain their self-care tasks.

Cognitively, infants develop awareness of objects, and they recognize familiar people. They begin to use toys and bring their hands to their mouths. The infant responds to his or her parent or caregiver. As infants begin to reach for and grasp objects, they learn cause and effect, an important concept for future learning. Infants learn by observing their surroundings and acquire the cognitive skills of object permanence (e.g., the object may be there even if it is out of sight). At this stage, infants begin to look for hidden objects.

Diagnoses and Settings

OT practitioners working with this age group work in neonatal intensive care units (NICU), hospitals, early intervention programs, and home health agencies. The NICU is a specialized environment with the main concern being the medical condition of the client. OT practitioners working in the NICU must receive advanced, specialized training. Pediatric hospitals serve children with numerous medical conditions for brief or extended times. Many pediatric hospitals offer outpatient care for children. This care is intended to maximize the child's development or monitor his or her progress. Some infants discharged from the hospital may receive periodic check-ups at outpatient clinics to monitor their development and growth. Early intervention programs provide services for children 0-3 years of age and may provide services at home or in specialized day care settings. Children may receive early intervention services from a team of professionals. The focus of early intervention is on family-centered care; therefore, empowering parents to advocate for their children is an emphasis of these programs. Infants may be also treated in the home by OT practitioners who work for home health agencies.

Because infants are developing, many OT practitioners work in diagnostic clinics to evaluate and provide input into the diagnoses of children. Diagnosing children early may help with payment, care, course of intervention, and support for parents. Diagnosing is meant to help parents and caregivers understand and consequently intervene on behalf of children. However, children will function at different levels despite being given particular diagnoses.

OT practitioners work with infants who may have experienced birth trauma, disease, or genetic conditions that affect their development. Infants with **cerebral palsy** continue to be the largest referral to OT practitioners working in pediatrics. These children experience motor abnormalities caused by an insult to the brain before, during, or soon after birth. Infants with cerebral palsy do not reach milestones as expected for their age. Their motor deficits may result in slow, awkward, or asymmetrical movements. Although the progression of the disorder does not worsen, the child may appear to be getting worse as he or she ages because more is expected as children age. Other diagnoses requiring occupational therapy services include Down syndrome, spina bifida, Erb's palsy, and a host of genetic disorders.

Infants may experience **developmental delays,** which refers to a general slowing of skills. Children with syndromes may be treated by OT practitioners and frequently exhibit developmental delays, cardiac difficulties, and intellectual delays (previously referred to as *mental retardation*). OT practitioners also work with infants who have failure to thrive, head injury, HIV, or congenital anomalies, such as cleft palate.

The OT practitioner does not treat the diagnosis but rather intervenes with infants and families to help the child function at the highest possible level and actively participate in infant occupations.

Intervention

The OT practitioner works with the infant and the family to facilitate development or, as Llorens suggests, "close the gap."[5] OT practitioners frequently use the developmental frame of reference to evaluate infants.[4,5] The **developmental frame of reference** postulates that practice in a skill set will enhance brain development and help the child progress through the stages. The OT practitioner using a developmental frame of reference begins by evaluating the current level of motor skill development. Once the practitioner has determined the skill level, the underlying client factors that may influence development are examined.[5] Such things as muscle tone, coordination, symmetrical movements, and posture may influence development. Intervention is aimed at improving the underlying factors so the infant may perform the desired skill.[3] Occupational therapy intervention with children is generally playful in nature, but it can include medically based intervention such as splinting, positioning, or cardiac rehabilitation.

OT practitioners working with infants provide **family-centered care,** entailing that they collaborate closely with the family. Family-centered care involves working with family members on goals that are considered important to them. This collaboration works best when members of the team respect and listen to each other. This philosophy of care supports parents as being the "expert" on their child and urges practitioners to listen and respond to family requests.

Although direct intervention using therapeutic use of self and therapeutic use of occupations and activity with infants frequently targets play, behavior regulation, feeding, motor skill development, and sensory regulation, practitioners also intervene through consulting and educating parents. Consulting with parents to address questions and concerns with the infant's development requires the expertise of an experienced OT practitioner. Consulting involves providing suggestions that the OT practitioner is not directly responsible for, such as suggesting an infant attend an infant massage program. The OT practitioner discusses strategies to enhance the infant's success in activity. The OT practitioners may consult with other programs to collaborate on strategies that will benefit the infant.

Parents may need education about caring for their infant and addressing the special needs of the infant. OT practitioners frequently teach parents how to hold, handle, and calm their infant. Education on feeding techniques and developmentally appropriate activities is common practice. Education may include providing parents with information on the infant's diagnosis, prognosis, and intervention strategies. OT practitioners are skillful at providing this information in a language and format that is understandable to the parents and sensitive to their emotional needs. OT practitioners may also have to educate parents on the data supporting a given intervention. This may involve teaching parents what to look for in terms of outcomes or service from providers. Not only do OT practitioners consult and educate others, but they also provide parents with resources. For example,

Box 10-2

Suggestions When Providing Home Programs

- Keep it simple; parents are busy and may be overwhelmed with demands.
- Provide playful, fun, and easy suggestions that can easily be incorporated into the day.
- Provide suggestions that will make things easier for the parent.
- Provide suggestions when asked.
- Limit suggestions.
- Write down home program suggestions.
- Be sure the parent will be successful when implementing the suggestion (adjust the activity so that it is easy to accomplish).
- Ask the parent to demonstrate the activity to you before suggesting it as a home program.
- Request that the parent demonstrate it to you when the family returns for the next session, and make sure you ask how it went. Let the parent show you how well the infant is doing. Praise the parent for being successful, and thank him or her for following through.
- If the parent did not follow through with the program, be sure to empathize and ask what interfered with the ability to do this. See if you can adapt the activity or provide a suggestion that will be more easily implemented.
- Try to provide the parent with activities for carry through, not activities that are therapy. If the child does not like doing something with you, do not give that as a home suggestion. However, you may give a portion of the activity (in which the child is successful) so that the child is more prepared for the next session.

OT practitioners may provide specialized equipment to help infants with positioning, feeding, bathing, and mobility. Infants may require adapted toys that make it possible for them to grasp or manipulate. Practitioners may help support parents by recommending support groups, respite care, and assistance in making things easy at home. OT practitioners must consider the demands of parents when providing home programs. Box 10-2 provides a list of suggestions for home programs.

Childhood

Childhood includes early childhood (1-6 years) and later childhood or school-aged children (6-12 years). Childhood represents a time of growth and refining of skills.[5] Children develop more coordination and strength and are therefore able to perform such skills as running, jumping, and more coordinated games. **Play** is the occupation of childhood; it is characterized as a spontaneous, enjoyable, rules-free, internally motivated activity in which there is no goal or purpose.[2] For example, children may spontaneously engage in playing and singing joyfully in the rain or at the beach (Figure 10-2, A and B). Furthermore, children progress from playing independently (solitary play), to playing alongside peers (parallel play) in early childhood. After parallel play, children gain more abilities and engage in cooperative play (play toward an end goal), and in later childhood, games with rules become important. The stages of childhood development are continuous and influenced by culture, family, and environmental variables (Box 10-3).

Developmental Tasks of Childhood

Motor skills develop during early childhood as children learn to sit, walk, run, climb, and jump. School-aged children refine motor coordination and develop strength and endurance for activities.

Play is the occupation of childhood and the manner in which children learn and practice social, cognitive, and motor abilities.[4,5] Early childhood is a time of intense play, and children move from parallel play to cooperative play activities. The nature of play changes as the child develops expertise. This is easily observed when comparing the difference between 2-year-olds trying to share toys (something that may not be easily accomplished) and the behavior of 4-year-olds (who are able to skillfully negotiate sharing). As children enter school, they begin to participate in cooperative play. For example, school-aged children spend large amounts of time working out the "rules" to games and developing elaborate themes and scenarios for their play.[2] Sports and competitive games become important as children begin to test their new skills.

Imaginative play develops around 3-5 years of age. This type of play involves "pretending" or make-believe scenarios, which requires cognitive problem-solving and sequencing. As children develop storylines, they may actually role-play concerns and consequently deal with stressful situations through play. Thus, imaginative play helps the child work through daily issues. Interestingly, children with special needs often do not exhibit imaginary play. Thus, the OT practitioner may want to promote the creativity and problem-solving skills that come with imaginative play.

As children go to school, they engage in the occupation of education, which involves interacting with others, following rules, reading, writing, playground activities, and socialization. Children must follow school routines and communicate their needs to a new authority figure (i.e., teacher). They must pay attention to verbal directions, take turns, and transition to new activities. Remembering the rules, routines, and tasks associated with learning may challenge children. Such tasks as remembering sneakers for gym, the note from the teacher, or the homework assignment may appear straightforward to an adult, but may be stressful to a child and difficult to remember. However, these tasks are part of childhood and, therefore, all children must have the opportunity to show they can complete them. In school, children must remember academic facts to participate in the cognitive processes entailed in learning.

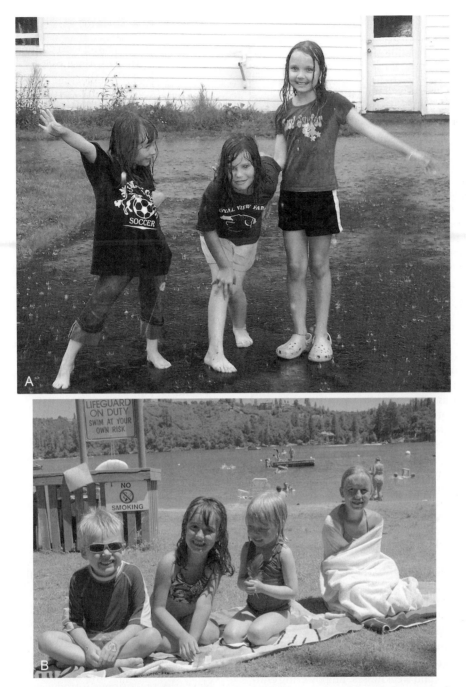

Figure 10-2 A, Children enjoy playing in the rain. **B,** Children enjoy a day playing at the beach.

Cognitive skills for learning require memory, attention, problem-solving, sequencing, calculation, categorizing, language, and communication. Children must be able to show their cognitive skills through verbal and written communication. In addition, sensory perception is necessary for making sense of one's environment. For example, children must not only identify the letters but also be able to use visual perception to ascribe meaning to them so that they can read.

Asserting one's needs is necessary to be successful in the classroom. Children need to ask questions when they are confused or curious. Furthermore, they need to hear answers and make sense of what they hear. Children with special needs are frequently passive, and often the OT practitioner helps them indicate their wants. Advocating for oneself is an important educational and life skill.

Along with the cognitive skills required for education, children engage in motor skills such as writing, tying their shoes, and carrying a book bag. Children move around the classroom. Motor requirements of gym or singing may pose difficulties for children. Children must be able to independently use the bathroom and eat in the lunchroom.

Box 10-3

Developmental Tasks of Childhood

Early Childhood (1-6 Years of Age)
Competency phase: children begin to regulate their behavior
Differentiates choices based upon inner images
Fluctuations in behavior ("terrible twos") may be observed as child tries to assert him or herself
Refinement of existing motor, cognitive, and social skills
Play is symbolic, dramatic, and constructive with pre-games
Fantasy play is a precursor for occupational choice; pretend play becomes more prevalent between the ages of 4 and 6
Learns sex differences
Learns concepts of social and physical reality
Learns to relate emotionally to parents, siblings, and others
Learns to distinguish right from wrong
Develops conscience

Late Childhood (6-12 Years of Age)
Achievement stage: children enter into the student role; there is a concern for standards of performance
Learns physical skills for ordinary games
Increases speed, accuracy, and coordination
Learns to get along with peers
Learns appropriate masculine or feminine social role
Develops wholesome attitude toward self
Develops skills in reading, writing, and calculating
Develops concepts necessary for everyday living
Develops conscience, morality, and scale of values
Achieves personal independence
Separates from family environment (toward school)
Develops attitudes toward social groups and institutions

Adapted from Llorens L: *Application of a Developmental Theory for Health and Rehabilitation*, Rockville, MD, 1982, American Occupational Therapy Association.

Frequently, adaptations are needed to allow all children to participate in these activities. OT practitioners help children in schools who may have difficulty with these tasks. Childhood can be an exciting time for children. Yet children may require support and assistance in learning how to work with their strengths and weaknesses. Empowering children through play and successful experiences lay the foundation for a strong sense of self and lead to positive self-esteem and self-concept.

Social participation is an important occupation of childhood. Children learn to get along with others through play as they express emotions, communicate, negotiate, and work out play issues. Children learn to take turns, listen to others, and express their needs. Through play, they begin to realize that everyone is different, with different strengths and weaknesses. In addition, children begin to figure out how the social systems work; consequently, children may be "best friends" one day and not speaking to each other the next day. These issues are important and emotional, and children may require support from the OT practitioner, parent, and teacher.

Diagnoses and Settings

OT practitioners working with children provide intervention to children with such diagnoses as cerebral palsy, autism, Down syndrome, intellectual disabilities, developmental coordination disorder, developmental delay, and others. Some children experience childhood illnesses, such as cancer, asthma, or sickle cell anemia, or have rare medical conditions such as William's, Angelman's, or Tourette's syndrome. Still others may experience physical disabilities such as spinal cord injuries, head injuries, amputations, burns, or orthopedic deformities. Finally, children may experience a host of behavioral and psychological disorders that may impact their ability to function in a school, such as attention deficit hyperactivity disorder, conduct disorder, learning disorder, or post-traumatic stress disorder.

Children receive occupational therapy in school systems, clinics, and hospitals.

Intervention

OT practitioners working with children focus intervention on play development.[2] Through play, children learn motor, cognitive, social, psychological, and language skills. Children who exhibit play deficits may have difficulty interacting with others, sharing toys, maneuvering around objects, and exhibiting signs of joy.

OT practitioners may use play as the end goal of therapy or as a means to improve motor, social, or cognitive skills.[2,6] When play is the goal of the therapy session, the practitioner is trying to improve the child's play skills. When play is the means used in the session, the practitioner is trying to reach another goal through play.[2,4,6]

Donovan is a 3-year-old boy whose parents are concerned that he does not play well with other children, does not share his toys, and frequently throws toys at others instead of manipulating them. The OT practitioner using play *as a means* may design a play session aimed at improving Donovan's ability to pick up objects and use them as they are intended. The practitioner begins by playing a game of catch with large balls, showing Donovan that this is fun. Next, the practitioner introduces a variety of large-sized Lego pieces and playfully tries to get Donovan to build. Play is the means used to improve Donovan's reaching and grasping skills. The OT practitioner may use play as the goal of the therapy session by focusing the session on improving Donovan's ability to engage in play. In another scenario, the goal of the session may be for Donovan to share his toys with the practitioner. The practitioner plays ball and a variety of games involving sharing of toys. Play is the goal of this session (specifically, sharing).

School-aged children must function in a school system. Therefore, OT practitioners help children obtain the necessary foundational skills for sitting at a desk, reading, writing, eating in the cafeteria, playing on the playground, and participating in music, gym, and other academic learning. Occupational therapy services provided in the schools are considered related services, and the role of the OT practitioner is to help the child function within the classroom in the **least restrictive environment.** The least restrictive environment is the classroom closest to a regular classroom in which the student can be successful. Inclusive environments, in which children are in regular classrooms as much as possible, are considered ideal for children with special needs, although some children require specialized classrooms for at least part of the academic day.

Practitioners working with children are creative, playful, and able to promote structure and limits. They are sensitive to the child's and parents' needs and attentive to the family. Intervention is aimed at play; school-aged tasks; and independence in playground behavior, handwriting, skills for learning (e.g., perception), and self-care skills.

OT practitioners working in schools are skillful at consulting with teachers, providing overall suggestions that may benefit all or one of the students. For example, the OT practitioner may suggest that the teacher promote handwriting warm-up exercises in the middle of the day prior to writing. The OT practitioner provides the warm-up exercises and reviews them with the teacher, but does not directly implement the intervention. An OT practitioner may work with children in the classroom or provide direct service to prepare children to be more successful.

Adolescence

Adolescence may be considered a time of turmoil as the person tries to develop a sense of self that is independent from his or her parents. Searching for one's identity is the primary role of adolescence (Box 10-4).[5,6] This period of striving for

---

Box 10-4

**Developmental Tasks of Adolescence
(12-20 Years of Age)**

Learns habits for adequate performance in adult roles
Role transition, ambiguity, and experimentation
Develops more mature relationships with peers
Masculine/feminine social roles are defined
Acceptance of one's physique and using body effectively
  occurs
Achieves assurance of economic independence
Selects and prepares for occupation
Prepares for marriage and family life
Develops intellectual skill and concepts necessary for civic
  competence
Desires and achieves socially responsible behavior
Acquires a set of values and ethics

Adapted from Llorens L: *Application of a Developmental Theory for Health and Rehabilitation*, Rockville, MD, 1982, American Occupational Therapy Association.

---

independence is characterized by peer group pressures to fit in or conform. Subsequently, adolescents focus on the peer group. Clothing, hair, and language may imitate other members of the peer group. Adolescents may engage in competitive games and enjoy group play and team activities (Figures 10-3A and 10-3B). The adolescent enjoys games with rules and is concerned with group standards rather than adult standards. Adolescents begin to show interest in town, state, and country, rather than just focusing on the family (as in childhood).[5]

Adolescence is a period of role confusion in relationships with adults and a time of developing a sexual identity.[5,6] In general, adolescents are striving to develop their own identity apart from their parents. Therefore, intense variability and insecurity occur during adolescence. Puberty occurs in early adolescence; and, with this change, adolescents demonstrate a strong desire for attention, an increased interest in the opposite sex, and frequent "crushes." They seek out support from their peers while trying to establish independence from their parents.

OT practitioners working with adolescents are aware of the challenges of this period of development when creating an intervention plan. OT practitioners work with adolescents who may have suffered disease, trauma, or a psychological event; they may require help to face the expected challenges of adolescence in addition to those presented by the disability.

Developmental Tasks of Adolescence

Physically, adolescents are growing and becoming stronger.[5,6] Children going through the awkward phase of puberty may be physically self-conscious and require assistance in understanding changes in their bodies. Postural changes, awkward motor movements, and rapid growth all make movements somewhat challenging. As the adolescent is concerned with how he or she is viewed by the peer group, the adolescent may spend more time on self-care, grooming, and hygiene issues. Girls will have to address menstruation issues. Boys will have to address the changes in their bodies as well. Furthermore, puberty is a time in which children develop a sexual identity.[4-6] Thus, parents and practitioners working with adolescents will need to address these issues. Adolescents can be self-conscious and egocentric. Safety issues may become important because an adolescent may make decisions that appear impulsive and immature. Leisure activities and social participation become very important to adolescents.

Adolescence is a period of self-identity. These children start thinking about what they want to be when they grow up. Peer groups are important and influence the adolescent's dress, behavior, habits, choices, and routines.[2,6] Adolescents who experience psychological disturbances beyond those that are typical of adolescence may need intervention to develop self-concept, identity, and social skills.[2,6]

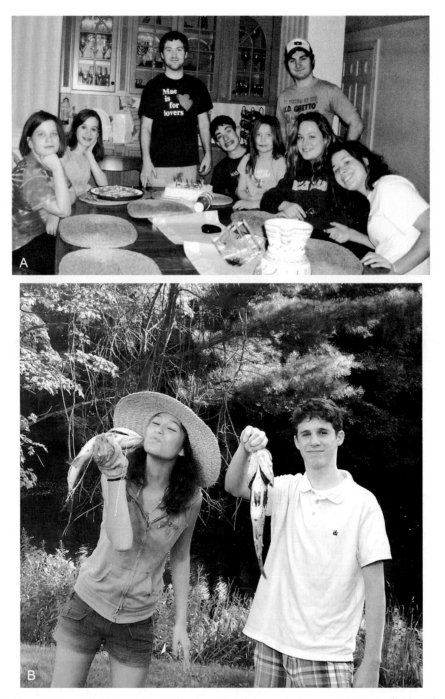

Figure 10-3 A, Teens enjoy socializing with each other. **B,** Adolescents "compete" over who has the biggest fish.

Diagnoses and Settings

OT practitioners work with adolescents in hospitals, day treatment centers, school systems, or rehabilitation centers. Because adolescence is a time of transition, the OT practitioner may assist adolescents in transitioning to high school or with work readiness such as vocational rehabilitation. Adolescents with whom OT practitioners work require firm limits, choice, understanding, and positive role models. The OT practitioner will want to relate to the adolescent without acting like a peer. Adolescents going through puberty may have questions about sexuality, which the OT practitioner may need to address.[5,6]

Mental health issues and psychological disorders such as bipolar or borderline personality disorder[4-6] may arise during puberty. Furthermore, adolescents may exhibit signs of anorexia, bulimia, or other eating disorders. They may become conflicted and show signs of suicidal depression. Finally, adolescents who experience physical disabilities may require special attention to deal with issues of sexuality, body image, and future goals and aspirations. The OT practitioner helps adolescents with all of these issues.

Intervention

OT practitioners working with adolescents must set firm yet fair limits. Because adolescents typically question authority figures, the OT practitioner must be firm about expectations and consequences.[6] Generally, adolescents with whom OT practitioners work are experiencing an emotional or physical trauma. This, along with the emotions associated with adolescence, may magnify feelings. Finding opportunities for the adolescent to express himself or herself appropriately (e.g., writing, reflection, small group, individual sessions) is beneficial.[6]

Teens may push limits and question authority. However, they must learn to trust the practitioner. Practitioners gain trust by following through with tasks and checking in with the adolescent. It is helpful to give the adolescent control where possible.[6] In occupational therapy practice, this may be as simple as providing the adolescent a choice of activities.

OT practitioners consider how adolescents will interact in a group situation.[6] Sometimes, involving teens in healthy group activities provides them with the support and mentoring they need. For example, Special Olympics provides teens with disabilities a feeling of competition and team membership. Adolescents with special needs may need help in self-care, leisure, and independence. OT practitioners may lead groups to teach teens the necessary skills for grooming, hygiene, and other self-care tasks. The practitioner may use an educational approach or may have to adapt the tasks so the teen with physical problems is able to complete them. For example, providing adaptive clothing may be a good solution when a teen is unable to button or zip. However, the OT practitioner should include the teen's clothing preferences in this intervention strategy. Perhaps the teen would prefer to struggle with regular clothing so that he or she could wear a special outfit. The clinician must be aware of the client's motivations.

Other interventions target work-related activities to prepare the teen for the workplace.[6] Perhaps the teen is in need of social skills for work, refined work habits, or skills in filling out a job application. OT practitioners examine all aspects of gaining employment by analyzing what is required and by determining areas in which the client may need assistance.

Other teens may participate in few leisure activities. In particular, troubled teens sometimes engage in unhealthy leisure activities. Exploring healthy leisure opportunities may open up new experiences for teens.

Young and Middle Adulthood

Where do you work? What do you do? Do you have a boyfriend or girlfriend? These questions represent the challenges of young and middle adulthood. Adults assume responsibility for their own development or deterioration. **Adulthood** is generally considered a time of achievement, a time when the adult makes employment decisions. Group affiliations continue to

be important (family, social, interest, civic). Adults are concerned with guiding the next generation, with creativity, and productivity.

Developmental Tasks of Young and Middle Adulthood

Adulthood can be separated into young (20-40 years), middle (40-65 years), and late adulthood (over 65 years). The developmental tasks may differ slightly among these stages of adulthood. In young adulthood, the developmental tasks include finding a significant relationship, securing employment, and developing a career path (Box 10-5). Adulthood includes establishing one's home—buying a home or renting an apartment. Typically, adults have an established identity, live independently, and may choose to marry and start a family.[4,5] Families can differ in configuration (Figure 10-4). For example, a "traditional" family consists of husband, wife, and children. Today, however, families may consist of two men raising children or two women raising children. Some children are raised by grandparents or aunts and uncles. Adults make these decisions about whether and how they will raise children, and what type of family configuration they wish to have.

Box 10-5

Developmental Tasks of Adulthood

Young Adulthood (20-40 Years of Age)
Ability to function independently
Selecting and establishing career; work is a major source of meaning
Formation of significant relationships
Development of self-identity
Acceptance of parents' limitations
Leaving home
Personal grooming and hygiene
Managing a home
Establishing a family
Child rearing

Middle Adulthood (40-65 Years of Age)
Achieving civic and social responsibility—legacy
Midlife crisis—reformulates direction
Establishing and maintaining an economic standard of living
Assisting teenaged children to become responsible, happy adults
Developing adult leisure time activity
Accepting and adjusting to physiological changes of middle age
Adjusting to aging parents
Emotional responsibilities as parents end as children leave home
Ongoing financial responsibility becomes finite and predictable
Women lose capacity to bear children

Adapted from Llorens L: *Application of a Developmental Theory for Health and Rehabilitation*, Rockville, MD, 1982, American Occupational Therapy Association.

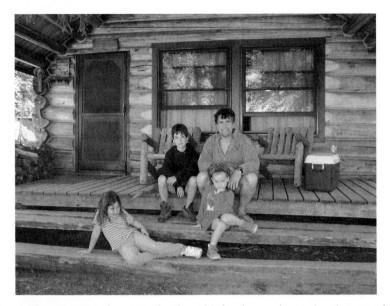

Figure 10-4 Adulthood is a time for raising families. This family spends vacation time together camping.

A major focus of adulthood is selecting and establishing a career. In young adulthood, individuals may be completing educational or other work requirements for their career. Middle adulthood is generally considered a time when the adult has met the requirements for the career or job and has an established track record. However, many adults will change careers, and seeking a new career is also considered a task of middle adulthood.

Middle adulthood is a time when the adult has maintained employment, established a satisfying lifestyle with loved ones, and is contributing to society. Successful adults may be financially secure and have friends and engage in leisure (Figure 10-5).

Interestingly, at some point many adults question decisions and examine their life progress. This is frequently referred to as the "midlife crisis." This may be a period when the adult changes jobs, goes back to school, or moves to another state. OT practitioners working with adults may encounter clients who have experienced a serious disruption due to illness, trauma, or a psychological event, and the practitioner helps the client reevaluate his or her abilities. Furthermore, later middle-aged adults must accept physical changes, such as decreased strength, decreased endurance, and signs of aging (e.g., wrinkles, weight gain, and hair loss).

Adults in this stage may be raising teenagers and adjusting to aging parents. This is sometimes referred to as the

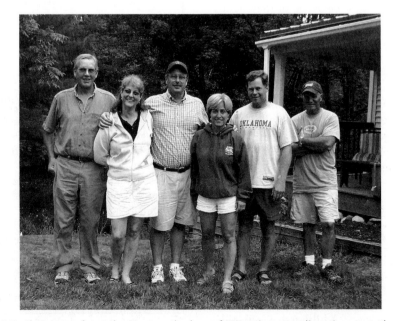

Figure 10-5 Classmates from the Yarmouth class of '77 enjoy spending time together during a recent reunion. The classmates (representing middle age) have established their own families and careers, and some have children entering college.

"sandwich generation" because adults may be caring for their children and their parents at the same time. Some middle adults may be experiencing the "empty nest syndrome," in which their children have all moved out of the house. One phenomenon today is that children who have left the house may return to live at home as young adults.

Diagnoses and Settings

Adults may experience a whole range of physical illnesses affecting functioning, including heart disease, neurological impairments, orthopedic disabilities, and psychological disturbances. Schizophrenia, bipolar disorder, borderline personality, obsessive-compulsive disorder, and a wide variety of psychiatric disorders may emerge during adulthood. Furthermore, clients may have such diagnoses as obesity, substance abuse, and other unhealthy life choices, which influence their occupational performance. Adults may have experienced physical or psychological trauma that has left them ill prepared to function in their various roles.

Intervention

The goal of occupational therapy intervention with adults is to help them re-engage in occupations that they find meaningful.[3-5] This involves examining the neuromusculoskeletal, social, psychological, and cognitive aspects of occupations within the contexts of the client's environment. Occupational therapy intervention may also focus on psychological functioning and take place in psychiatric settings, group settings, day treatment settings, or outpatient clinics. Clients with motor dysfunction may be treated at hospitals, clinics, rehabilitation settings, and specialized programs. Adults may also be served by OT practitioners at home or at work. Many work settings have ergonomic programs that employ an OT practitioner.

Later Adulthood

Later adulthood is a time of reflection and evaluation of one's life. Many physical changes occur during this period, and the older adult must adjust to physical changes. Older adults value group affiliations and may be concerned with what they will leave behind to the younger generation.

Developmental Tasks of Later Adulthood

Later adulthood is characterized by retirement and decrease in workload, and the emphasis shifts to community. Older adults deal with loss of spouse or peers, and this loss of others may result in depression, sadness, and prolonged grief. Some older adults have difficulty adapting to these changes; however, many healthy older adults are able to deal with loss and grief when supported by family and friends (Box 10-6).

Individuals struggle with physical declines, although this does not have to mean a loss of independence. Physical decline common with later adulthood includes impaired

---

Box 10-6

Developmental Tasks of Late Adulthood (Over 65 Years of Age)

Adjustment to decreasing physical strength and health
Adjustment to retirement and reduced income
Adjustment to death of spouse and peers
Adjustment to one's own impending death
Establishment of affiliations with one's own age group
Meeting social obligations
Volunteerism
Independent living

Adapted from Llorens L: *Application of a Developmental Theory for Health and Rehabilitation*, Rockville, MD, 1982, American Occupational Therapy Association.

---

hearing, poor balance and strength, and impaired vision. Adults in later adulthood may experience tactile changes or poor circulation issues interfering with their ability to feel changes in terrain.

Some older adults experience cognitive changes, such as difficulty with memory and attending to multiple stimuli. Remaining active physically and cognitively is important to staying independent and well.

Many older adults stay active in community activities and family events (Figure 10-6).[3] Those who continue to be physically and cognitively active live longer and with fewer hospitalizations.[3]

Diagnoses and Settings

OT practitioners working with older adults consider safety in the home and community. Wellness programs may be beneficial to older adults, such as those offered by senior citizen centers or local recreational leagues.[3-5] Clients with whom OT practitioners work may need assistance in modifying activities

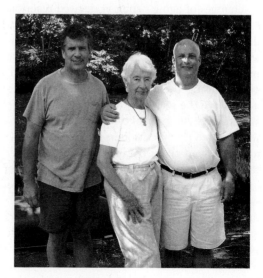

Figure 10-6 Older adults enjoy spending time with family and being active in the community.

and help in obtaining education on the various diseases, diagnoses, and prognoses associated with them.

The **aging** process provides older adults with challenges not found in the other age levels. For example, older adults experience sensory and physical declines. Older adults may lose social supports, and they frequently lose income due to retirement. The OT practitioner may work with older adults who are experiencing difficulty transitioning into new roles, or who have lost roles and are experiencing loss and grief. The OT practitioner working with older adults helps the client remain active and engaged in his or her occupations, despite physical limitations. Such diagnoses as Alzheimer's disease, Parkinson's disease, stroke, cardiac conditions, rheumatoid arthritis, and diabetes may take a toll on the older adult.

Some clients with terminal illnesses may be served through **hospice,** which provides services to help the client be comfortable during the last stages of life. OT practitioners may help clients be comfortable while others are caring for them. It may be that the practitioner provides adaptive equipment (e.g., specialized lift) so that a client may be cared for more easily.

Intervention

The OT practitioner is skilled at remediating dysfunction, compensating for lack of function, or adapting and modifying activities so that clients can be successful. Falls in the elderly and general safety issues are important concerns of occupational therapy. Practitioners may be called upon to conduct a home visit to analyze the safety of the environment. Practitioners search for unsafe walking areas, which may include stairs, scatter rugs, and uneven floors. Older persons may require changes in lighting to help with safety issues. The practitioner evaluates whether the person is able to contact someone in case of emergency and determines if extra precautions or accommodations need to be made in case of a fire or other home emergency.

Driving is important to older adults. Frequently, the physical changes of aging—such as delayed reaction time, slower movements, poor vision, and decreased hearing—make driving unsafe for older adults. Older adults who have suffered from cerebral vascular accidents (i.e., stroke) may have impaired physical abilities, such as decreased range of motion, causing them to have difficulty turning their heads to observe the road fully. They may have poor range of motion to depress the brake pedal adequately or a host of other issues. OT practitioners frequently analyze the numerous skills and client factors required for safe driving. The practitioner may help older adults regain skills for driving or address with the client how to use other means of transportation.

Because many older adults experience sensory changes, OT practitioners may help by providing instructions in large print and speaking loudly (although not infantilizing). Making visual accommodations, such as using contrasting materials, may be helpful to clients. Furthermore, limiting background noise, which may interfere with clarity of hearing, is beneficial to older adults. Older adults may experience difficulty maneuvering in crowded rooms with miscellaneous obstacles. Thus, the OT practitioner should ensure that the physical space in which the activity occurs is not cluttered.

Learned helplessness refers to a phenomenon that older adults experience as they begin to feel and act helpless and relinquish control over things that previously held value. This occurs when others do everything for the older individual and do not allow him or her to make decisions and engage in activities. Some elders are put into positions that do not feel comfortable to them. For example, if one spouse becomes ill, the other spouse may need to make financial and health decisions, which they have not done before. This can cause stress on the spouse and hinder his or her health. Keeping clients active and engaged is important, and it is the foundation of occupational therapy practice. For those older adults who do not want to participate, OT practitioners may ask them to help out a peer, which is frequently motivating for others. Furthermore, exploration of volunteer opportunities may prove rewarding for many older adults (e.g., reading programs, tutoring).

Summary

OT practitioners consider the stage of life of the client when conducting an evaluation and interventions. Each person enters different stages of life at different ages and for varied time periods. Clients may identify significant life events as turning points. Kielhofner suggests exploring the occupational profile of a client by examining the plots and trajectory of the person's life.[4] This provides the OT practitioner and client with a picture of a whole life to review. Understanding the developmental tasks over the life span provides important insight into the occupations associated with the period in a person's life.

Learning Activities

1. Divide the developmental stages among members of the class. Ask each group to present the developmental tasks for the respective developmental stage.
2. Divide the class into five groups and assign a developmental stage to each group. Ask each group to identify a variety of age-appropriate activities for their particular stage. Then have each group present their activities to the class, explaining why the activities are suited for their particular developmental stage.
3. Research some physical and psychological changes associated with a given age group. Summarize the findings in a short paper.
4. View movies such as On Golden Pond, Father of the Bride, and The Breakfast Club. Discuss the developmental issues displayed in each. Did the characters adjust to the tasks?
5. Develop a handout describing the expectations for each age group.

Review Questions

1. What are the developmental tasks associated with each age group (infancy, childhood, adolescence, adulthood, later adulthood)?
2. In what settings do OT practitioners who provide services to infants work?
3. What are some of the physical changes associated with later adulthood?
4. What are some suggestions for OT practitioners working with children or adolescents?
5. What are some of the occupational concerns of children, adolescents, adults, and older adults?

References

1. Anderson R, Boehme R, Cupps B: *Normal Development of Functional Motor Skills*, Austin, 1993, Therapy Skill Builders.
2. Bundy A: Assessment of play and leisure: Delineation of the problem, *Am J Occup Ther* 47:217, 1993.
3. Christiansen C, Baum C: *Occupational Therapy: Enabling Function and Well-Being*, ed 2, Thorofare, NJ, 1997, Slack Inc.
4. Kielhofner G, editor: *A Model of Human Occupation: Theory and Practice*, ed 4, Baltimore, MD, 2008, Lippincott Williams & Wilkins.
5. Llorens L: Application of a Developmental Theory for Health and Rehabilitation, Rockville, MD, 1982, American Occupational Therapy Association.
6. Vroman KD: Adolescent development: The journey to adulthood. In Solomon J, O'Brien J, editors: *Pediatric Skills for Occupational Therapy Assistants*, ed 3, St. Louis, 2010, Mosby.

I have always been interested in *why* and *when* people choose occupational therapy as their career. I chose occupational therapy early on, but it took years for me to realize that it was, indeed, the career for me. My first love was art. However, when I was nearing the end of my sophomore year, I ran out of funds and could not continue as a contemporary crafts major at the University of Kansas. My aunt, an occupational therapist at the Menninger Foundation in Topeka, was supervising a fieldwork student from Texas Woman's University, and in her observation, there was money for OT students at TWU, and in that era OT was synonymous with crafts.

I graduated with my BS in Occupational Therapy from TWU 2 years later, in 1964. I set out to be an artist/craftsman, financing my studio work by working as an occupational therapist. My next venture was graduate study in anthropology with an emphasis on American Indian textiles and textile conservation, then teaching fiber constructions in continuing education but also working as a part-time occupational therapist. The next degree was in counseling. As I moved from one discipline to another, I continued to work as a clinical occupational therapist across the country, and then as an educator. It was somewhere around 1982, when I had returned to TWU as an instructor and was preparing to teach an occupational therapy history course, I realized that my own personal evolution mirrored that of the profession. I didn't *discover* occupational therapy … for me, it was a process—not of immediate discovery and ownership but of entering through the "back door" without much fanfare. It took some time for me to realize that *occupation* was the consistent thread that connected all of my interests: art, crafts, anthropology, and counseling. People and their occupations, their engagement in meaningful activities, these were the things that interested me; no matter what path I took along the way … I *was an occupational therapist*, or, as I prefer, an *occupation-centered practitioner,* and continue to be, quite happily!

LINDA S. FAZIO, PhD, OTR/L, FAOTA
Professor of Clinical Occupational Therapy
Assistant Chair and Coordinator of the Professional Program
Department of Occupational Science and Occupational Therapy
University of Southern California
Los Angeles, California

CHAPTER 11

Treatment Settings and Areas of Practice

Key Terms
Acute care
Continuum of care
Diagnosis-related groups (DRGs)
Long-term care
Private for-profit agencies
Private not-for-profit agencies
Public agencies
Sociological sphere
Subacute care

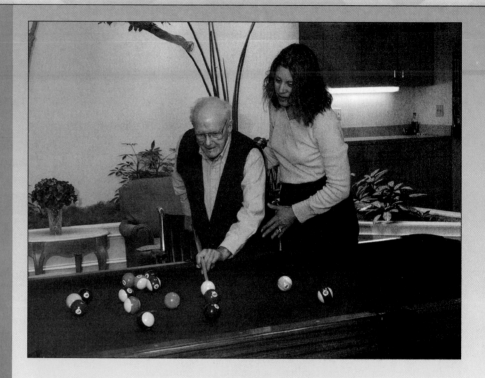

Objectives

After reading this chapter, the reader will be able to do the following:

- Characterize settings in which OT practitioners are employed by types of administration, levels of care, and areas of practice
- Identify the primary health problems addressed in different settings
- Describe how treatment setting influences the focus of OT intervention
- Describe workforce trends in occupational therapy

Occupational therapy practitioners examine the biological, social, and psychological aspects of a person to determine how to help him or her engage in meaningful occupations. Consequently, OT practitioners work with clients of all ages and disabilities, and in many different settings. This chapter provides an overview of the characteristics of settings, including the administration, levels of care, and areas of practice. The chapter also provides an overview of employment trends for OT practitioners.

Characteristic of Settings

The different types of settings in which OT practitioners are employed can be characterized according to (1) administration, (2) levels of care, and (3) areas of practice. Administration refers to the system's organization and management. Levels of care define the type of service and length of time a client receives services. Areas of practice relate to the types of conditions that the setting serves. Each of these characteristics influences the occupational therapy services provided to clients.

Administration of Setting

Health care agencies can be categorized as public, private not-for-profit, or private for-profit. This categorization affects the agency's mission and purpose, reimbursement mechanisms, and organizational structure.

Public agencies are operated by federal, state, or county governments. Federal agencies include the Veterans Administration Hospitals and Clinics, Public Health Services Hospitals and Clinics, and Indian Health Services. State-run agencies may include correctional facilities, mental health centers, and medical school hospitals, and their clinics. The county may operate county hospitals, clinics, and rehabilitation facilities that deliver services to clients in the same way as federal and state facilities. However, county administration must follow different rules and regulations than federal and state administrations, which may affect employment or method of reimbursement.

Private not-for-profit agencies receive special tax exemptions and typically charge a fee for services and maintain a balanced budget to provide services. These agencies include hospitals and clinics with religious affiliations, private teaching hospitals, and organizations such as the Easter Seal Society and United Cerebral Palsy.

Private for-profit agencies are owned and operated by individuals or a group of investors. These agencies are in business to make a profit. Large for-profit corporations may form multi-facility systems. These corporations may focus on one specific level of care (e.g., all hospitals or all skilled nursing facilities) or own multiple facilities across the continuum of care (e.g., a hospital, a skilled nursing facility, and an outpatient facility). A multi-facility system is able to buy supplies and equipment in bulk at a lower volume rate. Because these systems provide a wider range of services, they have an advantage when it comes to developing contracts with third-party payers to provide health care services.

Levels of Care

Another way of characterizing health care settings is by the level of care required by the client. Health care is provided to the consumer along a continuum, as the client's needs dictate, referred to as the **continuum of care. Acute care** is the first level on the continuum. A client at this level has a sudden and short-term need for services and is typically seen in a hospital. Services provided in the hospital are expensive because of the high cost of technology and the number of services provided.

The Prospective Payment System, introduced under Public Law 98-21 and passed in 1983, changed the way in which hospitals were paid through Medicare. Under this system, a nationwide schedule defines how much Medicare reimburses hospitals. Depending on the client's diagnosis, hospitals are paid a predetermined, fixed fee, based on **diagnosis-related groups (DRGs),** regardless of the services provided. The system provides an incentive for hospitals and physicians to reduce costs and to discharge clients from the hospital as soon as possible. As a result of the 1983 Prospective Payment System, the average length of a hospital stay has decreased.[8] The move to short hospital stays and the implementation of cost-cutting measures have resulted in a decrease in the number of OT practitioners working in hospital-based settings.[7-9] See Table 11-1.

Shorter hospital stays also created a need for an interim level of care, referred to as **subacute care.** At this level, the client still needs care but does not require an intensive level or specialized service, thereby reducing hospital costs. Typically these clients require 1 to 4 weeks more of rehabilitation. Hospitals with excess acute care beds have converted beds to less expensive subacute care beds, whereas skilled nursing facilities have upgraded some beds to the subacute level.[6] Freestanding subacute care facilities have been established to address client needs. The client typically served by a subacute care facility may be a person who has sustained a stroke or hip fracture, or one who has a cardiac condition or cancer. Rehabilitation services, including occupational therapy services, are a major component of subacute care.

Table 11-1 Employment Settings

Areas of Practice	Settings
Biological (medical)	Hospitals (general, state and federal, specialty)
	Clinics
	Work sites (industry)
	Home health
	Skilled nursing facilities
Sociological (social)	Schools (public, special—visual impairment, hearing impairment, cerebral palsy)
	Day treatment
	Hippotherapy centers
	Workshops
	Special Olympics
	Special camps (e.g., summer camps)
Psychological	Institutions (psychiatric, mental retardation)
	Community mental health
	Teen centers
	Supervised living
	After-school programs
All-inclusive	Long-term care
Private practice	Self-defined
Nontraditional	Correctional facilities
	Hospice
	National societies

Note: The categories do not indicate specialization. There are overlapping services in all areas; the classification highlights the setting's primary concern. Adapted from Reed K, Sanderson SR: *Concepts in Occupational Therapy,* ed 3, Baltimore, 1992, Lippincott Williams & Wilkins.

Long-term care serves clients who are medically stable but who have a chronic condition requiring services over time, potentially throughout life. Persons who have developmental disabilities, history of mental illness, age-related disabilities, or injury resulting in a severe disability may require this level of care. Services provided at this level may take place in an institution, skilled nursing or extended care facility, residential care facility, client's home, outpatient clinic, or community-based program.

Areas of Practice

Health care practice areas may be grouped into (1) biological (medical), (2) psychological, and (3) sociological (social). Health problems occurring in any of the areas affect a person's ability to engage in occupations. OT practitioners help clients make adjustments and find new ways to function by planning and guiding improvement of function in any or all of the three areas of practice. See Table 11-1.

Some settings address the **biological** nature of health. This refers to medical problems caused by disease, disorder, or trauma. The OT practitioner working in a setting addressing biological issues targets such things as loss of capacity, loss of sense, limitation in development or growth, limitation in movement, pain, damage to body systems, or neuromuscular disorders.

Other health organizations focus on helping clients manage **psychological** problems such as emotional, cognitive, and affective or personality disorders. These problems may be caused by an inability to cope with stress, biochemical imbalance, disease, or a combination of developmental and environmental factors. OT practitioners address psychological problems that affect thinking, memory, attention, emotional control, judgment, and self-concept.

Health care settings may also emphasize **sociological** issues to help clients meet the expectations of society. Social problems may result from severe physical or cognitive disability that limits functioning, developmental delays, intellectual disability, long-term emotional problems, or a combination of problems. OT practitioners address such things as the absence of the ability to take care of one's own needs, lack or loss of life skills, poor interpersonal skills, failure to properly adapt to environmental changes, lack of capacity for independent functioning, and improper or detrimental behavior patterns. In general, these problems require long-term life adjustments.

Jim receives OT to improve his work skills so he can return to work. The OT practitioner examines his work skills to determine if his lack of skills is due to biological (e.g., limited range of motion, loss of sensation, coordination, increased muscle tone), psychological (e.g., poor organization, intrusive thoughts, limited problem-solving, lack of motivation), or sociological (e.g., inability to follow directions, lack of awareness of social norms, limited life skills) problems. The goals, objectives, and techniques of intervention differ with regard to the types of problems the client possesses.

The above case study illustrates the overlap between practice areas. The OT practitioner employed in a medical setting must also address psychological and sociological factors when treating a client with biological limitations. Jim's work problems may be related to his condition and difficulties with organization and concentration or an inability to adhere to social norms in the workplace. All of these areas are important for success in the workplace.

An OT practitioner working in a community mental health clinic is teaching life skills to adults who have intellectual disabilities as a group. The practitioner helps clients engage in community activities, use the bus system, and understand basic social interactions (e.g., "please" and "thank you"). This setting generally addresses sociological aspects. However, the OT practitioner discovers specific upper extremity weakness in one client during a life skills group. The discovery of a weakness in the upper extremity requires further evaluation of and work on a goal that is considered biological—strengthening. Because decreased upper extremity functioning will interfere with the client's ability to complete life tasks, the clinician must also address this.

The above case shows how OT practitioners must evaluate all areas of performance. OT practitioners typically evaluate all areas and intervene as needed to help clients perform. In this case, helping a client develop upper extremity strength is key to improving life skills and, therefore, a necessary component of therapy sessions.

Settings

Occupational therapists primarily work in rehabilitation facilities, school systems, skilled nursing facilities, and acute care (Figure 11-1, A).[9] Occupational therapy assistants work primarily in skilled nursing facilities, rehabilitation facilities, and schools (Figure 11-1, B).[10]

Biological Focus

Medical facilities address biological or medical issues of clients. Intervention follows a medical model of identifying and addressing problems. These settings address clients' medical concerns including neurological, musculoskeletal, immunological, hematological, pulmonary, or cardiac systems. Many settings use a medical approach towards health care. Occupational therapists who work in these settings help clients perform daily occupations through remediation, restoration, rehabilitation, adaptation, or compensation techniques.

Hospitals

Clients in hospitals receive care for acute illnesses. Occupational therapy evaluation and intervention in hospitals generally focuses on medical and functional concerns.

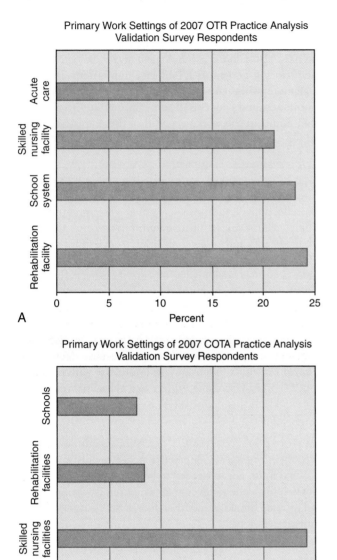

Figure 11-1 A, OTR® entry-level practice-setting trends, 2007. **B,** COTA® entry-level practice-setting trends, 2007. (From National Board for Certification in Occupational Therapy, Inc.: *Executive summary for the practice analysis summary occupational therapists: NBCOT 2008.* Retrieved March 6, 2011, from http://www.nbcot.org/pdf/Executive-Summary-for-the-Practice-Analysis-Study-OTR.pdf, p. 5) (From National Board for Certification in Occupational Therapy, Inc.: *Executive summary for the practice analysis summary of certified occupational therapy assistants: NBCOT 2008.* Retrieved March 6, 2011, from http://www.nbcot.org/pdf/Executive-Summary-for-the-Practice-Analysis-Study-COTA.pdf, p. 5.)

The OT practitioner evaluates feeding, dressing, bathing, and grooming, along with range of motion, muscle and perceptual functioning, problem solving, and thought processing. The practitioner may provide activities to increase strength, coordination, or self-care skills. The OT practitioner addresses concerns regarding the client's ability to return home (e.g., home equipment needs, family training).

In addition to inpatient acute care, some hospitals provide rehabilitation services over a longer period of time. Occupational therapy services in these specialty units occur within the general hospital. A typical rehabilitation unit provides services to clients who have sustained a disabling condition, such as stroke, head trauma, burns, or spinal cord injury. Rehabilitation services are also provided in the neonatal intensive care unit (NICU) for premature infants. The OT practitioner working in a NICU provides sensory stimulation, positioning, and feeding intervention. Training parents is also part of the intervention.

OT practitioners are employed at rehabilitation centers to provide services to a particular group of clients, such as those with spinal cord injuries, head traumas, burns, or childhood disorders. OT practitioners interact with a variety of medical professionals and, therefore, must learn to understand the roles of other professionals.

Clinics

Clinics generally serve clients with disabling conditions on an outpatient basis. These clients may have been recently discharged from a hospital setting but still need therapy services. Outpatient clinics may be affiliated with a hospital, or they may be a separate entity. The OT practitioner working in an outpatient clinic helps clients regain long-term occupational performance. Practitioners work to help clients engage in their occupations through remediation, rehabilitation, adaptation, and compensation. Rehabilitation clinics focusing on improving abilities include the Easter Seal Society, hand clinics, orthopedic clinics, and children's developmental clinics.

Home Health Agencies

OT practitioners working for home health agencies provide therapy in the client's home. The practitioner works on problems related to performance in self-care, home management, work and school, or play and leisure. Because clinicians working for home health agencies travel to clients, it may be difficult to communicate with team members. The practitioner maintains close communication with team members through documentation.

The OT practitioner may also work in the home of a person who receives hospice care. In this case, the emphasis of occupational therapy services is to maintain the person's abilities while making him or her comfortable and helping loved ones care for the client. When working with clients receiving hospice care, OT practitioners may provide modifications and compensations for decreased ability instead of trying to gain skills and improve functioning.

Settings with a Social Emphasis

Some clients experience functional limitations that impede their ability to satisfactorily interact with others. Frequently, these clients have long-term needs requiring that the OT practitioner help them improve social participation despite limitations. Intervention focuses on social skill development rather than medical. Settings with a social focus may include mental health centers such as day treatment settings or community agencies.

Schools and Special Education

In 1975, the Education for All Handicapped Children Act, known as Public Law (PL) 94-142, passed, making public school education available to all children, regardless of handicap or disability. Related services, such as occupational therapy, physical therapy, and speech and language pathology, are included in this law, which mandates that children have the services they need to be successful in the classroom. This law allows OT practitioners to work in school systems to help children engage in education. OT practitioners working in school settings may work with children who are mainstreamed or in specialty schools for children with autism, visual impairment (blind or low vision), hearing impairment (deaf), and cerebral palsy (CP).

To receive federal funding, every county in every state must provide therapy services to children with disabilities in schools. OT practitioners are either hired as an employee of the school district or contracted independently to provide services.

Day Treatment

Day treatment facilities serve people who need daytime supervision or are able to live in the community (rather than in an institution or full-care facility) but who require some assistance. Some individuals may live at home with families whose members work, whereas others live in boarding homes but cannot plan their own activities. OT practitioners are employed in day treatment settings to develop and provide structured programs of activities for clients. Day treatment programs may specialize in providing intervention activities for a variety of groups, including children with behavioral disorders, persons who have mental illness, persons with Alzheimer's disease, or older persons.

Workshops

Some communities provide special workshops for people who are not able to seek employment in a competitive job market. These workshops include sheltered workshops, training centers, or retirement workshops. Many clients in sheltered workshops have some type of developmental disability. OT practitioners may work on skill development, work hardening, environmental adaptations, or task modifications to help clients engage in work.

Settings with a Psychological Emphasis

A variety of settings focus on improving psychological functioning for occupational performance. These settings are regarded primarily as psychiatric or mental health settings but also address social difficulties.

Institutions

Deinstitutionalization, implemented in the 1970s, refers to moving clients who have mental illnesses from institutions (such as state mental hospitals) back into the community. Some state hospitals continue to provide services for those with severe developmental or emotional disabilities. These institutions (or state hospitals) may offer traditional psychiatric occupational therapy programs wherein the practitioner plans activities (e.g., crafts, recreation, outings) for the purposes of self-care, skill development, self-awareness, leisure exploration, and social participation.

Community Mental Health Centers

Community mental health centers emerged with the closing of institutions and are organized differently in regions and towns. Community mental health centers may offer medication clinics and counseling, crisis units, or day treatment programs. In community mental health settings, OT practitioners work with a client or group of clients to develop life skills, encourage social participation, explore leisure opportunities, and develop abilities to engage in areas of performance.

Supervised Living

Supervised living refers to partially or fully supervised housing for people whose problems do not warrant institutional care but who are not ready or able to manage on their own. Programming may vary from limited guidance to fully structured programs. Supervised living may include substance-abuse programs (often with a specific time limit) for alcoholics or drug addicts; halfway houses, which provide temporary living arrangements for someone leaving an institution before going to independent living; or group homes, which are more permanent living arrangements. In these settings, the OT practitioner may work with the client on general planning, (e.g., organizing household chores), participating in social events (e.g., outings, recreational activities), and engaging in life-skills training.

Older persons may live in assisted living facilities and may require occupational therapy services for physical, social, or psychological difficulties. OT practitioners may design activities for groups or individuals.

All-Inclusive Settings

All-inclusive settings include long-term care facilities that provide occupational therapy services that address biological, psychological, and sociological functions. An all-inclusive facility provides residence for people for long periods of time. The special skills needed by the OT practitioner in these settings depend on the nature of the facility.

Nontraditional Settings

OT practitioners work in correctional facilities, industrial settings, hospice, health maintenance organizations, and community transition settings. Practitioners work with therapeutic riding, aquatherapy, and in senior citizen centers. Some practitioners work with migrant workers, victims of disasters, or homeless people. The role of the practitioner varies according to the setting, but the aim is to help individuals function more fully in their lives. Practitioners may choose to work in wellness programs (such as those to help promote physical activity and nutrition for children or programs to promote healthy living in older persons).

Private Practice and Consulting

Self-employment, or private practice settings, address a variety of aspects of client functioning and include clients of all ages and diagnoses. Private practice settings in occupational therapy have increased since 1988, when the federal government, through the Health Care Financing Administration, implemented Medicare Part B coverage. This enabled OT practitioners to fully participate in Medicare programs by permitting qualified practitioners to apply for Medicare provider numbers. A provider number allows a practitioner to become an independent provider and to bill directly for services.

OT practitioners working in private practice may take individual referrals and administer treatment in private homes, or have clients come to their facilities. Other clinicians may contract with agencies to spend a specific number of hours at a school or at a nursing home. Some private practice companies employ practitioners from many disciplines and market therapy services as a business enterprise. Some practitioners in private practice consult with other agencies. Consultation requires highly developed professional expertise and management skills; the consultant and agency negotiate the parameters of service and set their own limits.[5] OT practitioners also consult with organizations in areas such as ergonomics, facility design, and wellness.[1,7,11]

Occupational Therapy Employment Trends

According to the Bureau of Labor Statistics (2010), occupational therapy and occupational therapy assistant employment opportunities are expected to grow "much faster than average" (increase 20% or more) between 2008 and 2018.[1,3,11] Job opportunities are good, especially for practitioners working with the elderly. Furthermore, occupational therapists are taking on supervisory roles, allowing OT assistants to work more closely with clients.[11]

Most occupational therapists (29%) are working in ambulatory health care services, followed by schools and early intervention centers (24%).[1,2,9] Other major employers are hospitals, offices of other health practitioners, public and private educational services, and nursing care facilities.[1,2,9] Some therapists are employed by home health care services, outpatient care centers, offices of physicians, individual and family services, community care facilities for the elderly, or government agencies. A small percentage of therapists are self-employed. The median annual wage of occupational therapists was $66,780 and for occupational therapy assistants was $48,230, in May 2008.[11]

Growth in the older population, the baby-boom generation's move into middle age, and medical advances continue to increase the demand for occupational therapy.[3,4,11] Furthermore, evidence-based practice supporting the effectiveness of occupational therapy intervention continues to support therapy.[4]

Future practice areas targeted for growth include: ergonomics, accessibility design, driver assessment and training, assisted living, technology, health and wellness, low vision, Alzheimer's, children and youth needs, and community service (see Chapter 4).[4,5,7]

AOTA reported "The number of practitioners in the 50-to 50-year-old group is at the highest level ever and the percentage of practitioners under age 30 is now just 7.9%."[2] This trend suggests a need for new practitioners. Furthermore, educational programs are in need of experienced faculty with earned doctoral degrees; only 45% of occupational therapy faculty held doctoral degrees in 2005.[2,3] Faculty shortages prevent programs from expanding.[3]

Summary

Settings in which OT practitioners are employed may be characterized according to (1) administration of the setting, (2) levels of care, and (3) areas of practice. OT practitioners view the biological, sociological, and psychological functioning of clients within the context of their environment. Thus, OT practitioners work in a variety of intervention settings with many types of clients who have varying abilities. As such, care is tailored to the client's needs and may take place in acute, subacute, long-term, and rehabilitation settings. OT practitioners work primarily in hospital and school settings. However, many OT practitioners are expanding services into nontraditional settings.

Occupational therapy is a growing profession with many career opportunities. Practitioners may choose from a variety of settings and work with clients of all ages and disabilities. OT practitioners may elect to practice and educate future practitioners or serve in supervisory roles. Practitioners are urged to take advantage of growth opportunities.

Learning Activities

1. Research occupational therapy employment settings in your area. Describe the types of settings, types of clients the practitioners serve, and the level of care provided.
2. Make salary comparisons for entry-level practitioners (OTs and OTAs) in different kinds of employment settings.
3. Observe occupational therapy in two different settings. Describe the clients and the services provided. Discuss how the practitioner worked with clients. Identify the area of practice.
4. Determine a need in your community, and define the type of services an OT practitioner could provide.
5. Review the job requirements for a particular setting that interests you. Present a brief description to the class.

Review Questions

1. What are the levels of care provided to clients?
2. What are the types of settings in which OT practitioners work?
3. What are the three areas of practice? Provide examples of the type of OT services considered within each area.
4. What are some nontraditional settings in which OT practitioners work?

References

1. American Occupational Therapy Association: *Workforce trends in occupational therapy*. Retrieved March 6, 2011, from http://www.aota.org/Students/Prospective/Outlook/38231.aspx?FT=.pdf.

2. American Occupational Therapy Association: Occupational therapy salaries and job opportunities continue to improve: 2006 AOTA Workforce and Compensation Survey, *OT Practice*. Retrieved March 6, 2011, from http://www.aota.org/Educate/EdRes/StuRecruit/Working/40691.aspx?FT=.pdf.

3. American Occupational Therapy Association: *Addressing health-care workforce issues for the future: Senate HELP testimony 2-27, 2008*. Retrieved March 5, 2011, from http://www.aota.org/Practitioners/Advocacy/Federal/Testimony/2008/Feb27.aspx.

4. Brachetesende A: The turnaround is here! *OT Practice*, January 24, 2005.

5. Jaffe EG, Epstein CF: *Occupational Therapy Consultation: Theory, Principles and Practice*, St. Louis, 1992, Mosby.

6. Joe B: Subacute care fills growing niche, *OT Week*, February 27, 1997. American Occupational Therapy Association.

7. Johansson C: Top 10 emerging practice areas to watch in the new millennium, *OT Practice*, January 31, 2000. Retrieved December 4, 2006, from www.aota.org.

8. Levy LL: Occupational therapy's place in the health care system. In Hopkins HL, Smith HD, editors: *Willard and Spackman's Occupational Therapy*, Philadelphia, 1993, JB Lippincott.

9. National Board for Certification in Occupational Therapy, Inc.: *Executive summary for the practice analysis summary occupational therapists: NBCOT 2008*. Retrieved March 6, 2011, from http://www.nbcot.org/pdf/Executive-Summary-for-the-Practice-Analysis-Study-OTR.pdf.

10. National Board for Certification in Occupational Therapy, Inc.: *Executive summary for the practice analysis summary occupational therapy assistants: NBCOT 2008*. Retrieved March 6, 2011, from http://www.nbcot.org/pdf/Executive-Summary-for-the-Practice-Analysis-Study-OTR.pdf.

11. U.S. Department of Labor, Bureau of Labor Statistics: *Occupational Outlook Handbook*, ed 2010–11. Retrieved March 5, 2011, from www.bls.gov/oco /oco20016.htm.

I was attracted to the profession when I realized the power of its medium—occupation. Life is, essentially, a chain of occupations. Occupation gives the context in which people build their skills, discover their interests, and reveal their hopes. Purposes in life are worked out through occupation. At the same time, occupation can influence and transform these purposes. The power of occupation lies in its intertwining of the person's body, mind, soul, and world. The work of the occupational therapist is to be an expert on the complexity of occupation and to use that knowledge artfully to help others achieve a life that is purposeful and meaningful. It is within this process that the therapist finds purpose and meaning; it is within this process that curiosity and wonder about how people create occupation grow.

RENÉ PADILLA, PhD, OTR/L, FAOTA
Associate Professor
Department of Occupational Therapy
Creighton University
Omaha, Nebraska

CHAPTER **12** — Occupational Therapy Process: Evaluation, Intervention, and Outcomes

Key Terms

Assessment procedures
Assessment instruments
Discharge plan
Interrater reliability
Intervention
Interview
Normative data
Nonstandardized tests
Observation
Occupational therapy process
Referral
Reliability
Screening
Standardized tests
Structured observation
Test-retest reliability
Transition services
Validity

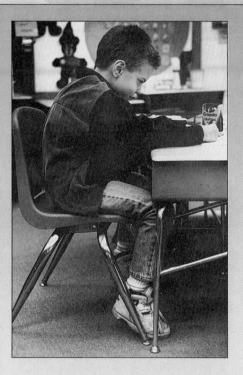

Objectives

After reading this chapter, the reader will be able to do the following:

- Describe the occupational therapy referral, screening, and evaluation process
- Identify the purpose of the occupational profile
- Describe the occupational performance analysis and how it is used in OT
- Discuss the steps in conducting an interview
- Understand the importance of observation skills in the evaluation process
- Identify the steps in the intervention process
- Describe the five general intervention approaches used in occupational therapy
- Characterize the roles of the occupational therapist (OT) and the occupational therapy assistant (OTA) as they engage in the occupational therapy process

The **occupational therapy process** involves the interaction between the practitioner *and* the client. The relationship between the practitioner and the client is a collaborative one that involves problem-solving to support the client's occupational performance. The process is dynamic and the focus is on occupation and the client as an occupational being.[2] The client may be an individual, caregiver, group, or population.

The occupational therapy process can be divided into the evaluation, intervention, and outcome (Figure 12-1).

The evaluation process includes referral, screening, developing an occupational profile, and analyzing occupational performance. The intervention process includes intervention planning, implementation, and review. The outcomes process includes measurement of outcomes and decision-making related to the future direction of intervention (i.e., continue, modify, or discontinue). In this chapter, we describe the components of each stage and delineate the roles of the OT and the OTA throughout the process.

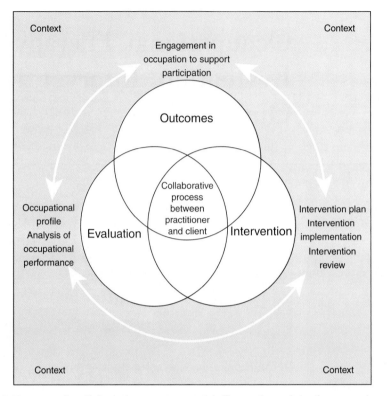

Figure 12-1 Framework collaborative process model. Illustration of the framework emphasizing the interactive nature of the client–practitioner relationship and of the service delivery process. (From American Occupational Therapy Association: Occupational therapy practice framework: Domain and process, ed 2, *Am J Occup Ther* 62:625–683, 2008.)

Evaluation Process

The purpose of the evaluation process is to find out what the client wants and needs, and to identify those factors that support or hinder occupational performance.[2] The OT practitioner develops an occupational profile of the client and analyzes the occupational performance to determine the client's skills and ability to carry out activities of daily living.

The OT practitioner bases the evaluation procedures on the client's age, diagnosis, developmental level, education, socioeconomic status, cultural background, and functional abilities. The steps of the evaluation process include referral, screening, and evaluation. Observation and interviewing are essential to this process.

Referral

The occupational therapy process begins when a **referral,** a request for service for a particular client, is made.[3] The OT is responsible for accepting and responding to the referral. Referrals may come from a physician, another professional, or the client. Referrals may range from a specific prescription for a dynamic orthosis to general suggestions to improve fine-motor problems. Federal, state, and local regulations and the policies of third-party payers determine the type of referral required (e.g., whether a physician's referral is necessary) and the role an OTA can have in the referral process.

Screening

Through **screening,** the OT practitioner gathers preliminary information about the client and determines whether further evaluation and occupational therapy intervention are warranted. Screening typically involves a review of the client's records, the use of a brief screening test, an interview with the client or caregiver, observation of the client, and/or a discussion of the client with the referral source. The practitioner investigates the client's prior and current level of occupational performance and determines the client's future occupational performance needs. The practitioner communicates the screening results to the appropriate individuals, including the party who made the referral.[1,3]

The OT initiates and directs the screening process, using methods that are appropriate to the client's developmental level, gender, cultural background, and medical and functional status.[1,3] The OTA contributes to the screening process under the direction of an OT. Before screening tasks are performed by an OTA, he or she must achieve service competency in the particular tasks.

If screening suggests the client is in need of services, a comprehensive evaluation is arranged. The OT identifies a model of practice (see Chapter 14) from which the evaluation is based. The model of practice helps organize the practitioner's thinking. From the model of practice, the practitioner selects a frame of reference and chooses **assessment instruments** consistent with the frame of reference.

Occupational Profile

The goal of this step is to gather information on the client so that an **occupational profile** can be developed. The OT practitioner obtains initial information about the client, including the client's age, gender, and reason for referral; diagnosis and medical history (including date of onset); prior living situation and level of function (e.g., independent at home or in a care home); and social, educational, and vocational background. The initial review may provide information regarding precautions that need to be adhered to during the occupational therapy process. This background information is usually recorded in the client's occupational therapy chart and on the evaluation form. Figure 12-2 illustrates an example of an evaluation form used in an occupational therapy setting.

An occupational profile provides the practitioner with a history of the client's background and functional performance with which to design intervention. The following questions from the *Occupational Therapy Practice Framework (OTPF)* help the practitioner develop the occupational therapy profile[2]:

- Who is the client (individual, caregiver, group, population)?
- Why is the client seeking service?
- What are the client's current concerns relative to engaging in occupations and daily life activities?
- What areas of occupation are successful, and what areas are causing problems or risks?
- What is the client's occupational history (i.e., life experiences, values, interests, previous patterns of engagement in occupations and in daily life activities, and the meanings associated with them)?
- What are the client's priorities and desired targeted outcomes?

Occupational Performance Analysis

From the information gathered during the occupational profile (e.g. client's needs, problems, and priorities), the practitioner makes decisions regarding the analysis of occupational performance. This information provides direction to the practitioner as to the areas that need to be further examined. The practitioner selects specific assessment instruments to collect further information.

The OT practitioner uses assessments to gather information on a client's occupational performance in regards to areas, skills, patterns, contexts, client factors, and activity demands (see Chapter 9).[2] The results are documented on a form typical to that shown in Figure 12-2. This evaluation information forms the basis for the intervention plan.

Occupational performance analysis involves analyzing all aspects of the occupation to determine the client factors, patterns, contexts, skills, and behaviors required to be successful. Once the practitioner has thoroughly analyzed the occupation, the practitioner can more easily determine what is interfering with the client's ability to engage in occupations.

Evaluation is an essential part of clinical decision-making requiring a depth of understanding of many factors. As a result, the final responsibility of evaluation rests with the OT. The OTA, though not responsible for the complete evaluation, may be delegated responsibility for certain procedures and thus may contribute to an evaluation under an OT's supervision. The OTA communicates the results of all evaluation procedures to the OT. As with the screening process, service competency for tasks performed by an OTA needs to be established. The overall evaluation, or the process of compiling all of the information to form a composite picture of the client, is the responsibility of an OT.

The evaluation requires that the OT gather accurate and useful information to identify the needs and problems of the client to plan intervention. The techniques used during the evaluation process can be classified into three basic procedures: (1) interview, (2) skilled observation, and (3) formal evaluation procedures.

Interview

The **interview** is the primary mechanism for gathering information for the occupational profile. The interview is a planned and organized way to collect pertinent information. The focus of occupational therapy is *occupations*, which include the activities in which a person engages throughout the day. Therefore, the practitioner gathers information related to the individual's occupations. The practitioner asks questions regarding the client's function in daily activities before the onset of the problem that resulted in the referral. The interview is also used as a means of developing trust and rapport with the client.

In some instances, the client is asked to fill out a checklist or questionnaire before the interview. For example, the interest checklist (Figure 12-3) developed by Matsutsuyu[8] has served as a model for others. Interest checklists enable clients to report on hobbies and interests. The activity configuration also provides information on how a client spends the day. The client compiles a list of all the different activities in which he or she participates and classifies activities according to the area of performance (e.g., activities of daily living, instrumental activities of daily living, education, work, play, leisure, and social participation). The client rates whether the activity is one he or she *has* to do or *wants* to do and how adequately the activity is performed. The practitioner uses the data to determine how the person spends his or her day and in what types of activities he or she is involved.

The interview takes place in a setting that is quiet and allows for privacy. Ideally, the interview should be relaxed and comfortable for both the interviewer and the client. The skill of interviewing involves blending the formal information gathering with informal person-to-person communication. The stages of an interview include: initial contact, information gathering, and closure.

Initial Contact

The skilled interviewer spends the first few minutes of the interview putting the subject at ease. Often, a person is worried and anxious at an interview. A client may experience

Occupational Therapy Initial Assessment

Name: _____ DOB: _____ Start of Service Date: _____

HICN: _____ Onset: _____

Medical Dx/ICD-9# _____Treatment Dx/ICD-9# _____

Past Medical History:_____

Occupational Profile:

Areas of Occupation:

ADL Status	dep	max	mod	min	sup	indep	comments:
Self-feeding							
Hygiene/grooming							
UB bathing							
UB dressing							
LB dressing							
Wet tub/shower							
Toilet transfer							
Toileting skills							
Functional mobility							
Personal device care							

IADL Status							
Kitchen survival skills							
Meal preparation							
Shopping							
Laundry							
Light housekeeping							
Community mobility							
Financial mgmt							
Care of others							
Work/Leisure/Social participation							

Figure 12-2 Sample occupational therapy evaluation form. *ADL,* Activities of daily living; *CGA,* contact guard assist; *dep,* dependent; *DOB,* date of birth; *DX,* diagnosis; *HICN,* health insurance carrier number; *IADL,* instrumental activities of daily living; *indep,* independent; *LB,* lower body; *LUE,* left upper extremity; *max,* maximum assist; *min,* minimum assist; *mod,* moderate assist; *OT,* occupational therapy; *ROM,* range of motion; *RUE,* right upper extremity; sup, supervised; *UB,* upper body. *(From Pendleton H, Schultz-Krohn W, editors:* Pedretti's Occupational Therapy: Practice Skills for Physical Dysfunction, *ed 6, St. Louis, 2006, Mosby.)*

Vocational:	
Avocational:	
Leisure participation:	
Social participation:	

Client Factors:	
Functional cognition	
Perceptual status	
Memory	
Vision/hearing	
Pain	
ROM:	
RUE:	
LUE:	
Motor control:	
RUE:	
LUE:	
Strength:	
RUE:	
LUE:	
Muscle tone	
Coordination/bilateral integration	
Body system function	

Performance Skills: Patient/family goals:

Posture	
Sit:	
Stand:	
Mobility	
Endurance/effort	

Short-term goals:	Long-term goals:

OT intervention plan:	Frequency/duration:

Therapist's Signature   Date

Figure 12-2—Cont'd.

stress related to the illness or trauma or he or she may feel threatened by the prospect of entering into therapy.

The practitioner begins the interview by introducing him or herself and informing the client about the clinic, the program, and standard procedures. It is important to convey general information but not burden the person with specific details that he or she may be afraid of forgetting.

Each OT practitioner develops his or her own interviewing style. Regardless, taking the time to create a relaxed and

NAME				UNIT		DATE		

Please check each item below according to your interest.

	INTEREST				INTEREST		
ACTIVITY	CASUAL	STRONG	NO	ACTIVITY	CASUAL	STRONG	NO
1. Gardening				41. Exercise			
2. Sewing				42. Volleyball			
3. Poker				43. Woodworking			
4. Languages				44. Billiards			
5. Social clubs				45. Driving			
6. Radio				46. Dusting			
7. Bridge				47. Jewelry making			
8. Car repair				48. Tennis			
9. Writing				49. Cooking			
10. Dancing				50. Basketball			
11. Needlework				51. History			
12. Golf				52. Guitar			
13. Football				53. Science			
14. Popular music				54. Collecting			
15. Puzzles				55. Ping pong			
16. Holidays				56. Leather work			
17. Solitaire				57. Shopping			
18. Movies				58. Photography			
19. Lectures				59. Painting			
20. Swimming				60. Television			
21. Bowling				61. Concerts			
22. Visiting				62. Ceramics			
23. Mending				63. Camping			
24. Chess				64. Laundry			
25. Barbeques				65. Dating			
26. Reading				66. Mosaics			
27. Traveling				67. Politics			
28. Manual arts				68. Scrabble			
29. Parties				69. Decorating			
30. Dramatics				70. Math			
31. Shuffleboard				71. Service groups			
32. Ironing				72. Piano			
33. Social studies				73. Scouting			
34. Classical music				74. Plays			
35. Floor mopping				75. Clothes			
36. Model building				76. Knitting			
37. Baseball				77. Hair styling			
38. Checkers				78. Religion			
39. Singing				79. Drums			
40. Home repairs				80. Conversation			

Figure 12-3 Neuropsychiatric Institute (NPI) Interest Checklist. (Courtesy of University of California at Los Angeles, from Matsutsuyu JS: The interest checklist, *Am J Occup Ther* 23:323, 1969.)

unthreatening atmosphere is beneficial to future therapy because the interview creates the "first impression" of the therapy process. The client who feels welcome will begin therapy prepared to become a partner in the therapy process.

Information Gathering

After discussing the purpose of therapy, the OT practitioner gathers information about the client. The skilled interviewer guides the conversation in a way that yields the desired data yet keeps the flow easy and comfortable. The OT practitioner explains before beginning the interview that he or she will be taking notes. He or she asks questions conversationally, while making eye contact, and does not read directly from notes. An unskilled interviewer may spend time interviewing only to discover he or she has not collected the needed information. To ensure that the desired information is secured, the OT practitioner works from an interview outline.

Closure

Effectively putting closure on the interview is also a learned skill. The OT practitioner guides the interview to collect needed data in a pleasant, conversational way. The interviewer signals when the interview is about to end by summarizing the information gathered and reviewing the next steps in the process. This technique avoids the discomfort of an abrupt "time is up" ending.

Developing Observation Skills

Observation is the means of gathering information about a person or an environment by watching and noticing. Observation may occur through a structured series of steps introduced by the OT practitioner, or it may be intentionally left unstructured to see what takes place. The OT practitioner obtains information about the client through observation. For example, the practitioner can observe the person's posture, dress, social skills, tone of voice, behavior, and physical abilities (i.e., use of the limbs and ambulation).

Observation is an important professional skill and can be developed through practice. Practitioners may develop observation skills by documenting findings and discussing this with an experienced practitioner. Examining skills by watching videotapes of clients is another technique to develop observational skills. Using observational questionnaires or worksheets may help guide an inexperienced practitioner and make it easier to identify important observations.

A **structured observation** involves watching the client perform a predetermined activity. OT practitioners frequently use structured observation to gain knowledge of what the person can or cannot do in relation to the demands of the task. If, for example, the OT practitioner wishes to evaluate a self-care activity like shaving, the client is asked to shave the way he usually does. While observing, the practitioner learns what is needed to improve function in this task. With information that identifies the extent of the limitation, the OT practitioner can make a plan for correction or improvement. OT practitioners examine the quality of performance through observation of the process, not just by examining the end product. For example, the clinician may observe how the person responds to directions, approaches the activity, interacts with others, deals with frustration, and engages in the task during the activity. Box 12-1 presents a guide for observation.

> ### Box 12-1
>
> #### Observation Guide
>
> 1. Describe how the client performs the activity in terms of the following client factors:
>   - Movement functions
>   - Specific mental functions (including thought, judgment, concept formation, emotional, language, motor planning, experience of self and others)
>   - Global mental functions (including consciousness, orientation, temperament and personality, energy, and drive)
> 2. Describe the client in terms of an overall impression during activities:
>   - Physical appearance
>   - Reaction to testing situation
>   - Response to examiner
>   - Approach to tasks
>   - Quality of production
>   - Communications with others
> 3. Gather information related to specific qualities:
>   - Attentiveness
>   - Independence
>   - Ability to follow verbal instructions
>   - Ability to follow written instructions
>   - Cooperativeness
>   - Initiative
>   - Response to authority
>   - Ability to read and write
>   - Timidity or aggressiveness
>   - Neatness
>   - Accuracy
>   - Distractibility
>   - Passive or active involvement
>   - Ease of movement
>   - Speed of performance
>   - Problem-solving
>   - Motor skills
>   - Adaptability
>   - Social skills
>   - Affect
>   - Interactions with others

Formal Assessment Procedures

Formal assessment procedures help determine the existing performance level of the client. Formal **assessment procedures** include tests, instruments, or strategies that provide specific guidelines.[4] This informs practitioners about what is to be examined, how it is to be examined, how data are communicated, and how the information is applied in clinical problem-solving. Formal assessment procedures have specific guidelines, and therefore they are easily duplicated and critically analyzed.

A test is said to have **validity** if research testing shows it to be a true measure of what it claims to measure. Test **reliability** is a measure of how accurately the scores obtained from the test reflect the true performance of the client. There are several different types of reliability with which the OT practitioner must be familiar. **Test-retest reliability** is an indicator of the consistency of the results of a given test from one administration to another. **Interrater reliability** is an indicator of the likelihood that test scores will be the same no matter who is the examiner. OT practitioners can place more confidence in instruments that have high validity and reliability.

A **standardized test** is one that has gone through a rigorous process of scientific inquiry to determine its reliability and validity. Each standardized test has a carefully established protocol for its administration. OT practitioners follow set procedures for administering and scoring the test. Some standardized tests require that clinicians say the exact same words to each client. Standardized tests may be based on **normative data,** often called *norms,* collected from a representative sample that can then be used by the examiner to make comparisons with his or her subjects. Normative data are compiled by administering the test to a large sample of subjects.[4] The Miller Assessment for Preschoolers (MAP)[9] and the Sensory Integration and Praxis Tests (SIPT)[5] are examples of standardized tests developed by OTs.

OT practitioners also use **nonstandardized tests** for measuring function. Nonstandardized tests have guidelines for administering and scoring but may not have established normative data, or established reliability and validity. The administration and scoring of nonstandardized tests are more subjective and rely on clinical skill, judgment, and experience of the therapist. For example, manual muscle testing and sensory testing are nonstandardized tests.

There is a broad range of assessment instruments available to OT practitioners. OT practitioners use frames of reference to guide the selection of a test instrument as well as consideration of the client's background, diagnosis, and needs.

OT practitioners administering a test instrument must be properly prepared. Before administering a test, the OT practitioner must become familiar with the procedures and know the correct way to administer items, score the test, and interpret the data. Comfort with any testing procedure is acquired through practice. Some tests even require special training or certification before they can be administered. Under the direction of an OT, an OTA may administer the test once service competency has been established.

Intervention Process

The aim of occupational therapy is to enable the person with a disability to function more independently in his or her environment. This requires problem-solving methods to improve occupational performance. The occupational therapy intervention process requires the practitioner develop goals for the client, select activities, direct intervention to guide the client to learn ways of engaging in occupational performance, and monitor the results of the intervention.

Intervention Planning: Problem Identification, Solution Development, and Plan of Action

The intervention plan is based on an analysis of the information accumulated during the evaluation. The initial step in developing the intervention plan is *problem identification.*[6] The OT reviews the results of the evaluation and identifies the client's strengths and deficits in occupational performance areas, performance skills, performance patterns, client factors, and contexts. From this, the OT determines the problem areas that need to be addressed through intervention. Problem identification also includes developing a hypothesis about the cause of the problem. Understanding the problem helps the OT practitioner select the most appropriate approach to treatment.

Solution development is the process of identifying alternatives for intervention and forming goals and objectives. Selecting a *model of practice* and *frame of reference* from which the OT practitioner operates is an important component of solution development. Several frames of reference are used in occupational therapy practice. Each frame of reference is based on a body of knowledge that identifies principles and processes of change (see Chapter 14 for more information on models of practice and frames of reference). The frame of reference selected provides the practitioner with guidelines for clinical reasoning and intervention planning. Exploring intervention strategies based on the different frames of reference will help the practitioner develop potential solutions.

Based on the problems and the identified frame of reference along with input received from the client, the practitioner determines a *plan of action* for intervention (expected outcomes). The first step in developing a plan of action is the creation of long- and short-term goals that address the problems identified. These goals are prioritized according to the needs of the client. Next, intervention methods that will help the client achieve the goals are determined. This involves a consideration of the tools or equipment needed, any special positioning, where the activity will take place, how it will be structured and graded, and whether it is to be performed in a group or individually.[2,7] The intervention methods are based on the selected frame of reference. The practitioner uses his or her knowledge of the disability and the intervention to predict which methods will likely achieve the desired results as stated in the goals. Chapter 15 discusses the types of therapeutic activities used in occupational therapy.

The outcome of this intervention planning process is a written report (or intervention plan). The written plan addresses the strengths and weaknesses of the individual, interests of the client and caregivers, estimate of rehabilitation potential, and expected outcomes (short- and long-term goals), along with frequency and duration of intervention, recommended methods and media, apparent environmental and time constraints, identification of a plan for reevaluation, and discharge planning (Figure 12-4).[2] The plan is formally entered in the client's records.

The OT is responsible for analyzing and interpreting the data from the evaluation and formulating and documenting the intervention plan.[1] The OTA contributes to this process.

Implementation of the Plan

Intervention involves working with the client through therapy to reach client goals. Five intervention approaches are used in occupational therapy: create/promote; establish, restore; maintain; modify; and prevent (see Appendix C).[2] The following examples describe how these approaches may be implemented in practice.

☐ Part A   ☐ Part B   ☐ Other _____   Room No. _____   ☐ F.F.S.   ☐ Direct Bill   Facility: _____

| **700 FORM   OCCUPATIONAL THERAPY PLAN OF TREATMENT** (Complete For Initial Claims Only) ☐ E.O.M.   ☐ D/C Sum |

1. Patient's Last Name | First Name | M.I. | ☐ M ☐ F | 2. Provider No. | 3. Provider Name

4. HIC# | 5. Medical Record No. | 6. Onset Date | 7. SOC Date

8. DOB | 9. Primary Diagnosis (Pertinent Medical DX) (ICD-9) | 10. Treatment Diagnosis (ICD-9) | 11. Visits From SOC

12. Functional Goals (Short Term) - In ___ weeks, patient will:
1.

2.

3.

4.

☐ Evaluation

PLAN OF TREATMENT
☐ Self Care/Home Management Training   ☐ Cognitive Retraining
☐ Therapeutic Activities   ☐ Orthotics Fitting Training/UE Splinting
☐ Neuromuscular Re-education   ☐ Other _____
☐ Therapeutic Exercise   ☐ Other _____
☐ *In Individual and/or Group Treatment*

OUTCOME (Long Term Goal) - In ___ weeks, patient will:

I have reviewed this Plan of Treatment and certify the need for service.
13. **PHYSICIAN SIGNATURE**   DATE   ☐ N/A

14. Frequency/Duration (e.g., 5x/wk x 4 wks)

15. Certification   From   Through   ☐ N/A

16. Physician's Name

18. INITIAL ASSESSMENT :
Reason for Referral:

Prior Level of Function:

History/Medical Complications:

Precautions/Contraindications:

Check and document with skilled objective data, on the areas that impact function.
☐ Cognition/Safety Judgment:

☐ Visual Motor/Perception:

☐ Neuromotor:

☐ Sensorimotor:

☐ Balance: Sitting Static: Dynamic:

☐ Balance: Standing Static: Dynamic:

17. Prior Hospitalization   From   Through   ☐ N/A

Scoring Key: *MDS ADL Self Performance:* 0=Independent 1=Supervision→Supervision(SBA)
2=Limited →C.G.A.   3=Extensive →Min, Mod, Max Assist   4=Total →Dependent
Support (SUP): 0=No Set-up   1=Set-up help only   2=1 person assist   3=2 person assist

☐ ROM:

☐ Strength:

☐ Activity Tolerance:

☐ Other/Comments:

Clinical Impressions:

Positive Prognostic Indicators:

Rehab Potential: ☐ Good ☐ Excellent   Patient aware of prognosis: ☐ Yes ☐ No
Admit Cond: ☐ Mild ☐ Mod ☐ Sev ☐ Dep   Patient aware of diagnosis: ☐ Yes ☐ No

ADL Status	0 Ind	1 Sup	2 CGA	3 Min	3 Mod	4 Max	Total	SUP
Self Feeding								
Hygiene / Grooming								
Dressing-Upper Body								
Dressing-Lower Body								
Toileting								
Toilet Transfers								
Bathing-Upper Body								
Bathing-Lower Body								
Functional Mobility								

19. SIGNATURE (professional establishing POT, including credentials)   DATE

Document Impairments and Reason to: ☐ Continue Services   *or*   ☐ D/C Services

20. FUNCTIONAL LEVEL (End of Billing Period)
Skilled Interventions:

Resident/Caregiver Training:

Recommendations:

ADL Status	0 Ind	1 Sup	2 CGA	3 Min	3 Mod	4 Max	Total	SUP
Self Feeding								
Hygiene / Grooming								
Dressing-Upper Body								
Dressing-Lower Body								
Toileting								
Toilet Transfer								
Bathing-Upper Body								
Bathing-Lower Body								
Functional Mobility								

D/C Prognosis to Maintain Function: ☐ Good   ☐ Fair   ☐ N/A
D/C Condition: ☐ Goals Met   ☐ Improved   ☐ Declined   ☐ No Change
D/C Location: ☐ Home ☐ ALF ☐ LTC ☐ SNF ☐ Hospital ☐ Other ☐ Expired

21. THERAPIST SIGNATURE:
Service Dates: From: Through:

REHABWORKS
A Division of Symphony Health Services   Modified OT 700 Form   **RW5904** OT Plan of Treatment 11/2004

Figure 12-4 Modified Medicare 700 form—occupational therapy plan of treatment. (Courtesy of RehabWorks, a division of Symphony Rehabilitation, Hunt Valley, MD. From Pendleton H, Schultz-Krohn, editors: *Pedretti's Occupational Therapy: Practice Skills for Physical Dysfunction*, ed 6, St. Louis, 2006, Mosby.)

These examples are just a few of the many intervention strategies employed by OT practitioners.

Consulting is also an important part of intervention. Practitioners frequently consult with other professionals, family members, and clients regarding intervention strategies. When the OT practitioner consults with others, he or she is not directly responsible for the implementation and subsequent outcome of the intervention. For example, the practitioner may consult with a teacher on how to facilitate handwriting skills in the classroom. A practitioner may consult in a work setting about ergonomically correct lifting techniques or workspace arrangements. Consultation requires advanced knowledge, the ability to communicate clearly with others, and knowledge of the context in which the consultation occurs.

Create/Promote: The OT practitioner organizes an afternoon handwriting group for school-aged children. The practitioner recommends the group to children in his or her caseload who have difficulty with handwriting.

Establish, restore: The OT practitioner works with Galen, a 67-year-old man who has lost use of his right side since his cerebral vascular accident. The clinician works to help Galen return to his typical morning routine.

Maintain: After performing a home visit, the OT practitioner makes recommendations so 90-year-old Harry can stay at home.

Modify: The OT practitioner provides 35-year-old Karen, who has cerebral palsy, with adapted feeding equipment so that she can feed herself.

Prevent: The OT practitioner explains proper lifting techniques to a group of workers at the blanket factory with the goal of preventing injuries.

Another important aspect of intervention is **education.**[2] OT practitioners educate the client, family, and caregivers about activities that support the intervention plan. When caregivers are responsible for implementing treatment, they need to be aware of the risks and benefits of intervention as well. Education may be formal or informal in nature. For example, the OT practitioner may provide an educational workshop to a parent group regarding a particular frame of reference. The practitioner may educate the client in a session, by providing a demonstration and handout. Education must be tailored to the client's level. The OT practitioner should speak clearly and avoid the use of jargon. OT practitioners teaching clients to re-engage in occupations need to make sure that the client understands the lesson and can provide a demonstration of the targeted techniques. The OT practitioner answers any questions and follows up at the next visit.

The interaction between the practitioner and client is an essential element of therapy. A therapeutic relationship should always have the interest of the client as its central concern. The practitioner's role is to choose the interaction style that best supports the goals of the intervention plan and to help the client move toward independence. Setting the tone of interaction will be a decision based on the overall cognitive ability and attitude of the client. Chapter 16 describes in detail the development of a therapeutic relationship.

Although the implementation of the intervention plan is the responsibility of both OT and OTA, it is the *central* responsibility of the OTA. Educational programs are designed to ensure that OTAs develop an understanding of the philosophy and skills of occupational therapy to enable them to interpret and implement intervention plans. The OTA conducts intervention under the supervision of the OT.

Intervention Review

As intervention is implemented, the OT practitioner reevaluates the client's progress in therapy. The practitioner continually monitors the client's needs, circumstances, and conditions to identify whether any permanent or temporary change in the intervention plan is required. Reevaluation may result in changing activities, retesting, writing a new plan, or making needed referrals.

The OT practitioner assesses the client each treatment session by monitoring the influence of intervention and evaluating whether the activity has the desired therapeutic effect. For example, if the activity becomes too easy for the client, the OT practitioner may increase the level of difficulty by adding resistance or by changing the demands of the activity. The OT practitioner reevaluates the plan and how it is being carried out and achieving outcomes targeted for the client; modifies the plan as needed; and determines the need for continuation, discontinuation, or referral to another service.[2] Intervention services change as the needs of the client change.

Transition Services

Transition services are the coordination or facilitation of services for the purpose of preparing the client for a change. Transition services may involve a change to a new functional level, life stage, program, or environment. The OT practitioner is involved in identifying services and preparing an individualized transition plan to facilitate the client's change from one place to another.[1] In other words, the transition plan needs to be individualized to meet the goals, needs, and environmental considerations of the individual client.

The following cases provide an example of the importance of transition services.

Mr. G, a 75-year-old married man, was hospitalized for a total hip replacement. Because he is able to return home to a spouse willing to cook, clean, and assist him with self-care, he requires little outside assistance. His children who live nearby also will help out. His transition service plan includes training Mr. G and his spouse to safely move around the house, transfer to the toilet safely, and perform basic self-care.

Mr. W, a 75-year-old single man, was also hospitalized for a total hip replacement. However, he lives alone and has no family nearby. Mr. W will require a different transition plan. His transition plan includes a daily visit by the home health nurse, meals-on-wheels, and a home evaluation by the OT practitioner. The OT practitioner will work on mobility through the house, simple meal preparation, and home safety.

These two cases demonstrate the differences in transition services required. Some clients may need to be transferred to a lower level of care (e.g., a skilled nursing facility) before returning home. Careful planning is the key to preparing the client for the transition home.

Discontinuation of Services

The last step of the intervention process is the discontinuation of the client from occupational therapy services. The client is discharged from occupational therapy when he or she has reached the goals delineated in the intervention plan, when he or she has realized the maximum benefit of occupational therapy services, or when he or she does not wish to continue services.[1,2] The **discharge plan** is developed and implemented to address the resources and supports that may be required upon discharge. The discharge plan includes recommendations for continued services (including occupational therapy, if necessary), equipment recommendations, and any therapy the client is required to follow after discharge. In addition, the plan may include training family members and caregivers.

The OT writes a discharge summary of the client's functional level, changes that were made throughout the course of occupational therapy intervention, plans for discharge, equipment and services recommended, and follow-up. The OT prepares and implements the discharge plan with input from the OTA.[1]

Outcomes Process

OT practitioners use outcome measures to determine whether goals have been met and to make decisions regarding future intervention.[2] Outcome measures provide objective feedback to the client and practitioner. Thus, selecting measures that are valid, reliable, and appropriately sensitive to change is important. OT practitioners are interested in selecting measures early and using measures that may predict future outcomes.[2] Because the broad outcome of occupational therapy is engagement in occupation to support participation, measures that evaluate this outcome should be selected. OT practitioners are also interested in measuring occupational performance, client satisfaction, adaptation, quality of life, role competence, prevention, and health and wellness.[2] These outcomes and their measurement are discussed in detail in Chapter 9.

Summary

The occupational therapy process is a dynamic ongoing interactive process. Generally, the process includes referral, screening, evaluation, intervention planning, implementation of the intervention plan, transition services, and discontinuation of services. Each stage requires that the OT practitioner observe carefully and listen to the client's needs. Intervention is continually monitored and adjusted as needed. As a client meets his or her goals, new goals may be developed. The OT practitioner is skillful at creating, promoting, maintaining, rehabilitating, or modifying activities for the client.

Learning Activities

1. Provide the class with a case study. Randomly assign students (or teams) with one of the five treatment approaches (e.g., create, establish, maintain, modify, or prevent). Ask students to provide examples of how this treatment approach would be used with the case. Compare and contrast the benefits of each in class.

2. Interview a classmate for a few minutes to determine the occupations in which he or she engages. Write a page summary of the interview. Submit a page reflection of the interview process by discussing what you could have done differently and what you did well. Ask your partner for feedback.

3. Help students improve their observation skills by writing down everything they see while watching a fellow classmate perform a simple activity (e.g., making a cup of cocoa). After they have made a list, have them use the *Occupational Therapy Practice Framework* as a guide to examine the activity. Discuss the findings.

4. Review a journal article that examines the effectiveness of a given intervention. Summarize the intervention techniques the researchers used and the results of the study. What did you learn about occupational therapy intervention?

5. Interview an OT practitioner to find out about a particular case that the practitioner finds interesting. Find out the intervention approach and context(s) in which the intervention took place. Present this to your classmates.

Review Questions

1. What are the five general treatment approaches used in occupational therapy practice?
2. What are some techniques for successful interviewing?
3. What are the stages of the occupational therapy process?
4. Compare and contrast the roles of the OT and the OTA in the occupational therapy process.
5. What type of information is included in an occupational profile?
6. What is included in a discharge summary?
7. What are the steps to intervention planning?

References

1. American Occupational Therapy Association: Standards of practice for occupational therapy, *Am J Occup Ther* 64(6):415–420, 2010.
2. American Occupational Therapy Association: Occupational therapy practice framework: Domain and process, ed 2, *Am J Occup Ther* 62:625–683, 2008.
3. American Occupational Therapy Association: Scope of practice, *Am J Occup Ther* 64(6):389–396, 2010.
4. Asher IE: *Occupational Therapy Assessment Tools: An Annotated Index*, ed 3, Bethesda, MD, 2007, American Occupational Therapy Association Press.
5. Ayres J: *Sensory Integration and Praxis Tests (SIPT)*, Los Angeles, CA, 1988, Western Psychological Services.
6. Early MB: *Mental Health Concepts and Techniques for the Occupational Therapy Assistant*, ed 2, New York, 1993, Raven Press.
7. Hopkins HL: Tools of practice: Section 4, problem-solving. In Hopkins HL, Smith HD, editors: *Willard and Spackman's Occupational Therapy*, ed 8, Philadelphia, 1993, JB Lippincott.
8. Matsutsuyu J: The interest checklist, *Am J Occup Ther* 23:323, 1969.
9. Miller L: *Miller Assessment for Preschoolers (MAP)*, San Antonio, 1982, Psychological Corporation.

On plucking thistles and planting flowers . . .

How one lives life or chooses an occupation can be simple and straightforward or a long journey. As an undergraduate student, I wanted to be in premed—convinced that my calling was to be a physician. During undergraduate school, I explored two directions.

My first job was as a genetics technician in a university-based medical center. My days were spent centrifuging and fixing samples on slides, counting chromosomes, and photographing and creating karyotypes. When I closed my eyes each night, all I could visualize was chromosomes floating in emulsion. I would briefly meet people when they gave a sample in the laboratory, but I never got to know them or know what having the test meant to the greater scheme of their lives.

My second exploration was as a volunteer in an occupational therapy department in a psychiatric hospital. Suddenly, I was fascinated by people and their stories—intrigued by what went wrong and how their lives could be reorganized, allowing them to return to some sense of normalcy in their day-to-day lives. Occupational therapy seemed less scientific yet so very meaningful—listening while we were doing. I found that change and growth can be found through doing. I was a potential "agent of change"—the very meaning of the word "therapist" directed me to choose occupational therapy. The process of occupational therapy reminds me of Abraham Lincoln's words, which I have embraced: "I want it said of me by those who knew me best that I always plucked a thistle and planted a flower where I knew one would grow." I chose occupational therapy and have been plucking and planting. What a garden has grown and continues to grow each and every day!

ANN BURKHARDT, OTD, OTR/L, BCN, FAOTA
Director, Division of Occupational Therapy
Associate Professor of Occupational Therapy
School of Health Professions
Long Island University
Brooklyn Campus
Brooklyn, New York

Key Terms

Accreditation
Diagnosis codes
Documentation
Emergency procedures
Evidence-based practice
Individualized education plan
Outcome measures
Private funding sources
Problem-Oriented Medical Record
Procedure codes
Program evaluation
Program process
Program structure
Public funding sources
Service management functions
SOAP note
Universal precautions

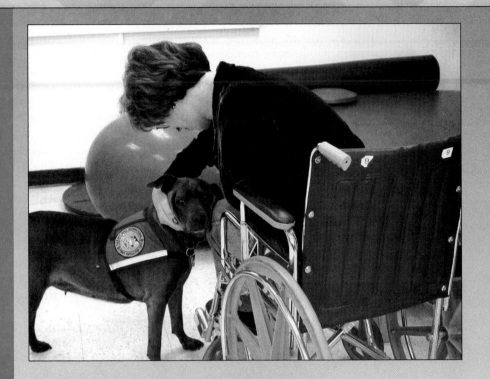

Objectives

After reading this chapter, the reader will be able to do the following:

- Explain the various service management functions
- Identify factors in a safe and efficient clinical environment
- Describe how the spread of infection is prevented in the workplace
- Define the three major categories of funding sources that reimburse for occupational therapy (OT) services
- Recognize the importance of program planning and evaluation as service management functions
- Understand the purpose of documentation
- Describe the documentation that occurs at various stages in the occupational therapy process
- Identify the fundamental elements in a client record
- Understand the integration of professional development and research into practice
- State the importance of marketing and public relations as a professional responsibility

Occupational therapy practitioners work with clients in a variety of environments. Along with evaluating and intervening with clients, practitioners are involved in service management functions. **Service management functions** include maintaining a safe and efficient workplace, documenting occupational therapy services, getting reimbursed for services, planning programs and evaluating them, integrating professional development activities and evidence-based practice into the workplace, and engaging in marketing and public relations. These functions are essential components of professional practice.

Maintaining a Safe and Efficient Workplace

Occupational therapy practitioners provide services to clients in an orderly and safe environment to ensure the safety of clients and efficiency of intervention and work procedures. The space in which practitioners work must accommodate clients with disabilities. For example, therapy settings must be wheelchair accessible, be free of clutter, have good lighting and ventilation, and have proper storage for equipment. The setting must be large enough to carry out intervention procedures.

Each practitioner assumes responsibility for maintaining a safe and efficient work environment. He or she is responsible for reporting problems to the occupational therapy administrator or to the maintenance department. Practitioners are directly responsible for putting away equipment and supplies that they use during a session and for cleaning the work area. The department operates more effectively and with less stress when everyone participates and cooperates in maintaining a safe and efficient work environment. The following sections describe specific factors considered in the work setting.

Safe Environment

Accreditation refers to a form of regulation that determines whether an organization meets a prescribed standard. Occupational therapy clinics must adhere to accreditation standards set by specific accreditation bodies. Many of these standards relate to establishing a safe work environment. For example, rehabilitation settings must meet CARF (Commission on Accreditation of Rehabilitation Facilities) standards. Each setting develops written policies and procedures in accordance with the accreditation standards. Practitioners are responsible for following the written policies and procedures of their setting.

In general, clinical settings need to be large enough so that staff and consumers can move without bumping into equipment or objects. Equipment and furniture should be out of traffic areas. Sharp corners on cabinets should not protrude into areas where people may walk. The clinic should have non-slip floor surfaces and grab bars in bathrooms, with emergency call buttons.

The clinical setting must have proper storage for items that may potentially be a safety hazard. This may require items be placed in locked cabinets. For example, in certain settings scissors, knives, and other sharp objects may be considered potentially harmful and need to be monitored carefully and stored securely.

Some materials used in occupational therapy clinics may pose a health hazard. For example, some therapy clinics use toxic paints or stains, which need to be stored and used carefully. Toxic chemicals and flammable substances must be stored in a special cabinet for flammables. The Occupational Safety and Health Administration (OSHA) requires that manufacturers of such materials provide a material safety data sheet (MSDS), which outlines information on the proper procedures for working with the material and describes procedures for storage and disposal. The data sheet describes the type of protective equipment required to work with the material. The data sheet outlines the procedures to follow in case of a spill or accident. MSDS sheets should be read carefully before a practitioner uses any hazardous material; they are kept in a readily accessible area of the clinic. All staff must be trained in the proper use of equipment and supplies that are found in the occupational therapy clinic. Practitioners may have to use protective goggles or masks when working with materials.[13]

Many OT clinics have kitchen areas which must be maintained according to health standards. Guidelines are provided for how food is handled and stored in occupational therapy clinics. Practitioners should inquire about the policies and procedures for their clinical setting, including how to ensure cleanliness of the clinic space, dishes, and materials.

OT practitioners are frequently involved in lifting and moving clients (e.g., from bed to wheelchair). It is important that practitioners use proper body mechanics to avoid injury. Employers are required to provide training on the use of proper body mechanics for lifting or transferring clients.

Each setting of practice has established **emergency procedures** in the case of an injury or accident in the clinic. All staff must be aware of the emergency procedures and emergency call system. Everyone must stay aware of who is in the clinic at all times. These procedures include who to contact and what to do. Many settings require OT practitioners maintain current certification in cardiopulmonary resuscitation (CPR) and first aid. Some settings require practitioners know how to determine blood pressure and pulse rate, manage a seizure, and intervene when someone is choking.[13] Practitioners document any injury, accident, or incident in a report (usually a standard form) and submit it to the administration in accordance with the procedures for that clinic. Box 13-1 summarizes safety considerations in the occupational therapy clinic.

Ordering and Storing Supplies

Maintaining an efficient therapy setting requires having appropriate equipment and supplies. The amount of supplies ordered and stored varies among facilities, depending on the size of the occupational therapy department, and its storage capacity.[13] Staff use an inventory system to track the supply. This responsibility is often part of an occupational therapy assistant (OTA)'s job.

Infection Control

The Centers for Disease Control and Prevention (CDC) is a federal agency that works to "protect people's health and safety, provide reliable health information, and improve health through strong partnerships."[9] The CDC developed

Box 13-1

Safety Considerations in the Occupational Therapy Setting

Sharp objects should be properly stored in a locked cabinet or drawer.

Keep flammables in a locked metal cabinet.

The clinical environment needs to be free of clutter so that staff and clients can move safely. Sharp corners on cabinets should not protrude into traffic areas. Equipment and furniture must be kept out of traffic areas.

Bathroom areas that are used by clients must have securely anchored grab bars.

The emergency call system should be readily available, and all staff must understand emergency procedures.

Flooring must be nonslip, and the staff must alert others to anything that changes this condition (i.e., water).

All staff are required to have proper training in the safe use of equipment and supplies found in the occupational therapy clinic.

In kitchen areas, foods must be safely stored and handled.

Staff need to be trained in the use of proper body mechanics when lifting or moving clients, equipment, and supplies.

Staff must be aware of who is in the clinic at all times and report suspicious persons.

universal precautions, a set of guidelines designed to prevent the transmission of HIV, HBV, and other blood-borne pathogens to health care providers.

The CDC recommends that health care personnel consider blood and body fluids of all clients as potentially infectious and follow universal precautions.[8] Universal precautions involve using protective barriers (e.g., gloves, gowns, aprons, masks, or protective eyewear) to reduce the risk of exposure to blood and other body fluids.[8] For example, OT practitioners following universal precautions wear protective gloves while addressing activities for daily living (ADL), such as grooming, personal hygiene, toileting, and dressing. The practitioner changes his or her gloves and washes his or her hands after contact with each client. In many clinical settings, a notice is placed in the client's medical record of the need for health care workers to use precautions. See Box 13-2 on Universal Precautions.

Box 13-2

Universal Precautions

1. Wash hands before and after each session.
2. Wear gloves whenever there is the possibility of coming into contact with body fluids (i.e., saliva, blood, urine).
3. Wear full-body gowns, face masks, and eye protection whenever there is the possibility of blood splashing.
4. Dispose of contaminated sharp objects in a puncture-proof container.
5. Dispose of all contaminated personal protective equipment in a bio-hazardous waste container.

Adapted from http://www.udsmr.org/WebModules/FIM/Fim_About.aspx.

Hand washing is the most effective method for preventing the transfer of disease. The OT practitioner washes his or her hands before and after each treatment session and before and after eating. Practitioners wash hands after using the toilet, sneezing, coughing, or coming in contact with oral and nasal areas. Procedures for hand washing are provided in Box 13-3.

Federal agencies, employers, and employees are responsible for controlling the spread of infection.[16] The regulations are established and monitored by the CDC and by the Occupational Safety and Health Association (OSHA). OSHA monitors compliance of employers and fines those settings that do not follow the regulations, whereas the CDC monitors individuals' exposure to disease in the workplace.

OSHA standards define the responsibilities of the employer to provide education on universal precautions and to provide the necessary protective barriers, hand washing facilities, and supplies needed by employees. Employers must provide employee health services to conduct mandatory annual testing for TB, HBV vaccine, and to maintain employee health records (i.e., tests and vaccines given and any exposure to infectious disease).[16]

Box 13-3

Techniques for Effective Hand Washing

1. Remove all jewelry, except plain band rings. Remove watch, or move it up the arm. Provide complete access to area to be washed.
2. Approach the sink, and avoid touching the sink or nearby objects.
3. Turn on the water, and adjust it to a lukewarm temperature and a moderate flow to avoid splashing.
4. Wet wrists and hands with fingers directed downward, and apply approximately 1 teaspoon of liquid soap or granules.
5. Begin to wash all areas of hands (palms, sides, backs), fingers, knuckles, and between each finger, using vigorous rubbing and circular motions. If wearing a band, slide it up or down the finger and scrub skin underneath it. Interlace fingers, and scrub between each finger.
6. Wash for at least 30 seconds, keeping hands and forearms at elbow level or below and hands pointed down. Wash longer if a patient known to have an infection was treated.
7. Rinse hands well under running water.
8. Wash as high up wrists and forearms as contamination is likely.
9. Rinse hands, wrists, and forearms under running water.
10. Thoroughly dry hands, wrists, and forearms with paper towels. Use a dry towel for each hand. Water should continue to flow from tap as hands are dried.
11. Use another dry paper towel to turn water faucet off. Discard all towels in an appropriate container.

Modified from Zakus SM: *Clinical Procedures for Medical Assistants*, ed 3, St. Louis, 1995, Mosby.

Employees are responsible for attending educational programs that are offered and following universal precautions guidelines. Employees must have an annual TB test and report any exposures to the employee health services department. The employee may decide whether to take the HBV vaccine or to sign a waiver.[16]

Scheduling

Each clinic maintains a schedule of appointments for each practitioner. Schedules include the time for direct service and the time to complete service management functions, attend meetings or conferences, complete paperwork, and bill for services.

The schedule for each client varies, depending on the type of facility and the client's needs. For example, in some mental health outpatient programs, intervention may be performed in groups that meet once a week. Conversely, a practitioner treating hand injuries in an outpatient setting may schedule clients two to three times a week.

Third-party payers may influence the frequency and duration of scheduled sessions. For example, Medicare requires clients in acute rehabilitation settings receive therapy twice a day. Clients who cannot complete two daily sessions may be transferred to a setting that provides a lower level of care (e.g., skilled nursing facility). Many health maintenance organizations (HMOs) limit the number of outpatient OT visits. This along with family routines and commitments are considered when scheduling clients for intervention.

The supervising occupational therapist usually assigns clients to staff for scheduling. This decision-making step considers the client's needs, staff expertise, and cost effectiveness. Occupational therapy departments adhere to productivity standards to be successful. Practitioners manage and adhere to the schedule to ensure that everything is completed as planned.

Documenting Occupational Therapy Services

Documenting provides an accurate record of service. **Documentation** provides a justification for occupational therapy intervention. The practitioner's professional judgment and clinical reasoning are reflected in documentation. Therefore, documentation is used to communicate to other health care professionals, third-party payers, and administrators. Documentation is a record of the status of the client, techniques used, and progress the client makes in therapy. Consequently, documentation is essential to intervention planning and communication between team members. Documentation provides a chronological record of the client's status, the services provided, and the outcomes of those services. See Box 13-4. Common types of documentation at the various stages of the occupational therapy process are shown in Table 13-1.

The *evaluation or screening report* contains information on the referral source and data gathered during the evaluation process.[3] This report provides a client's occupational profile, an analysis

---

Box 13-4

Purpose of Documentation

- Justification of services
- Record of services
- Description of client's journey
- Record of outcome of intervention
- Billing
- Communication

Table 13-1 **Types of Documentation**

Process Areas	Types of Reports
I. Evaluation	A. Evaluation or Screening Report
	B. Reevaluation Report
II. Intervention	A. Intervention Plan
	B. Occupational Therapy Service Contacts
	C. Progress Report
	D. Transition Plan
III. Outcomes	A. Discharge/Discontinuation Report

From American Occupational Therapy Association: Guidelines for documentation of occupational therapy, *Am J Occup Ther* 62(6):684, 2008.

---

of the client's occupational performance, factors that support or inhibit performance, and the expected outcomes of intervention. The *reevaluation* provides recommendations for changes to services, goals, frequency, and referral to other sources.

During the intervention stage, practitioners complete an intervention plan, service contacts, progress reports, and a transition plan. The *intervention plan* documents the client's goals and approaches used to reach those goals.[3] It identifies frequency and duration of service, service provider, and location of service. Documentation of *service contacts* records the specific interactions between the client and OT practitioner.[3] It is an ongoing log of therapy and includes date, length of time, interventions, and the client's response. Telephone contacts, interventions, and meetings with others are also documented. An example of a daily narrative note describing a service contact (intervention session) with a client is shown in Box 13-5.

A *progress report* summarizes the intervention and the client's progress towards the goals.[3] It summarizes new data and modifications to the intervention plan, and concludes

---

Box 13-5

Sample Narrative Daily Note

Client actively participated in eating retraining and right upper extremity strengthening program. Client ate 75% of meal with adapted utensils and required minimal assistance for cutting meat. Established treatment plan should continue.

Modified from Early MB: *Physical Dysfunction Practice Skills for the Occupational Therapy Assistant*, ed 2, St. Louis, 2006, Mosby.

Box 13-6
Sample Weekly Progress Note
Client has been treated daily for eating retraining and right upper extremity functional strengthening program. Using adapted utensils, client ate 75% of meal with minimal assistance for cutting meat. Previously, client ate 50% of meal and required moderate assistance for cutting meat. Client will eat independently with no assistive devices in 1 week.

Modified from Early MB: *Physical Dysfunction Practice Skills for the Occupational Therapy Assistant*, ed 2, St. Louis, 2006, Mosby.

with recommendations (e.g., continue or discontinue services or be referred to another source). Progress reports vary between settings and reimbursement mechanisms. An example of a weekly progress report is shown in Box 13-6.

A *transition plan* describes the client's progression from one type of setting to another within the same delivery system. For example, a transition plan must be completed when a client transfers from a rehabilitation setting to a skilled nursing facility. The transition plan provides information regarding the client's current status; the reason for the transition; a time frame for transition; and recommendations and rationale for occupational therapy services, modifications, or assistive technology.

The *discharge/discontinuation report* is completed during the outcomes stage. This report summarizes the changes in the client's ability to participate in occupations between the initial evaluation and the discontinuation of services. Recommendations for further services and follow-up are documented.

There are many types and methods of documentation. Public policy, accreditation bodies, third-party payers, and the practice setting determine documentation practices. For example, school settings funded by the federal and state governments require each child to have an **individualized education plan** (IEP) completed by a multidisciplinary team. The problems, goals, and interventions reflect behaviors and skills necessary for the child's success in school.[19]

There are specific documentation requirements mandated by the federal government for clients who are covered by Medicare. One common method of documentation that is used in medical settings is the **Problem-Oriented Medical Record** (POMR). This format is based on a list of problems identified by the treatment team during the assessment of the client. Subsequent progress notes relate to the problem(s) identified in the list. The format used for writing the progress note is referred to as the **SOAP note.** S stands for *subjective* (information reported by the client); O is for *objective* (clinical findings or measurable, observable data); A represents *assessment* (OT practitioner's professional judgment or opinion); and P is for *plan* (specific plan of action to be followed). See Box 13-7.

Each client receives a permanent record. The record is organized, legible, concise, accurate, complete, grammatically

Box 13-7
Sample SOAP Note
Problem 1: Dependence in wheelchair mobility
S: Client stated that his hands often slip on the metal hand rims when propelling his wheelchair.
O: Friction tape was placed on rims of wheelchair to improve client's ability to grasp and propel chair. Wheelchair mobility training outside over grass and asphalt was provided. Client participated for 30 minutes in wheelchair training with only 5-minute rest period. He experienced no difficulty propelling wheelchair over varied terrain.
A: Friction tape on rims helped improve client's ability to propel wheelchair. Client's endurance for wheelchair mobility improved over yesterday.
P: Continue OT training in wheelchair mobility. Increase time and distance for wheelchair mobility. Teach client how to maneuver wheelchair in and out of doors and up and down ramps.

Box 13-8
Fundamental Elements of Documentation
1. Client's full name and case number (if applicable) on each page of documentation
2. Date and type of occupational therapy contact
3. Identification of type of documentation, agency, and department name
4. Occupational therapist's or occupational therapy assistant's signature with a minimum of first name or initial, last name, and professional designation
5. When applicable on notes or reports, signature of the recorder directly at the end of the note without space left between the body of the note and the signature
6. Countersignature by an occupational therapist on documentation written by students and occupational therapy assistants, when required by law or the facility
7. Acceptable terminology defined within the boundaries of setting
8. Abbreviations usage as acceptable within the boundaries of setting
9. When no facility requirements are listed, errors corrected by drawing a single line through an error and by initialing the correction (liquid correction fluid and erasures are not acceptable)
10. Adherence to professional standards of technology, when used to document occupational therapy services
11. Disposal of records within law or agency requirements
12. Compliance with confidentiality standards
13. Compliance with agency or legal requirements of storage of records

From American Occupational Therapy Association: Guidelines for documentation of occupational therapy, *Am J Occup Ther* 62(6):689, 2008.

correct, and objective.[3] Even though the format of the documentation varies among settings, there are certain elements present in all documentation (Box 13-8). Good planning and regular documentation make record keeping easier, and, ultimately, lead to better quality intervention.

Reimbursement for Services

To stay in business, occupational therapy departments need to produce revenue by collecting fees for services provided. Each OT practitioner is responsible for submitting accurate charges that are reflected in either units based on the amount of time spent with the client or a set fee based on services provided.[13] Determining charges involves a complex process, usually performed by the administration of the facility. Third-party payers have different amounts that they will pay in "allowable charges" for a particular client. The charges set by the facility do not reflect what is actually paid by the third-party payer for an individual client but rather for the client population as a whole.

Occupational therapy services are reimbursed by a number of sources, which can be categorized into three groups: (1) public sources that include federal, state, and local government agencies; (2) private payers that include insurance companies; and (3) other sources that include service agencies and volunteer organizations. Each source of payment has different regulations and guidelines that identify the services for which it will pay (number of visits and equipment) and the amount of reimbursement. Because these regulations and guidelines often change, the OT practitioner must stay informed on current policies. The administration of the facility typically informs staff members of any changes in funding regulations.

Public Funding Sources

Public funding sources include federal, state, and local sources, such as Medicare, Veteran's Administration, Medicaid, Maternal and Child Health programs, Department of Education, vocational rehabilitation services, and Social Security benefits. Typically, Congress authorizes funding through legislation and designates a federal agency to determine the scope and criteria for the program. An agency is designated in each state to ensure compliance with the programs mandated by the federal government.[11] The funds are then distributed to the local agencies or programs, which are responsible for ensuring that mandated services are provided. Chapter 2 discusses federal legislation that has mandated occupational therapy as a reimbursable service.

Private Funding Sources

Private funding sources include health insurance, worker's compensation, casualty insurance, and disability insurance. A growing number of individuals are paying for health care services personally because they either do not have health insurance or their plan does not provide for a specific service. Private insurance companies have a variety of plans with different benefits and restrictions. Health insurance policies stipulate whether occupational therapy services are covered and whether there are any limitations on those services (e.g., maximum number of visits, maximum amount of dollars).

Worker's compensation benefits cover expenses incurred from work-related injuries. Worker's compensation benefits are regulated by state agencies and managed by private insurance companies. For that reason, allowable occupational therapy services vary from state to state.

Other Funding Sources

Other sources of funding of OT services or equipment include service clubs, private foundations, and volunteer organizations. (e.g., Kiwanis, Rotary Club). In some cases, private foundations, specific to a disability, will provide funding for an individual with that disability.[11] Some volunteer agencies also provide funding. OT practitioners may need to be creative to get equipment for clients. For example, many colleges and universities require students complete service projects that may benefit clients.

Coding and Billing for Services

To receive payment for occupational therapy services, the provider (either a facility or individual) submits a claim form using the correct billing codes. Services provided in occupational therapy are either billed by diagnosis codes or procedure codes. **Diagnosis codes** are based on the client's medical condition or the medical justification for services. The most frequently used coding system is the *International Classification of Diseases, Ninth Revision, Clinical Modification (ICD-9-CM)*.[17] Diseases are categorized in *ICD-9-CM* according to anatomical systems. Mental health providers use the *Diagnostic and Statistical Manual of Mental Disorders, Fourth Edition, Text Revision (DSM-IV-TR)*.[4]

Procedure codes are based on the specific services performed by health care providers. The most commonly used procedure coding system is the *Current Procedural Terminology (CPT)*, which is published and updated annually by the American Medical Association.[1] OT practitioners select the codes that most accurately define the services performed and bill to these codes by relative value units. Payers may limit the number and range of codes that a specialty may use to bill services; therefore, OT practitioners must be aware of the allowable codes for each insurer.

There are two types of claim forms commonly used in occupational therapy to bill third-party payers: (1) the Uniform Bill (UB-92; CMS-01450), which is used by hospitals, skilled nursing facilities, and home health agencies; and (2) the CMS-1500 claim form, used primarily by physicians or OT practitioners in private practice.

OT practitioners educate third-party payers continually regarding the benefits of occupational therapy services. Practitioners advocate for including occupational therapy as a reimbursable service. It is important to keep abreast of proposed changes in state and federal legislation and regulations that have the potential to affect payment for occupational therapy services. This can be done on an individual basis and also by supporting local and national occupational therapy associations that provide lobbying efforts for the purpose of influencing legislation that may affect the profession.

Program Planning and Evaluation

Program planning and evaluation are primarily the responsibilities of the administrator, although staff provides input into both processes. In an occupational therapy department, the administrator is involved in planning things such as space utilization, equipment needs, staff levels, effective use of staff, the annual budget, department policies and procedures, and new programs and services.

Health care professionals measure the effectiveness of programming. This is referred to as **program evaluation,** and it involves "determining the extent to which programs are achieving the goals and objectives established for them and using that information as necessary to modify activities."[5] Program evaluation is not only important for ensuring client satisfaction, but it is also necessary for accreditation by outside agencies. **Accreditation** is a form of regulation that determines whether an organization or program meets a prescribed standard. Organizations seek to be accredited in order to be reimbursed by third-party payers. Many of the organizations in which OT practitioners are likely to work are influenced by some type of accreditation. In health care, the two most widely known accreditation bodies are the Joint Commission (TJC) and the Commission on Accreditation of Rehabilitation Facilities (CARF).

TJC develops standards and accredits health care organizations including hospitals, health care networks, and organizations that provide long-term care, behavioral care, and laboratory and ambulatory services.[12]

CARF sets standards and accredits organizations that deliver rehabilitation services. CARF's standards and guidelines are separated into three areas: behavioral health, employment and community services, and medical rehabilitation. The CARF accreditation process is aimed at improving the quality of services provided to individuals with disabilities.[20] CARF is also involved in research related to outcomes measurement and management.

Accreditation requires a detailed program evaluation including a written report of self-study. Following the completion of the self-study, a team representing the accrediting body visits the facility. The program evaluation includes examination of program structure, program process, and outcome measures. **Program structure** refers to the system in which the services are delivered (e.g., staff levels and expertise, equipment, budget, and range of services). The **program process** refers to the stages of referral, evaluation, and intervention. This examines such things as how timely the evaluation was performed. **Outcome measures** refer to the results of the intervention.

OT practitioners use a number of tools to measure outcomes. One tool is the Functional Independence Measure (FIM™).[22] The FIM™ measures an individual client's functional ability for 18 items across the domains of self-care, motor, and cognitive.[22] The person is given a separate score for each item and also a total score. The FIM™ scores a client at different points in the rehabilitation process (e.g., at time of referral and at discharge) and provides an objective measure of how the individual is progressing. Program evaluation looks at a compilation of client data. For example, the program could compile data over the last fiscal year that portrayed the average percentage of change in client scores from time of admission to time of discharge. Program evaluation is an ongoing process that helps ensure that quality services are provided by the occupational therapy program.

Integrating Professional Development Activities and Evidence-Based Practice into the Workplace

Practitioners must maintain competence in the field through participation in educational programs and professional development activities (see Chapter 6). OT practitioners participate in educational opportunities at their workplace through in-service presentations. Another way that OT practitioners can be involved in professional development in the workplace is by supervising Level I or Level II fieldwork students. OTs and OTAs with a minimum of 1 year of work experience are eligible to supervise students. Clinical internships are critical to the profession. Not only is fieldwork an important component of the student's training, but is a valuable experience for the supervisor, who learns and grows professionally from the mentoring experience.

Evidence-based practice enhances occupational therapy practice by supporting practice through research. Consumers, practitioners, and third-party payers benefit from knowing that occupational and therapy is provided based on the best available evidence.[6,15]

Evidence-based practice refers to "finding, appraising, and using research findings as the basis for clinical decisions."[21] Research evidence is used by the OT practitioner in conjunction with clinical knowledge and reasoning to determine the interventions that are effective for a particular client.[14] There are four steps in evidence-based practice: (1) forming a clinical question that can be researched; (2) searching the literature for best evidence on the question; (3) appraising the evidence for validity and applicability to practice; and (4) applying the evidence to practice.[10] Applying research to practice does not always mean changing the intervention approach. It may mean providing clients with more specific and current information about the efficacy of the approaches used.[7] In some situations, the research may provide information on interventions to facilitate a client's outcomes.[7]

Resources are available to assist the OT practitioner in retrieving research findings (e.g., Rehabilitation Reference Center, Cochrane Reviews). AOTA's *Evidence Briefs* is a series of literature reviews of occupational therapy research with particular health conditions (e.g., brain injury, attention deficit hyperactivity disorder, substance use).[2] Each brief presents a summary of a selected article that outlines the study's key features, methods, procedures, findings, and application to practice.

The *Evidence-Based Practice (EBP) Resource Directory*[2] provides links to Internet sites related to the use of evidence-based practice in occupational therapy. Students and practitioners are urged to use a variety of resources to critically appraise and incorporate evidence into their daily practice.

The Accreditation Council for Occupational Therapy Education (ACOTE) requires that students be able to:

- Articulate the importance of professional literature/research for practice and the continued development of the profession.
- Use professional literature to make informed practice decisions.
- Know when and how to find and use informational resources, including appropriate literature within and outside of occupational therapy.

Marketing and Public Relations

Marketing and public relations help increase the visibility of occupational therapy. Many departments plan and implement public relations activities during the month of April, which is designated as National Occupational Therapy Month. For example, a booth set up in the facility's cafeteria that demonstrates adaptive equipment may provide good publicity for occupational therapy. AOTA is committed to increase the visibility of occupational therapy and has materials available for members to promote the profession.

Marketing differs slightly from public relations in that it involves the development and implementation of a marketing plan. This plan requires consideration of (1) the clients who are served, (2) the sources who refer or have the potential to refer clients to occupational therapy, (3) the administration (or internal source of funding for the department) of the facility, and (4) the third-party payers who reimburse (or have the potential to reimburse) for occupational therapy services.[18]

Summary

Service management functions are activities performed by the OT practitioner outside of direct service delivery to the client. These functions include maintaining a safe and efficient workplace, documenting occupational therapy services, getting reimbursed for services, planning programs and their evaluations, integrating professional development activities and evidence-based practice into the workplace, and engaging in public relations and marketing. For an occupational therapy department to operate effectively, it is important that each practitioner take the responsibility for being involved in these activities.

Learning Activities

1. Visit an occupational therapy department. Describe the service management functions. Describe the environment of the department. Is the storage adequate? Does there appear to be an adequate amount of equipment and supplies? Does the clinic appear cluttered, or is it neat with everything safely put away? Are there any obvious safety hazards that you noticed during your visit?
2. Interview either an OTA or an OT about the types of service management functions they perform. Compare notes with your classmates. Are there differences between the jobs OTs and OTAs do?
3. In a group of two or three students, develop several public relations activities to promote National Occupational Therapy Month. Conduct one activity during OT Month.
4. Visit an occupational therapy department and discuss the type of documentation used by the OT practitioners. Review examples of the different types of documentation (e.g., assessment reports, progress notes, treatment plans, and discharge summaries).

Review Questions

1. What are the various service management functions in which the OT practitioner participates?
2. What are some factors for safety in the clinic?
3. What are universal precautions?
4. What do each of the areas of the SOAP method of documentation mean?
5. Why is research important in practice?
6. How is program evaluation used in practice?

References

1. American Medical Association: *Current Procedural Terminology 2010*, Chicago, 2010, American Medical Association.
2. American Occupational Therapy Association: *Evidence-based practice and research*. Retrieved February 26, 2011, from http://www.aota.org/ebp (must be an AOTA member).
3. American Occupational Therapy Association: Guidelines for documentation of occupational therapy, *Am J Occup Ther* 62(6):684–690, 2008.
4. American Psychiatric Association: *Diagnostic and Statistical Manual of Mental Disorders*, ed 4, *Text Revision (DSM-IV-TR)*, Arlington, VA, 2000, American Psychiatric Association.
5. Bair J, Gray M, editors: *The Occupational Therapy Manager*, Rockville, MD, 1985, AOTA.
6. Canadian Association of Occupational Therapists, the Association of Canadian Occupational Therapy University Programs, the Association of Canadian Occupational Therapy Regulatory Organizations, and the President's Advisory Committee: *Joint position statement on evidence-based occupational therapy* (1999). Retrieved August 23, 2006, from http://www.caot.ca.
7. Arbesman M, Lieberman D: Using AOTA evidence-based practice resources, *OT Practice* 11(21):CE1-CE8.
8. Siegel JD, Rhinehart E, Jackson M, et al, the Healthcare Infection Control Practices Advisory Committee: *2007 Guidelines*

for Isolation Precautions: Preventing Transmission of Infectious Agents in Healthcare Settings. Retrieved February 26, 2011, from http://www.cdc.gov/ncidod/dhgp/pdf/isolation2007.pdf.

9. Centers for Disease Control and Prevention: *Vision, mission, core values, and pledge.* Retrieved February 26, 2011, from http://www.cdc.gov/about/organization/mission.htm.

10. KT (Knowledge Transition) Centre for Evidence-Based Medicine: *Centre for Evidence-Based Medicine.* Retrieved February 26, 2011, from http://ktclearinghouse.ca/cebm.

11. Cook AM, Hussey SM: *Assistive Technologies: Principles and Practice,* St. Louis, 1995, Mosby.

12. The Joint Commission: *About the Joint Commission.* Retrieved February 26, 2011, from http://www.jointcommission.org/about_us/about_the_joint_commission_main.aspx.

13. Jones RA: Service operations. In Ryan SE, editor: *Practice Issues in Occupational Therapy: Intraprofessional Team Building,* Thorofare, NJ, 1993, Slack Inc.

14. Law M, Baum C: Evidence-based occupational therapy, *Canad J Occup Ther* 65(3):131–135, 1998.

15. Lieberman D, Scheer J: AOTA's evidence-based literature review project: An overview, *Am J Occup Ther* 56(3):344–349, 2002.

16. Meriano C: Universal precautions. In Sladyk K, editor: *OT Student Primer: A Guide to College Success,* Thorofare, NJ, 1997, Slack Inc.

17. National Center for Health Statistics: *International Classification of Diseases, Ninth Revision, Clinical Modification,* Hyattsville, MD, 2005, National Center for Health Statistics.

18. Olson TS, Urban C: Marketing. In Bair J, Gray M, editors: *The Occupational Therapy Manager,* Rockville, MD, 1985, AOTA.

19. Perinchief JM: Documentation and management of occupational therapy services. In Crepeau EB, Cohn ES, Schell BB, editors: *Willard and Spackman's Occupational Therapy,* ed 10, Philadelphia, 2003, Lippincott Williams & Wilkins.

20. Commission on the Accreditation of Rehabilitation Facilities: *Quick facts about CARF.* Retrieved February 26, 2011, from www.carf.org.

21. Rosenberg W, Donald A: Evidence-based medicine: An approach to clinical problem-solving, *Br Med J* 310(6987):1122–1126, 1995.

22. Uniform Data System for Medical Rehabilitation: *FIM™ Instrument.* Retrieved February 26, 2011, from http://www.udsmr.org/WebModules/FIM/Fim_About.aspx.

My debut into the occupational therapy career happened by chance. After high school, I was trying to figure out what I wanted to do with my life. I was interested in studying psychology. However, in the country of Kenya, Africa, where I grew up, there was no psychology major at the time in any of the institutions of higher education. My sister had just completed her studies at the Kenya Medical Training College and had been awarded a diploma in radiography. She informed me that there was a program at the college called occupational therapy. She did not know much about the program, except that she saw occupational therapists doing much basket weaving and seemingly having lots of fun. However, she also knew that they studied a lot of psychology. So, I applied and got into the program.

Since graduating way back in 1985, my progress in the profession has been fortuitous. For some time, I left the profession all together and studied, and for a while I practiced counseling psychology. However, I realized that "doing" meaningful things (meaningful occupations) with clients is far more therapeutic than just talking about issues. So, I came back to the profession, hopefully much wiser and with more commitment based on insight. My experiences have led me to believe that the way to strengthen occupational therapy and ensure its survival far into the future is by therapists being very clear of their origin (which in my view is mental health), and staying true to the original principles, even while making progressive and useful innovations. That is why one of my favorites pastimes is discussing with students (future occupational therapists) occupational therapy theory and its origins, and speculating about its future development.

MOSES N. IKIUGU, PhD, OTR/L
Associate Professor and Director of Research
Department of Occupational Therapy
University of South Dakota
Vermillion, South Dakota

CHAPTER 14   Models of Practice and Frames of Reference

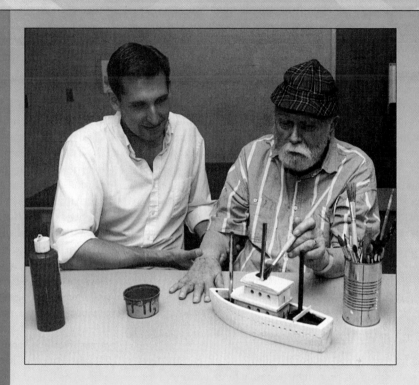

Objectives

After reading this chapter, the reader will be able to do the following:

- Define theory, model of practice (MOP), and frame of reference (FOR)
- Discuss the importance of using a model of practice and frame of reference
- Understand how research supports practice
- Identify the components of a frame of reference
- Summarize selected occupational therapy (OT) models of practice
- Identify the principles guiding selected frames of reference

---

Occupational therapy practitioners help clients engage in occupations. They work with clients of all ages, from numerous cultures, and clients who have a variety of conditions and circumstances. Practitioners base intervention on knowledge of the underlying conditions and evidence to support the intervention techniques.

A model of practice helps organize one's thinking, whereas a frame of reference is a tool to guide one's intervention.[13,15] A frame of reference tells you what to do and how

to evaluate and intervene with clients. Furthermore, frames of reference have research to support the principles guiding evaluation and intervention. Thus, using a frame of reference to guide one's practice is essential to **evidence-based practice.** Evidence-based practice refers to choosing intervention techniques based upon the best possible research. This chapter will outline selected occupational therapy models of practice and frames of reference and describe how they are applied in practice.

Understanding Theory

A **theory** is a set of ideas that helps explain things. Research is used to support or refute theories. Occupational therapy borrows theories from other disciplines such as psychology, medicine, nursing, and social work. Theory is the analysis of a set of facts in their relation to one another.[14] There are two major structural components to theory: concepts and principles.[24,25] **Concepts** are ideas that represent something in the mind of the individual. These range from simple concrete ideas to complex, abstract ideas. Concepts are expressed through the use of symbols and language. Children develop categories for different concepts. For example, a child learns that clothing is a category that can be divided into shoes, pants, dresses, and shirts, among others. **Principles** explain the relationship between two or more concepts.[24] For instance, once the concept of color is learned, such as blue and yellow, a child learns the principle that mixing these two colors produces green.

Theory is defined as "a set of interrelated assumptions, concepts, and definitions that presents a systematic view of phenomena by specifying relationships among variables, with the purpose of explaining and predicting the phenomena."[19] Theories range in scope and complexity along a continuum. Theories may be broad in scope and attempt to cover many aspects of a discipline, or they may have a narrow focus and concern only a small portion of the field.[24] Figure 14-1 provides an illustration of how these concepts fit together.

Why Is It Important to Know About and Use Theory in Occupational Therapy Practice?

Students frequently resist theory. They prefer to "get in there and do something" rather than discuss why it is done. Not applying theory to practice is similar to taking a trip without a road map. The trip will be disorganized and lack structure. The traveler may eventually find a way to the final destination but may not know exactly how he or she got from point A to point B. Consequently, it is difficult to give directions to anyone else or to replicate the journey in the future. OT practitioners appreciate theory, because it is required to clinically reason and develop effective intervention. Theory provides the basis for practice.

Parham states, "Theory is a key element in problem setting and in problem solving. It is a tool that enables the practitioner to 'name it and frame it.' Both language and logic are needed to identify a problem (name it) and to plan a means for altering the situation (frame it). Theory provides these by giving us words or concepts for naming what we observe and by spelling out logical relationships between concepts."[16] Theory allows the OT practitioner to structure and organize his or her intervention.

Theory also serves to (1) validate and guide practice, (2) justify reimbursement, (3) clarify specialization issues, (4) enhance the growth of the profession and the professionalism of its members, and (5) educate competent practitioners.[24]

Theories specific to occupational therapy practice originated in science-based disciplines such as biology, chemistry, physics, psychology, and occupational science. The practitioner may use a number of theories during intervention and combine parts of theories. To do so, the practitioner must be knowledgeable about the theories to be sure that they are compatible with one another. Theories used in occupational therapy include those developed by Mosey, Kielhofner, Ayres, Reilly, Llorens, and Fidler. It is beyond the scope of this introductory text to describe the various theories used. Theory is linked to clinical practice through models of practice and frames of reference.

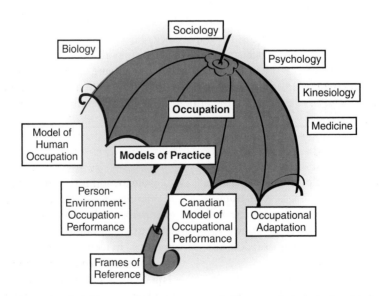

Figure 14-1 The umbrella of occupation: a conceptual diagram of the relationship between theories, occupation, models of practice, and frames of reference. (From MacRae N, O'Brien J: OT 301 Foundations of occupational therapy, unpublished lecture notes, 2001, University of New England.)

Model of Practice

The terms *model of practice, conceptual model, practice model,* and *frame of reference* have been used interchangeably. In this text, we distinguish between model of practice and frame of reference. However, this is just one way to organize the content.

A **model of practice** takes the philosophical base of the profession and organizes the concepts for practice. As such, occupational therapy models of practice help OT practitioners organize their thinking around occupation,[13] which is the central unifying feature of the occupational therapy profession. A model of practice provides practitioners with terms to describe practice, an overall view of the profession, tools for evaluation, and a guide for intervention.[8,13,15]

By reading and critically analyzing current literature, practitioners who use a model of practice to guide their practice find a depth of information, which allows them to better understand practice and intervention to the benefit of clients. Using a model of practice ensures a systematic examination of the client and is an important step in providing evidence-based practice.

The **Model of Human Occupation** (MOHO)[9] is the best-researched model of practice in occupational therapy. Kielhofner and colleagues have published extensively on all aspects of this model, and thus this model provides well-supported evidence to support its use in practice. The Model of Human Occupation views occupational performance in terms of volition, habituation, performance, and environment. Volition refers to the person's motivation, interests, values, and belief in skill. Habituation refers to one's daily patterns of behaviors, one's roles (the rules and expectations of those positions), and one's everyday routine. Performance refers to the motor, cognitive, and emotional aspects required to act upon the environment.[9] Environment refers to the physical, social, and societal surroundings in which the person is involved. Each system is divided into components with many well-researched instruments to operationalize the terms for practice.[9] Working with the assessment tools designed to operationalize the concepts of the model helps practitioners understand the concepts more fully for practice.

The **Canadian Model of Occupational Performance** (CMOP)[10,22] has also generated a wealth of research to support its design. The core of this model is spirituality, which is defined broadly as anything that motivates or inspires a person.[10,22] Person, environment (which includes institutions), and occupations are the other parts of the model. This model emphasizes client-centered care,[10,22] which refers to understanding the client's desires and wishes for intervention and outcome. Getting to know the client is crucial to this model. The *Canadian Occupational Performance Measure*[11] is a semi-structured interview based on this model and provides practitioners with a tool to organize their thoughts.

The **Person-Environment-Occupation-Performance** (PEOP) model[6] developed by Christiansen and Baum provides definitions for each term and describes the interactive nature of the human being. This model provides generic, broad terms for each area (e.g., person, environment, occupation, performance). *Person* includes the physical, social, and psychological aspects of the individual. *Environment* includes the physical and social supports, and those things that interfere with the individual's performance. *Occupation* refers to the everyday things people do and in which they find meaning. *Performance* refers to the actions of occupations.[6]

Occupational Adaptation, articulated by Schkade and Schultz, proposes that OT practitioners examine how they may change the person, environment, or task so the client may engage in occupations. In this model, occupation is viewed as the primary means for the individual to achieve adaptation. Individual adaptation is seen as both a state of being and a process that can be examined at a given time, over a specified time period, or over a lifetime.[20] This model focuses on the person, the occupational environment, and the interaction. It supports compensatory techniques if necessary.

Other models of practice exist in occupational therapy practice, such as the Ecological model by Dunn and Spatiotemporal Adaptation by Gilfoyle and Grady.

Case Application

The following case studies provide an overview of the use of the different models of practice.

> Raven is a 37-year-old woman who was hospitalized with a brain aneurysm, which affected her speech, right-sided movement, and cognitive abilities. Raven is unable to remain standing for long periods of time, and she needs frequent breaks during seated activities. Raven experiences difficulty with memory and poor concentration.
>
> The occupational therapist (OT) meets with Raven on her first day on the rehabilitation unit. The following comparison describes the type of information she will collect about Raven from each model of practice.

Model of Human Occupation

Volition: Raven enjoys family events, singing, and cooking. Raven lives close to her family and sees her mother, three children, and many other family members daily. Furthermore, the family attends church services on Sunday and then gathers at Raven's for a potluck supper. She is active in the church choir.

Habituation: Raven works 5 days a week from 8 AM to 5 PM in a local grocery store, where she is the assistant manager. She attends her grandchildren's school events and periodically helps her daughters with child care and transportation. Raven attends church Wednesday evenings and Sundays.

Performance: Prior to her aneurysm, Raven was able to complete all occupations without difficulty. Currently, she is unable to use her right side, slurs her speech, has difficulty maintaining a conversation, and becomes easily confused. Raven is unable to remain active for over 20 minutes, showing obvious signs of fatigue.

Environment: Raven lives in a small apartment building in the city with her husband. She has been married for 20 years. They live on the third floor. The building has elevators, but Raven is afraid to use them. Raven's family members live close by and frequently visit her. She holds many family gatherings at her house.

Canadian Model of Occupational Performance

Spirituality: Raven attends church Wednesday nights and Sundays. She is active in her church and enjoys the family camaraderie of the church. Raven sings in the choir and defines herself as a very devoted Christian.

Person: Raven is a 37-year-old married woman who suffered an aneurysm and is in a rehabilitation hospital. She is unable to use her right side, slurs her speech, and shows poor memory and concentration.

Environment: Raven works for the institution of a grocery chain. As such, she must follow institutional policy and procedures. She has medical insurance. She also follows the church's institutional policies.

Occupations: Raven enjoys spending time with family; she is active in the church and a member of the choir. Raven works at a local grocery store. She attends her grandchildren's school events when possible.

Person-Environment-Occupation-Performance

Person: Raven lives with her husband. She has been married for 20 years. She has many family members whom she sees regularly. Raven enjoys family events, singing, and cooking.

Environment: Raven lives in a small apartment building in the city. She lives on the third floor. Raven's family live close by.

Occupations: She works 5 days a week from 8 AM to 5 PM in a local grocery store. Raven attends church and sees her family frequently. Raven attends her grandchildren's events.

Performance: Raven slurs her speech and has difficulty using her right side. She fatigues easily.

Occupational Adaptation

Occupation: Raven works as an assistant manager at a grocery store. She takes care of her family and is involved in the church. She enjoys socializing with others. Currently, she is unable to engage in these occupations, due to right-sided weakness, slurred speech, and fatigue.

Adaptation: The OT practitioner changes the demands of the occupation of socializing, by allowing Raven to sit in a chair and visit with family members for short periods of time. The OT practitioner provides Raven with short projects in which she can participate with her grandchildren when they visit. This helps Raven continue her nurturing occupations, while helping her gain function.

Conclusion

The above case study applications illustrate the subtle discrepancies of each model of practice. Although the information gathered may be similar, the focus differs. Readers should explore the complexities, definitions, and explanations of each of the terms because they provide insight into how to analyze human occupation. Furthermore, readers are encouraged to examine the available assessment tools and measures that more specifically define the concepts of the various models. For example, the Volitional Questionnaire designed under the Model of Human Occupation (MOHO) examines one's interests, values, and personal causation. Understanding this assessment tool helps practitioners more completely understand the concept of volition to better serve their clients.

Frames of Reference

Williamson states that "Frames of reference are produced from the body of knowledge of the profession and address a specific aspect of the profession's domain of concern."[25] A frame of reference describes the process for change in the client and the principles for moving a client along a continuum from dysfunction to function. Depending on the focus of intervention, the practitioner may use several frames of reference at one time or use them sequentially over time.[25]

One of the most efficient and practical ways to conduct evidence-based practice is to examine frames of reference, which apply theory and put principles into practice. As such, frames of reference provide practitioners with specifics about how to treat specific clients. A **frame of reference** includes a description of the population, theory regarding change, function and dysfunction, principles of intervention, role of the practitioner, and evaluation instruments. The parts of a FOR are listed in Box 14-1 and are described in the following sections.

Population

The frame of reference identifies the types of diagnoses or population that would benefit from the intervention. It also describes the age, type of condition, and type of deficit addressed in intervention. For example, clients who experience decreased strength and endurance are typically treated

---

Box 14-1

Necessary Parts of a Frame of Reference

- Population
- Continuum of function/dysfunction
- Theory regarding change
- Principles
- Role of the practitioner
- Assessment instruments

using the biomechanical FOR. Research supports the use of repetitive exercise in strengthening muscles. Practitioners using a biomechanical FOR do not have to conduct their own research on how to strengthen muscles; instead, they use the research from this FOR, which states that providing repetitive movements, increasing the weight, and providing gradual resistance are all techniques that improve strength.[17,18,23]

Continuum of Function and Dysfunction

The FOR defines characteristics and behaviors on the continuum of function and dysfunction based on available research. The therapist evaluates these behaviors, which vary according to the frame of reference, during the assessment process. For example, according to the biomechanical FOR, function includes strength, endurance, and range of motion (ROM) that is adequate to perform occupations. Dysfunction is measured in limitations to strength, range of motion, and endurance.[17,18,23]

Conversely, the behavioral frame of reference defines function as the absence of abnormal behaviors, and dysfunction is the presence of behaviors that interfere with function. According to a behavioral frame of reference, abnormal behaviors may be socially unacceptable behaviors or those defined by the team as interfering with function. Research provides guidelines to determine "typical" function. Practitioners use the available research to determine if occupational therapy services are warranted.

Theories Regarding Change

The FOR describes the theory and hypotheses regarding change. For example, many of the neurological frames of reference (e.g., neurodevelopmental theory [NDT], sensory integration [SI], motor control) are based upon the theory of **brain plasticity,** which refers to the phenomenon that the brain is capable of change and through activity one may get improved neurological synapses, improved dendritic growth, or additional pathways. Therefore intervention is aimed at improving neuronal firing and generating improved brain activity through repetition. Understanding the theory regarding change according to the FOR is important to providing evidence-based intervention.

Principles

The FOR defines the underlying principles guiding the evaluation and intervention. These statements relate back to the theoretical base and describe how an individual is aided to make changes and progress from a state of dysfunction to one of function. Understanding the principles of the FOR allows practitioners to use clinical reasoning to determine whether the FOR may benefit their client (although it may not be originally intended for that population). The principles are based upon theory and research. OT practitioners critique the evidence and rationale to decide if the FOR supports its claims. The FOR should clearly describe the principles surrounding the techniques. For example, the principle of strengthening is that by repetitive muscle contractions, more fibers are recruited and the muscle is able to lift more.[18] Practitioners benefit from knowing that the principle behind strengthening is the recruitment of more muscle fibers.

Role of the Practitioner

The role of the practitioner is based upon the principles and theory of the FOR. These statements provide a guide as to how the practitioner will interact with the client and the environment. This is based upon research evidence that supports the expectation that if a practitioner employs a certain technique the client's function will improve. Subsequently, OT practitioners can be assured when using a FOR that it worked for someone else. However, a careful analysis is still required to determine whether the technique is well founded or supported. Evidence-based practice suggests that the OT practitioner examine the rigor of the study, including the methodology, rationale, results, and design. Examining the research of a FOR helps the practitioner fully understand the intricacies of the FOR and as such the role of the practitioner.

Importantly, the FOR describes how practitioners interact with clients. For example, practitioners using a behavioral frame of reference are to reward positive behaviors and ignore negative ones. The behavioral FOR provides insight into the type of cues that may be provided to clients. The neurodevelopment FOR requires that the practitioner touch the client throughout the movement and facilitate a normal movement pattern.[4,21] Thus, knowledge and investigation into the FOR provide practitioners with a wealth of information for practice.

Assessment Instruments

The FOR also provides the OT practitioner with a variety of instruments to operationalize the principles. For example, Allen's Cognitive Levels was designed to identify the level of cognitive functioning for clients and to be used with the cognitive disability frame of reference.[1,2]

The Sensory Integration and Praxis Tests, Miller Assessment for Preschoolers, Adult Sensory Profile, and clinical observations are based upon SI principles and designed to assist the practitioner in determining how the client would benefit from the FOR.[3,5] The *Occupational Self-Assessment, Volitional Questionnaire,* and *Model of Human Occupation Screening Test* are some examples of the assessments designed to operationalize concepts associated with MOHO theory and practice.[9]

Numerous instruments have been developed to examine a client's functioning in relation to the principles of a specific FOR.

Why Use a Frame of Reference?

Students frequently return from fieldwork convinced that their supervisor did not use a FOR. However, if that is the case, did the supervisor develop the principles of range of motion by himself or herself? In fact, the principle of gradual stretch to elongate the muscle fibers was developed under the biomechanical FOR. Many researchers evaluated the changes in muscle tension through passive stretch before developing the principle. Today, range of motion is a standard occupational therapy intervention; few practitioners stop to think about the theory behind it. However, if range of motion is not working for a client, the OT practitioner may find it helpful to review the principles and previous research. This is all part of critically analyzing the research and explaining what OT practitioners do, and it is considered essential to evidence-based practice.

If OT practitioners do not use a FOR, then how do they justify their practice? They are basing their results on someone's work. Certainly, they are not coming up with the entire practice on their own. OT practitioners need to articulate what they are doing. Occupational therapy professionals are being asked to justify their practice and to contribute new knowledge. It is not sufficient to do things just because someone says. Instead, OT practitioners must become critical consumers of research so they can critique and analyze current practices.

Application of Two Frames of Reference

Several frames of reference can be found in occupational therapy. For illustration purposes, two different frames of reference are described using the above components. The first is the **biomechanical frame of reference.** This frame of reference is derived from theories in kinetics and kinematics (sciences that study the effects of forces and motion on material bodies).[23]

On the function-dysfunction continuum, the biomechanical frame of reference is used with individuals who have deficits in the peripheral nervous, musculoskeletal, integumentary (e.g., skin), or cardiopulmonary system. These individuals, however, have a central nervous system that is intact.[17,18,23] The deficits may cause posture and mobility problems, impairment in range of motion and strength, and decreased endurance. Disabling conditions that may benefit from the biomechanical approach include rheumatoid arthritis and osteoarthritis, fractures, burns, hand traumas, amputations, and spinal cord injuries.

The practitioner evaluates the client's range of motion, muscle strength, and endurance through the use of a variety of tools. Through exercise, activity, and physical agent modalities, change in the person's range of motion, strength, and endurance can be demonstrated.[7]

Another frame of reference used for illustrative purposes is the **cognitive disability frame of reference** proposed by Claudia Allen. This frame of reference is based on the premise that cognitive disorders in those with mental health disabilities are caused by neurobiological defects or deficits related to the biologic functioning of the brain.[1,2] Its theoretical base is derived from research in neuroscience, cognitive psychology, information processing, and biologic psychiatry.[7]

Along the function-dysfunction continuum, function exists when an individual is able to process information to perform routine tasks demanded by the environment.[7] Dysfunction results when the person's ability to process information is restricted in such a way that carrying out routine tasks is impossible. Allen defines six cognitive levels, which are organized in a hierarchy along a continuum. Level 1 represents the individual who has a profound disability in information processing, whereas level 6 represents the normal ability to acquire and process information. Each cognitive level represents information processing behaviors indicative of function-dysfunction. Two specific tools used by practitioners to evaluate an individual's level of functioning are the Allen Cognitive Level (ACL) Test and the Routine Task Inventory Test.[7] The cognitive disability frame of reference proposes that change occurs because of (1) the capacity of the client and (2) the environment. Change in the capacity of the client may be influenced by medical intervention and psychotropic medications, as well as occupational therapy intervention, which teaches the client how to perform routine tasks (cognitive levels 4 and 5). Occupational therapy intervention can also produce change in the environment through modification of task procedures, amount of assistance offered, directions, and setting.[7] Environmental changes may allow the client to experience greater success in performing activities.

Using Multiple Frames of Reference

Although organizing one's thoughts around one model of practice makes sense in occupational therapy, there are many FORs for different clientele. OT practitioners may use multiple FORs, depending on the setting and clientele. The practitioner must examine the theory, principles, and techniques used according to the FOR before deciding if the FOR would work with a given client and setting. If the practitioner is going to modify the FOR, the practitioner must be mindful of the reasons why and critically examine the rationale and research. Using a FOR in a different way may result in less dramatic changes, but may be more practical in certain situations.

Sometimes, a practitioner may decide to combine FORs. For example, combining a sensory integration and behavioral frame of reference may work with some clients. However, the OT practitioner must carefully observe how this blend is working and understand the principles behind each FOR to determine if the blending is appropriate.

Some FORs do not fit together, and using them together may result in less progress toward the stated goals.

Evaluating Frames of Reference

The OT practitioner is responsible for evaluating the client's progress towards his or her goals. If progress is slow or not being made, the OT practitioner re-examines the goals and the FOR. A careful examination of the techniques provided by the FOR may reveal other techniques to help the client reach the goals. Furthermore, the FOR may provide more insight into the role of the practitioner. The practitioner may change how he or she is working with the client, or modify some techniques. It may be necessary to consult with a more experienced practitioner.

The practitioner explores the principles of the FOR to understand the reasoning behind the lack of progress. Could something else be going on that has been missed? The practitioner may re-examine the literature to determine if others have found this FOR successful with the given population. If so, what techniques were used? How did the service differ from what the therapist is currently doing? It may be that the practitioner needs more time or needs to treat the client with more intensity.

When the FOR is not working, the OT practitioner may decide to change FORs. He or she considers the principles, goals, role of the therapist, and the client's motivations. Changing the FOR may provide the right momentum to spur progress.

Case Application

George is a 34-year-old man who experienced a head trauma from a motor vehicle accident. He currently walks with a wide-based gait and shows uncoordinated movement patterns. He leans to the right and drags his left leg. George has poor lip closure (right facial droop) and difficulty chewing some foods. George has a poor right-handed grasp. He shows impaired long-term and short-term memory. Frequently, George is tearful during the session and he has difficulty reading other's cues.

The following examples show how the OT practitioner might view this case from different frames of reference.

Behavioral: Work on George's ability to complete activities and engage in social conversation without inappropriate affect or comments. The practitioner provides positive reinforcements when positive behavior is noted.

Biomechanical: Improve George's strength and endurance through repetitive activity. The OT practitioner provides George with activities that are increasingly difficult. The sessions focus on strength, endurance, and range of motion.

Cognitive-behavioral: Help George identify his own goals and behaviors in hopes that through self-reflection he may make the changes. The OT practitioner allows George to complete an activity and discusses how it went afterwards and how they would improve his behavior next time. The theory behind this frame of reference is that clients will make more significant changes when they are able to cognitively acknowledge them.

Developmental: Identify the highest level of motor, social, and cognitive skills in which George can engage, and facilitate improvements in function from that starting point. Grade activities so that he can achieve them, but is slightly challenged. Help "close the gap" in the areas in which he is unable to perform.[12]

Model of Human Occupation: Explore George's previous interests, motivations, routines, habits, and occupations and determine what he wants to return to doing. Consider how his environment supports or hinders his goals. Help him develop the motor skills to return to his previous occupations, by remediating skills, adapting and modifying tasks along the way. Work to develop feelings of self-efficacy.

Motor control: Work on George's impaired motor skills through activities in the natural environment. Allow George to make mistakes and learn from them. The motor control frame of reference suggests that the practitioner provide verbal and physical cues as necessary. Practice should take place in short sessions with frequent breaks.

Neurodevelopmental: Work on George's motor skills by inhibiting abnormal muscle tone and facilitating normal movement patterns. The OT practitioner requests that George complete activities while the practitioner facilitates the movement at selected "key points of control" (i.e., hand, shoulders, and waist).

Perceptual motor training: Work with George on improving his memory, cognitive skills, safety awareness, and visual perception through a variety of tabletop activities. Perceptual motor training may include many computer-type games and strategies.

Sensorimotor: Work on improving George's motor skills through practice of occupations. The OT practitioner sets up activities in which George practices his coordination.

The above examples provide a brief summary of how intervention differs when using selected frames of reference. The OT practitioner relies on clinical reasoning, experience, judgment, current research, and a thorough understanding of the occupational profile of the client, including the contexts in which the occupations occur. Together, this information forms the basis for the occupational therapy intervention.

Summary

Models of practice help organize one's thinking, whereas frames of reference tell practitioners what to do in practice. Organizing one's practice around the concepts of occupation is central to the profession. Thus, selecting a model of practice developed by OTs provides the best assurance that the practitioner is "thinking" like an OT practitioner. This is helpful in educating the public, clients, and consumers about the profession.

Frames of reference are important in ensuring that practitioners are using evidence-based practice. By critiquing the research on the effectiveness of the selected frame of reference, practitioners are able to fully understand the principles, intervention procedures, and techniques. This helps practitioners adapt the frame of reference if necessary for clients and diagnoses in which the research has not been conducted so that other clients may benefit. Practitioners with knowledge of the subtleties of the frames of reference are able to skillfully work with clients. Articulating the rationale behind intervention techniques is important in today's health care environment. Furthermore, understanding the frames of reference helps OT practitioners better serve clients.

Learning Activities

1. Use a selected model of practice to analyze your occupational performance. Summarize the findings in a report format.
2. Compare and contrast two models of practice in a short paper.
3. Have each member of the class present findings from at least three intervention studies on a given frame of reference. Discuss the effectiveness of this FOR on a selected population.
4. Ask students to provide their rationale for selecting a specific FOR for a given population. Use at least three research studies to justify the selection.
5. Identify the theory for change, principles, and intervention strategies for a specific frame of reference. Present the findings in class.
6. Visit an occupational therapy department and determine which models of practice and frames of reference are used at this setting. Ask to observe an OT practitioner during a treatment that implements one of the frames of reference.

Review Questions

1. What is a theory, model of practice, and frame of reference?
2. Why is it important to use a model of practice? Frame of reference?
3. What are the parts to a frame of reference?
4. How does research on frames of reference support occupational therapy practice?
5. What are some occupational therapy models of practice? Describe them in general terms.

References

1. Allen CK: Activity, occupational therapy's treatment method, *Am J Occup Ther* 41:563, 1987.
2. Allen CK: *Occupational Therapy for Psychiatric Diseases: Measurement and Management of Cognitive Disabilities*, Boston, 1985, Little Brown.
3. Ayres JA: *Sensory Integration for the Child*, Los Angeles, 1979, Western Psychological Services.
4. Bobath B: Sensorimotor development, *NDT Newsletter* 7:1, 1975.
5. Case-Smith J, O'Brien J: *Occupational Therapy for Children*, ed 6, St. Louis, 2010, Mosby.
6. Christiansen CH, Baum CM, editors: *Occupational Therapy: Performance, Participation and Well-being*, Thorofare, NJ, 2005, Slack Inc.
7. Crepeau EB, Cohn ES, Boyt Schell BA, editors: *Willard and Spackman's Occupational Therapy*, ed 10, Philadelphia, 2003, Lippincott Williams & Wilkins.
8. Kielhofner G: *Conceptual Foundations of Occupational Therapy*, ed 4, Philadelphia, 2009, FA Davis.
9. Kielhofner G: *A Model of Human Occupation: Theory and Application*, ed 4, Baltimore, 2008, Lippincott Williams & Wilkins.
10. Law M, Cooper B, Stewart D, et al: The person-environment-occupation model: A transactive approach to occupational performance, *Canad J Occup Ther* 63(1):9–23, 1996.
11. Law M, Baptiste S, Carswell A, et al: *Canadian Occupational Performance Measure*, ed 2, Toronto, 1994, Canadian Association of Occupational Therapists Publication.
12. Llorens LA: *Application of a Developmental Theory for Health and Rehabilitation*, Rockville, MD, 1976, American Occupational Therapy Association.
13. MacRae N, O'Brien J: *OT 301 Foundations of occupational therapy*, unpublished lecture notes, 2001, University of New England.
14. Mish F, editor: *Merriam-Webster's Collegiate Dictionary®*, ed 10, Springfield, MA, 1994, Merriam-Webster.
15. O'Brien J, Solomon J: Scope of practice. In Solomon J, O'Brien J, editors: *Pediatric Skills for Occupational Therapy Assistants*, ed 3, St. Louis, 2010, Mosby.
16. Parham D: Toward professionalism: The reflective therapist, *Am J Occup Ther* 41:555, 1987.
17. Pedretti LW, Paszuinielli S: A frame of reference for occupational therapy in physical dysfunction. In Pedritti LW, Zoltan B, editors: *Occupational Therapy: Practice Skills for Physical Dysfunction*, ed 3, St. Louis, 1990, Mosby, pp 1–17.
18. Pendleton H, Schultz-Krohn W, editors: *Pedretti's Occupational Therapy: Practice Skills for Physical Dysfunction*, ed 6, St. Louis, 2006, Mosby.
19. Reed KL: Understanding theory: The first step in learning about research, *Am J Occup Ther* 38:677, 1984.
20. Schkade JK, Schultz S: Occupational adaptation: Toward a holistic approach in contemporary practice, Part I, *Am J Occup Ther* 46:829–837, 1992.
21. Schoen S, Anderson J: Neurodevelopmental treatment frame of reference. In Kramer P, Hinojosa J, editors: *Frames of Reference for Pediatric Occupational Therapy*, ed 3, Baltimore, 2009, Lippincott Williams & Wilkins.
22. Townsend E, Brintnell S, Staisey N: Developing guidelines for client-centered occupational therapy practice, *Canad J Occup Ther* 57:69–76, 1990.

23. Trombly CS, Radomski MV: *Occupational Therapy for Physical Dysfunction*, ed 5, Philadelphia, 2002, Lippincott Williams & Wilkins.

24. Walker KF, Ludwig F, editors: *Perspectives on Theory for the Practice of Occupational Therapy*, ed 3, Austin, TX, 2004, Pro-Ed.

25. Williamson GG: A heritage of activity: Development of theory, *Am J Occup Ther* 36:716, 1982.

Occupational therapy provides me with the unique opportunity to observe and to share my knowledge and my experiences in order to affect the well-being of another person. The potential to observe makes life interesting. It provides an opportunity to stand aside, note, and experience reality within its context, be it beautiful or painful. Observation further provides an opportunity to stand still and acknowledge. It provides the occupational therapist with an opportunity to apply activity analysis—the main method of occupational therapy—to detect function or dysfunction of task performance, as well as the performance components; but task performance is the focus of the human being. Observation thus allows the occupational therapist to view the human through activities or tasks, these tasks being crucial forces responsible for shaping the human being. In other words, an occupational therapist is an observer with a powerful tool, "activity analysis." Through observation, the therapist can assess performance, set goals, treat the individual with the set goals in mind, and critically evaluate its impact, all by applying different forms of clinical reasoning.

The human being evolves around task performance. The human is shaped by what he or she performs, and life is meaningless without the ability and the motivation to perform at whatever small capacity. The smallest gains can be as rewarding and worthwhile for those involved as are the bigger accomplishments or achievements for others.

Occupational therapy has further allowed me to share my knowledge regarding occupational performance that could, in some instances, affect the quality of life of those involved. It has provided me with an opportunity to challenge limitations at different levels of performance, in a very exciting way, as some of these limitations have been at a level that I would have thought would be impossible to influence. Limitations have the potential to develop maturity in life, and many limitations not only bring about frustrations and negative aspects but the inner beauty of the person involved and the unknown potentials that may flourish and thereby enhance maturity.

Task performance is, therefore, the force that molds the human being into an occupational being. It is a privilege to be an occupational therapist and to be involved with that powerful driving force.

GUðRÚN ÁRNADÓTTIR, MA, BOT
Private Practitioner
Reykjavík, Iceland

The art of therapy involves reading the client's cues within the context of the setting and the client–therapist relationship. Artistic reasoning requires skill in the therapeutic relationship, creativity, reflection, and self-awareness (see Chapter 16).

Thought Process During Clinical Reasoning

Clinical reasoning is a cognitive thought process in which many diverse bits of information are gathered together (evaluation), many outside factors are considered (e.g., life space, prognosis, and desires), the demands of activities are analyzed (activity analysis), time investment choices are made (plan), and identifiable goals are organized (intervention). Clinical reasoning used throughout the therapy process requires analysis of data, use of specific knowledge bases, and synthesis of the process and information. The OT practitioner must actively think and process information from multiple sources.

Rogers and Holm[13] describe the steps in the thought process of clinical reasoning that is used during the occupational therapy evaluation and intervention process. During each step, the OT practitioner gathers, organizes, analyzes, and synthesizes information.[13] See Box 17-1.

Box 17-1

Steps in the Thought Process of Clinical Reasoning

1. *Formation of preassessment image:* Practitioner gathers initial information regarding the client, including information on diagnosis, age, and prior level of function. The practitioner asks, "What am I going to consider in regard to this client?" and "What do I know about this condition (in general and how it affects this person)?"
2. *Cue acquisition:* Practitioner gathers the data regarding the client's functional status and occupational roles.
3. *Hypothesis generation:* Practitioner organizes the data that have been gathered and makes tentative assumptions, which will serve as the basis for therapeutic action.
4. *Cue interpretation:* Practitioner gathers further cues and continues the search for data. Each cue is compared with the hypothesis being considered to determine relevancy. The practitioner interprets whether the cue confirms the hypothesis, does not confirm the hypothesis, or does not contribute in either way to the hypothesis.
5. *Hypothesis evaluation:* Practitioner examines the data that have been collected and weighs the evidence for and against each of the diagnostic hypotheses. The hypothesis with the most supporting evidence is selected and forms the basis for intervention.

Adapted from Rogers JC, Holm MB: Occupational therapy diagnostic reasoning: A component of clinical reasoning, *Am J Occup Ther* 45: 1045, 1991.

In the first step, the OT practitioner forms a *preassessment image* of the client, an initial outline that will be used for further assessment of the client. The practitioner considers the client's diagnosis, age, and contexts (e.g., time in life). The OT practitioner seeks to find out information related to the diagnosis, client's life roles, and functional status prior to the injury or trauma. At this stage, the practitioner is forming a general picture of the person.

The OT practitioner uses the preassessment image to begin the *cue acquisition* step. This step involves gathering the data regarding the client's current functional status, occupational roles, and past experiences. The purpose of this stage is to gather data, or *cues*, to inform the intervention planning.

The practitioner generates a *hypothesis* using the cues regarding the client's needs. The practitioner organizes the data that have been gathered and makes tentative assumptions, which serve as the basis for therapeutic action. The hypotheses generated are based on all available data, knowledge of models or practice and frames of reference, and the practitioner's experience.

In evaluating a female client's ability to feed herself, the OT practitioner notices that the client is having difficulty and does not eat all of the food on her plate. The food spills out of her mouth. The client is unable to use her left hand. The practitioner's hypothesis in this situation is that the difficulty is the result of poor oral motor skills caused by the client's stroke. The practitioner could also hypothesize that the client's difficulty is due to the fact that she must use her non-dominant hand to feed herself, which makes it hard to get the food on the utensil and tires her out easily.

The process continues with step four, *cue interpretation*, where the practitioner continues the search for data based on the hypothesis being considered. During this stage, the practitioner may conduct intervention on a given hypothesis and collect more data to verify the relevancy. This leads to the *hypothesis evaluation* in which the practitioner interprets whether the cues confirm the hypothesis, do not confirm the hypothesis, or do not contribute in either way to the hypothesis.[12] The hypothesis with the most supporting evidence forms the basis for intervention.

This clinical reasoning process leads to an assessment of the client's occupational therapy performance deficits and an intervention plan based on available data. The process considers the cause of the deficit, the signs and symptoms, knowledge of the condition, and a definition of the problems.[13] OT practitioners use clinical reasoning during all aspects of the occupational therapy process. They select from a variety of intervention approaches and make decisions on goals, modalities, and activity selection. They use clinical reasoning to evaluate the effectiveness of intervention.

The practitioner closely monitors and evaluates the intervention to determine whether the modalities that were selected achieve the intended goal(s). Importantly, the OT practitioner collaborates with the client throughout the process to confirm that therapy is proceeding on a track that is meaningful to the client. The process of clinical reasoning is a dynamic process.

Clinical Reasoning Strategies

Therapists who understand and employ a range of clinical reasoning strategies are able to adapt their interventions to meet individuals' needs. Several types of clinical reasoning strategies are described in Table 17-1.

Mattingly and Fleming discovered that OT practitioners used three distinct strategies, or tracks, for clinical reasoning: procedural, interactive, and conditional tracks.[3,8] Practitioners shift easily and frequently among the three tracks, depending on what they are addressing in therapy with a specific client.

Procedural reasoning is a strategy used by the OT practitioner when he or she focuses on the client's disease or disability and determines what will be the most appropriate modalities to use to improve functional performance. Central tasks for the OT practitioner during procedural reasoning are problem identification, goal setting, and treatment planning.[3] The problem-solving skills discussed in Chapter 12 may be employed during procedural reasoning. This track is similar to the scientific element of clinical reasoning.

> The OT practitioner working with a new client examines the diagnosis, etiology, characteristics, prognosis, and suggested interventions. The practitioner determines the most commonly used approach for clients with this diagnosis and begins intervention based upon this knowledge.

Interactive reasoning is a strategy used by the OT practitioner to understand the client as a person. This type of reasoning takes place during face-to-face interactions between the practitioner and the client. OT practitioners use interactive reasoning strategies to (1) understand the disability from the client's point of view, (2) engage the client in treatment, (3) individualize the intervention setting by matching goals and procedures to the particular client and his or her life experiences and disability, (4) impart a sense of trust and acceptance to the client, (5) relieve tension by using humor, (6) develop a common language of actions and meanings, and (7) determine whether the intervention is working.[3]

> The OT practitioner learns that the client lives at home with his wife of 20 years and three teenage children. The client hopes to return to his job as a certified public accountant (CPA); he enjoys biking with his family and hiking in the country. The OT practitioner uses this information along with the information about the diagnosis, prognosis, etiology, and intervention strategies when designing the intervention plan.

Table 17-1 Strategies Used by Occupational Therapy Practitioners in Clinical Reasoning

Strategy	Description
Procedural reasoning	Strategy used by the OT practitioner to focus on the client's disease or disability and determine what will be the most appropriate modalities to use to improve the client's functional performance. Central tasks include problem identification, goal setting, and treatment planning.
Interactive reasoning	Strategy used by the OT practitioner when he or she wants to understand the client as a person; takes place during face-to-face interactions between the practitioner and the client.
Conditional reasoning	Involves consideration by the practitioner of the client's condition as a whole, including the disease or disability and what it means to the person, the physical context, and the social context; consideration of how the client's condition may change, depending upon level of participation in treatment.
Narrative reasoning	Use of storytelling wherein practitioners tell "stories" about clients to each other. Use of story creation, wherein the practitioner envisions how the future may be for the client so that he or she may guide the intervention process.
Pragmatic reasoning	The practitioner takes into account how factors in the context of the practice setting and his or her personal context might affect intervention. Factors in the practice setting relate to the availability of resources (i.e., reimbursement or availability of equipment). Factors in the personal context of the practitioner might include repertoire of therapeutic skills and personal motivation.

Adapted from Mattingly C, Fleming M: *Clinical Reasoning: Forms of Inquiry in a Therapeutic Practice*, Philadelphia, 1994, FA Davis.
Neistadt ME: Teaching strategies for the development of clinical reasoning, *Am J Occup Ther* 50:676, 1996.
Rogers JC, Holm MB: Occupational therapy diagnostic reasoning: A component of clinical reasoning, *Am J Occup Ther* 45:1045, 1991.
Schell BA, Cervero RM: Clinical reasoning in occupational therapy: An integrative review, *Am J Occup Ther* 47:605, 1993.

Interactive reasoning takes into account the client's identity, goals, and environment. While OT practitioners use procedural reasoning to form a foundation for intervention, they personalize the intervention through interactive reasoning.

The third type of strategy used by OT practitioners is **conditional reasoning.** Conditional reasoning has several aspects.[3] The practitioner considers the client's condition as a whole, including the disease or disability and what it means to the person—the physical context and the social context. The practitioner motivates the client to participate in intervention by sharing the same vision for the outcome of intervention.[3] With these images in mind, the practitioner implements intervention and compares changes observed in the client with the client's future goals.[3] The practitioner using conditional reasoning examines all aspects of the client's circumstances. In particular, the practitioner evaluates the context of the intervention in relation to the client's goals and desires.

Anna, the OT practitioner, evaluates Sam's progress in therapy and decides to change the focus of intervention from remediation to compensation. Anna believes that Sam has worked hard in therapy, but based upon the severity of his condition and the progress to date, Anna decides that compensation techniques will enable Sam to return to his occupations earlier.

Anna used conditional reasoning to change the focus of the intervention and to allow Sam to return to his occupations. She analyzed multiple factors contributing to Sam's progress and reasoned that changing the intervention may allow him to return to his occupational goals faster.

Another clinical reasoning strategy described in the literature is called **narrative reasoning.** Mattingly describes two different ways in which OT practitioners use narrative reasoning—storytelling and story creation.[7] In storytelling, OT practitioners tell stories about clients to other practitioners to better understand and reason through concepts. This type of storytelling may be observed during case study presentations.

Mattingly states, "Narratives make sense of reality by linking the outward world of actions and events to the inner world of human intention and motivation."[7]

Clients also use storytelling to reframe their own narrative and make sense of events. Telling one's story about their past is a helpful way to create a future story. Thus, storytelling can be therapeutic for clients and families. For example, a young athlete who sustained a spinal cord injury may tell stories about his past successes as an athlete. As he progresses through therapy, he may develop new stories about successes and re-invent his athlete image by engaging in adapted sport activities, such as wheelchair races, adapted sailing programs, or wheelchair basketball. He may use storytelling to redefine who he is in his current body. Storytelling can help clients understand their occupational performance and develop a new identity.

Pragmatic reasoning takes into consideration such factors as the context of the practice setting and the personal context of the OT practitioner that may inhibit or facilitate intervention. Factors related to the context of the practice setting include reimbursement and the availability of equipment and space.[14] For example, a practitioner considers reimbursement and available resources when developing an intervention plan. The OT practitioner must also consider personal factors, including his or her repertoire of therapeutic skills, knowledge, and experience. Other pragmatic factors include time/habits, costs, resources, environment, setting, and personnel.

Nick, the OT practitioner, is treating Carlos, a 63-year-old client who has had a stroke. Nick and Carlos are working toward improving movement in Carlos's affected arm and hand so that he can return to his occupation as a car mechanic. Carlos creates a vision for his future by explaining to the therapist the many tasks he performs at work and identifying the pride he receives from his co-workers and family. Nick explains that the projects he completes in occupational therapy require concentration, design, problem solving, and fine motor skills which are also skills Carlos needs when working as a mechanic. Together, Nick helps Carlos understand that he has heard his story and will help him return to his job as car mechanic.

From Novice to Expert: Development of Clinical Reasoning Skills

Clinical reasoning develops over time with practical experience. Generally, authors describe five different stages of career development: novice, advanced beginner, competent, proficient, and expert[15] (Table 17-2).

The focus of the **novice** practitioner is on learning procedural skills (e.g., assessment, diagnostic, and treatment planning procedures) necessary to practice.[3,15] The novice practitioner feels most comfortable performing and refining the techniques and procedures learned in school. Novice practitioners do not feel comfortable using interactive reasoning strategies. The **advanced beginner** recognizes additional cues and begins to view the client as an individual.[15] However, the advanced beginner still does not see the whole picture.

The **competent practitioner** sees more facts and determines the importance of these facts and observations.[15] At this stage, practitioners have a broader understanding of the client's problems and are more likely to individualize treatment. However, flexibility and creativity are still lacking. The **proficient practitioner** views situations as a whole instead of as isolated parts.[15] Practical experience allows him or her to develop a direction and vision of where the client should be going. If the initial plans do not work, the proficient therapist is easily able to modify them.

Expert practitioners recognize and understand rules of practice; however, for this group of practitioners, the rules shift to the background.[15] The expert practitioner often uses

Table 17-2 **Development of Clinical Reasoning Skills**		
Stage of Development	Name	Type of Functioning
1	Novice	Uses procedural or scientific reasoning, knowledge from coursework
2	Advanced beginner	Recognizes additional cues and begins to see client as an individual
3	Competent	Sees more facts, understands client's problems, individualizes treatment, may lack creativity and flexibility
4	Proficient	Views situations as whole instead of in isolated parts, able to develop a vision of where the client should go, able to modify easily
5	Expert	Recognizes and understands rules of practice, uses intuition to know what to do next, uses conditional reasoning

Adapted from Benner PE: *From Novice to Expert: Excellence and Power in Clinical Nursing Practice*, Menlo Park, CA, 1984, Addison-Wesley.
Dreyfus HL, Dreyfus SE: *Mind over Machine, the Power of Human Intuition and Expertise in the Era of the Computer*, pp. 101–121, New York, 1986, The Free Press.
Neistadt ME, Atkins A: Analysis of the orthopedic content in an occupational therapy curriculum from a clinical reasoning perspective, *AJOT* 50:669–675, 1996.

intuition to know what to do next. "This intuitive judgment is based on correct identification of relevant cues at a particular time in the patient's therapy and a variety of medical, physical, and psychosocial factors."[15] Expert practitioners use procedural, interactive, and conditional skills without difficulty.[3] They rely on past clinical situations to help process imagined outcomes for the client.

Techniques to Develop Clinical Reasoning Skills

Occupational therapy educators realize the importance of facilitating and fostering clinical reasoning skills in students and clinicians. Problem-based learning is one technique used by educational programs to encourage clinical reasoning skills. Other closely related techniques include case-based integration courses and assignments requiring students to complete evaluation and intervention protocols in a simulated manner. The intent of these courses and assignments is to help the students participate in clinical reasoning, reflect on their learning, and advance in their ability to consider multiple factors. In a comparison of clinical reasoning skills in occupational therapy students in the United States and Scotland, McCannon et al. found that the predominant form of clinical reasoning by students in a problem-based learning course was

procedural.[9] Vroman and MacRae reported similar findings in their work.[18] Overall, educational programs provide students with the tools to clinically reason and should continue to provide authentic experiences for students.[5] Bailey and Cohn suggest that faculty help students learn from clients.[1] They provided students opportunities to interview clients with disabilities and discuss the process. Reflection and introspection are key factors in developing clinical reasoning. Students and practitioners must be able to seek and receive feedback.

Unsworth suggested in her study of expert and novice practitioners that novice practitioners could benefit from more time reflecting on the therapy process and discussing their therapy with expert clinicians.[17] Interestingly, she found, as did Taylor[16] and Mattingly,[6] that expert clinicians were able to self-critique their work and showed willingness to change. Liu et al. found that more experienced therapists used conditional reasoning, whereas junior therapists relied on procedural reasoning.[5]

Novice practitioners and students gather information using individual cues, whereas experts use chunking to sort and record information. Chunking is a strategy that is used to remember several units of information. For example, it is easier to remember a phone number if it is divided into chunks (e.g., 501-555-9487) instead of trying to remember individual numbers (e.g., 5015559487). Expert practitioners use the technique of chunking to categorize information about clients and apply it to practice.[12]

The student or novice practitioner can enhance his or her clinical reasoning skills through coaching, reflecting, analyzing, and role modeling.[2,10,15] Reading and reflecting on the personal experiences of individuals with disabilities can help a practitioner develop clinical reasoning skills.[10] The student can analyze case studies to develop reasoning. The novice practitioner can observe expert practitioners and examine the clinical reasoning processes and strategies that the expert uses. Furthermore, discussions and systematic analysis of fieldwork experiences may help novice practitioners develop clinical reasoning skills.

The students trying to advance their clinical reasoning abilities benefit by exploring the literature, critically analyzing data, and reflecting on their own performance. Requesting feedback from more advanced practitioners helps the novice understand approaches and reasoning.

Practitioners develop skills by discussing specific cases and problem solving through the clinical reasoning process.

Practitioners are encouraged to seek education and knowledge and remain reflective of their own practice. Clinical reasoning skills may be further developed through new knowledge and careful analysis of one's practice skills and thinking. Practitioners may improve clinical reasoning skills by seeking feedback from others on intervention approaches and reasoning.

Conducting research through case study analysis may enhance a practitioner's clinical reasoning skills as this requires a careful examination of the intervention process. Following a specific frame of reference can help practitioners develop clinical reasoning skills. For example, in separate studies, O'Brien et al.[11] and Keponen and Launiainen[4] examined he therapeutic reasoning process using the Model of Human Occupation. Finally, remaining current and critically examining available research enhances a practitioner's clinical reasoning skills and abilities, thereby benefiting clients.

Summary

Clinical reasoning provides the foundation for making choices and helping improve clients' ability to function and engage in occupations. The elements of science, ethics, and art are combined in the therapy process. OT practitioners skillfully design intervention to make a difference in the lives of the clients they serve. Knowledge of science provides data on the condition, diagnosis, prognosis, and client factors that may be involved. The art of therapy involves designing creative intervention to address occupational performance deficits. The art of therapy involves the therapeutic use of self and refers to how practitioners relate to clients. Finally, ethical considerations may influence the course of the intervention and outcomes.

OT practitioners use a variety of strategies to effectively integrate the scientific, artistic, and ethical elements into intervention plans. These reasoning strategies include procedural, interactive, conditional, narrative, and pragmatic reasoning. The strategies are seldom used in isolation, and, in fact, expert practitioners intertwine the strategies to provide the most effective and intuitive intervention. Novice practitioners may be limited in the strategies they use.

Practice, reflection, education, supervision, research, and critical analysis of practice provide excellent techniques for increasing a practitioner's ability to use clinical reasoning. OT practitioners must always remain mindful of the clinical reasoning strategies they are employing so that intervention remains beneficial to clients.

Learning Activities

1. Provide students with a case study. Provide examples of the type of clinical reasoning strategies based on the specific client. Share examples in class.
2. View a videotape of a case study of a client in a therapy session. Analyze the clinical reasoning strategies used by the practitioner. Were the strategies effective? What would you have done differently?
3. Write a short story about someone who has a disability. Report how this individual's past and present may reflect on his or her possible future.[5]
4. Read a literary work about an individual who has experienced a disabling condition. Using the narrative reasoning strategy, analyze the person's experiences. Describe the person's story. (Your instructor can provide suggestions for books to read.)
5. Use clinical reasoning strategies to develop an intervention plan for a given case study, in which the only information available is the client's age, diagnosis, and living situation. Discuss the findings in class. What would be the next step in the process?

Review Questions

1. What is clinical reasoning?
2. What is the clinical reasoning thought process?
3. Provide an example of the scientific, ethical, and artistic elements of clinical reasoning.
4. What are the three types of clinical reasoning as described by Mattingly and Fleming?
5. What are the stages of clinical reasoning? Provide a description of each.

References

1. Bailey DM, Cohn ES: Understanding others: A course to learn interactive clinical reasoning, *Occup Ther Health Care* 15(1/2):31–46, 2001.
2. Benamy BC: *Developing Clinical Reasoning Skills: Strategies for the Occupational Therapist*, San Antonio, 1996, Therapy Skill Builders.
3. Fleming MH: The therapist with the three-track mind, *Am J Occup Ther* 45:1007, 1991.
4. Keponen R, Launiainen H: Using the model of human occupation to nurture an occupational focus in the clinical reasoning of experienced therapists, *Occup Ther Health Care* 22(2/3):95–104, 2008.
5. Liu KPY, Chan CCH, Hui-Chan CWY: Clinical reasoning and the occupational therapy curriculum, *Occup Ther Int* 7(3):173–183, 2000.
6. Mattingly C, Fleming M: *Clinical Reasoning: Forms of Inquiry in a Therapeutic Practice*, Philadelphia, 1994, FA Davis.
7. Mattingly C: The narrative nature of clinical reasoning, *Am J Occup Ther* 45:998, 1991.
8. Mattingly C: What is clinical reasoning? *Am J Occup Ther* 45:979, 1991.
9. McCannon R, Robertson D, Caldwell J, et al: Comparison of clinical reasoning skills in occupational therapy students in the USA and Scotland, *Occup Ther Int* 11(3):160–176, 2004.
10. Neistadt ME: Teaching strategies for the development of clinical reasoning, *Am J Occup Ther* 50:676, 1996.
11. O'Brien J, Asselin L, Fortier K, et al: Using therapeutic reasoning to apply the Model of Human Occupation in pediatric occupational therapy practice, *J Occup Ther Schools Early Interv* 3(4):348–365, 2010.
12. Rogers JC: Clinical reasoning: The ethics, science and art, *Am J Occup Ther* 37:601, 1983.
13. Rogers JC, Holm MB: Occupational therapy diagnostic reasoning: A component of clinical reasoning, *Am J Occup Ther* 45:1045, 1991.
14. Schell BA, Cervero RM: Clinical reasoning in occupational therapy: An integrative review, *Am J Occup Ther* 47:605, 1993.
15. Slater DY, Cohn ES: Staff development through analysis of practice, *Am J Occup Ther* 45:1038, 1991.
16. Taylor RR: *The Intentional Relationship: Use of Self and Occupational Therapy*, Philadelphia, 2008, FA Davis.
17. Unsworth G: The clinical reasoning of novice and expert occupational therapists, *Scand J Occup Ther* 8:163–173, 2001.
18. Vroman KE, MacRae N: How should the effectiveness of problem-based learning in occupational therapy education be examined? *Am J Occup Ther* 53:533–536, 1999.

Occupational Therapy Code of Ethics and Ethics Standards (2010)

Preamble

The American Occupational Therapy Association (AOTA) *Occupational Therapy Code of Ethics and Ethics Standards (2010)* ("Code and Ethics Standards") is a public statement of principles used to promote and maintain high standards of conduct within the profession. Members of AOTA are committed to promoting inclusion, diversity, independence, and safety for all recipients in various stages of life, health, and illness and to empower all beneficiaries of occupational therapy. This commitment extends beyond service recipients to include professional colleagues, students, educators, businesses, and the community.

Fundamental to the mission of the occupational therapy profession is the therapeutic use of everyday life activities (occupations) with individuals or groups for the purpose of participation in roles and situations in home, school, workplace, community, and other settings. "Occupational therapy addresses the physical, cognitive, psychosocial, sensory, and other aspects of performance in a variety of contexts to support engagement in everyday life activities that affect health, well being, and quality of life" (AOTA, 2004). Occupational therapy personnel have an ethical responsibility primarily to recipients of service and secondarily to society.

The *Occupational Therapy Code of Ethics and Ethics Standards (2010)* was tailored to address the most prevalent ethical concerns of the profession in education, research, and practice. The concerns of stakeholders, including the public, consumers, students, colleagues, employers, research participants, researchers, educators, and practitioners, were addressed in the creation of this document. A review of issues raised in ethics cases, member questions related to ethics, and content of other professional codes of ethics was utilized to ensure that the revised document is applicable to occupational therapists, occupational therapy assistants, and students in all roles.

The historical foundation of this Code and Ethics Standards is based on ethical reasoning surrounding practice and professional issues, as well as on empathic reflection regarding these interactions with others (see e.g., AOTA, 2005, 2006). This reflection resulted in the establishment of principles that guide ethical action, which goes beyond rote following of rules or application of principles. Rather, *ethical action* is a manifestation of moral character and mindful reflection. It is a commitment to benefit others, to virtuous practice of artistry and science, to genuinely good behaviors, and to noble acts of courage.

While much has changed over the course of the profession's history, more has remained the same. The profession of occupational therapy remains grounded in seven core concepts, as identified in the *Core Values and Attitudes of Occupational Therapy Practice* (AOTA, 1993): *altruism, equality, freedom, justice, dignity, truth,* and *prudence. Altruism* is the individual's ability to place the needs of others before their own. *Equality* refers to the desire to promote fairness in interactions with others. The concept of *freedom* and personal choice is paramount in a profession in which the desires of the client must guide our interventions. Occupational therapy practitioners, educators, and researchers relate in a fair and impartial manner to individuals with whom they interact and respect and adhere to the applicable laws and standards regarding their area of practice, be it direct care, education, or research (*justice*). Inherent in the practice of occupational therapy is the promotion and preservation of the individuality and *dignity* of the client, by assisting him or her to engage in occupations that are meaningful to him or her regardless of level of disability. In all situations, occupational therapists, occupational therapy assistants, and students must provide accurate information, both in oral and written form (*truth*). Occupational therapy personnel use their clinical and ethical reasoning skills, sound judgment, and reflection to make decisions to direct them in their area(s) of practice (*prudence*). These seven core values provide a foundation by which occupational therapy personnel guide their interactions with others, be they students, clients, colleagues, research participants, or communities. These values also define the ethical principles to which the profession is committed and which the public can expect.

The *Occupational Therapy Code of Ethics and Ethics Standards (2010)* is a guide to professional conduct when ethical issues arise. Ethical decision-making is a process that includes awareness of how the outcome will impact occupational therapy clients in all spheres. Applications of Code and Ethics Standards Principles are considered situation-specific, and where a conflict exists, occupational therapy personnel will pursue responsible efforts for resolution. These principles apply to occupational therapy personnel engaged in any professional role, including elected and volunteer leadership positions.

The specific purposes of the *Occupational Therapy Code of Ethics and Ethics Standards (2010)* are to

1. Identify and describe the principles supported by the occupational therapy profession.
2. Educate the general public and members regarding established principles to which occupational therapy personnel are accountable.
3. Socialize occupational therapy personnel to expected standards of conduct.
4. Assist occupational therapy personnel in recognition and resolution of ethical dilemmas.

The *Occupational Therapy Code of Ethics and Ethics Standards (2010)* defines the set of principles that apply to occupational therapy personnel at all levels.

Definitions

Recipient of service: Individuals or groups receiving occupational therapy.

Student: A person who is enrolled in an accredited occupational therapy education program.

Research participant: A prospective participant or one who has agreed to participate in an approved research project.

Employee: A person who is hired by a business (facility or organization) to provide occupational therapy services.

Colleague: A person who provides services in the same or different business (facility or organization) to which a professional relationship exists or may exist.

Public: The community of people at large.

Beneficence

Principle 1. Occupational Therapy Personnel Shall Demonstrate a Concern for the Well-Being and Safety of the Recipients of Their Services.

Beneficence includes all forms of action intended to benefit other persons. The term *beneficence* connotes acts of mercy, kindness, and charity (Beauchamp & Childress, 2009). Forms of beneficence typically include altruism, love, and humanity. Beneficence requires taking action by helping others, in other words, by promoting good, by preventing harm, and by removing harm. Examples of beneficence include protecting and defending the rights of others, preventing harm from occurring to others, removing conditions that will cause harm to others, helping persons with disabilities, and rescuing persons in danger (Beauchamp & Childress, 2009).

Occupational Therapy Personnel Shall

A. Respond to requests for occupational therapy services (e.g., a referral) in a timely manner as determined by law, regulation, or policy.
B. Provide appropriate evaluation and a plan of intervention for all recipients of occupational therapy services specific to their needs.
C. Reevaluate and reassess recipients of service in a timely manner to determine whether goals are being achieved and whether intervention plans should be revised.
D. Avoid the inappropriate use of outdated or obsolete tests/assessments or data obtained from such tests in making intervention decisions or recommendations.
E. Provide occupational therapy services that are within each practitioner's level of competence and scope of practice (e.g., qualifications, experience, the law).
F. Use, to the extent possible, evaluation, planning, intervention techniques, and therapeutic equipment that are evidence-based and within the recognized scope of occupational therapy practice.
G. Take responsible steps (e.g., continuing education, research, supervision, training) and use careful judgment to ensure their own competence and weigh potential for client harm when generally recognized standards do not exist in emerging technology or areas of practice.
H. Terminate occupational therapy services in collaboration with the service recipient or responsible party when the needs and goals of the recipient have been met or when services no longer produce a measurable change or outcome.
I. Refer to other health care specialists solely on the basis of the needs of the client.
J. Provide occupational therapy education, continuing education, instruction, and training that are within the instructor's subject area of expertise and level of competence.
K. Provide students and employees with information about the Code and Ethics Standards, opportunities to discuss ethical conflicts, and procedures for reporting unresolved ethical conflicts.
L. Ensure that occupational therapy research is conducted in accordance with currently accepted ethical guidelines and standards for the protection of research participants and the dissemination of results.
M. Report to appropriate authorities any acts in practice, education, and research that appear unethical or illegal.
N. Take responsibility for promoting and practicing occupational therapy on the basis of current knowledge and research and for further developing the profession's body of knowledge.

Nonmaleficence

Principle 2. Occupational Therapy Personnel Shall Intentionally Refrain from Actions That Cause Harm.

Nonmaleficence imparts an obligation to refrain from harming others (Beauchamp & Childress, 2009). The principle of nonmaleficence is grounded in the practitioner's responsibility to refrain from causing harm, inflicting injury, or wronging others. While beneficence requires action to incur benefit, nonmaleficence requires non-action to avoid harm (Beauchamp & Childress, 2009). Nonmaleficence also includes an obligation to not impose risks of harm even if the potential risk is without malicious or harmful intent. This principle often is examined under the context of *due care*. If the standard of due care outweighs the benefit of treatment, then refraining from treatment provision would be ethically indicated (Beauchamp & Childress, 2009).

Occupational Therapy Personnel Shall

A. Avoid inflicting harm or injury to recipients of occupational therapy services, students, research participants, or employees.

B. Make every effort to ensure continuity of services or options for transition to appropriate services to avoid abandoning the service recipient if the current provider is unavailable due to medical or other absence or loss of employment.

C. Avoid relationships that exploit the recipient of services, students, research participants, or employees physically, emotionally, psychologically, financially, socially, or in any other manner that conflicts or interferes with professional judgment and objectivity.

D. Avoid engaging in any sexual relationship or activity, whether consensual or nonconsensual, with any recipient of service, including family or significant other, student, research participant, or employee, while a relationship exists as an occupational therapy practitioner, educator, researcher, supervisor, or employer.

E. Recognize and take appropriate action to remedy personal problems and limitations that might cause harm to recipients of service, colleagues, students, research participants, or others.

F. Avoid any undue influences, such as alcohol or drugs, that may compromise the provision of occupational therapy services, education, or research.

G. Avoid situations in which a practitioner, educator, researcher, or employer is unable to maintain clear professional boundaries or objectivity to ensure the safety and well-being of recipients of service, students, research participants, and employees.

H. Maintain awareness of and adherence to the Code and Ethics Standards when participating in volunteer roles.

I. Avoid compromising client rights or well-being based on arbitrary administrative directives by exercising professional judgment and critical analysis.

J. Avoid exploiting any relationship established as an occupational therapist or occupational therapy assistant to further one's own physical, emotional, financial, political, or business interests at the expense of the best interests of recipients of services, students, research participants, employees, or colleagues.

K. Avoid participating in bartering for services because of the potential for exploitation and conflict of interest unless there are clearly no contraindications or bartering is a culturally appropriate custom.

L. Determine the proportion of risk to benefit for participants in research prior to implementing a study.

Autonomy and Confidentiality

Principle 3. Occupational Therapy Personnel Shall Respect the Right of the Individual to Self-Determination.

The principle of autonomy and confidentiality expresses the concept that practitioners have a duty to treat the client according to the client's desires, within the bounds of accepted standards of care and to protect the client's confidential information. Often *autonomy* is referred to as the *self-determination* principle. However, respect for autonomy goes beyond acknowledging an individual as a mere agent and also acknowledges a "person's right to hold views, to make choices, and to take actions based on personal values and beliefs" (Beauchamp & Childress, 2009, p. 103). Autonomy has become a prominent principle in health care ethics; the right to make a determination regarding care decisions that directly impact the life of the service recipient should reside with that individual. The principle of autonomy and confidentiality also applies to students in an educational program, to participants in research studies, and to the public who seek information about occupational therapy services.

Occupational Therapy Personnel Shall

A. Establish a collaborative relationship with recipients of service, including families, significant others, and caregivers in setting goals and priorities throughout the intervention process. This includes full disclosure of the benefits, risks, and potential outcomes of any intervention; the personnel who will be providing the intervention(s); and/or any reasonable alternatives to the proposed intervention.

B. Obtain consent before administering any occupational therapy service, including evaluation, and ensure that recipients of service (or their legal representatives) are kept informed of the progress in meeting goals specified in the plan of intervention/care. If the service recipient cannot give consent, the practitioner must be sure that consent has been obtained from the person who is legally responsible for that recipient.

C. Respect the recipient of service's right to refuse occupational therapy services temporarily or permanently without negative consequences.

D. Provide students with access to accurate information regarding educational requirements and academic policies and procedures relative to the occupational therapy program/educational institution.

E. Obtain informed consent from participants involved in research activities, and ensure that they understand the benefits, risks, and potential outcomes as a result of their participation as research subjects.

F. Respect research participant's right to withdraw from a research study without consequences.

G. Ensure that confidentiality and the right to privacy are respected and maintained regarding all information obtained about recipients of service, students, research participants, colleagues, or employees. The only exceptions are when a practitioner or staff member believes that an individual is in serious foreseeable or imminent harm. Laws and regulations may require disclosure to appropriate authorities without consent.

H. Maintain the confidentiality of all verbal, written, electronic, augmentative, and nonverbal communications, including compliance with HIPAA regulations.

I. Take appropriate steps to facilitate meaningful communication and comprehension in cases in which the recipient of service, student, or research participant has limited ability to communicate (e.g., aphasia or differences in language, literacy, or culture).

J. Make every effort to facilitate open and collaborative dialogue with clients and/or responsible parties to facilitate comprehension of services and their potential risks/benefits.

Social Justice

Principle 4. Occupational Therapy Personnel Shall Provide Services in a Fair and Equitable Manner.

Social justice, also called *distributive justice*, refers to the fair, equitable, and appropriate distribution of resources. The principle of social justice refers broadly to the distribution of all rights and responsibilities in society (Beauchamp & Childress, 2009). In general, the principle of social justice supports the concept of achieving justice in every aspect of society rather than merely the administration of law. The general idea is that individuals and groups should receive fair treatment and an impartial share of the benefits of society. Occupational therapy personnel have a vested interest in addressing unjust inequities that limit opportunities for participation in society (Braveman & Bass-Haugen, 2009). While opinions differ regarding the most ethical approach to addressing the distribution of health care resources and the reduction of health disparities, the issue of social justice continues to focus on limiting the impact of social inequality on health outcomes.

Occupational Therapy Personnel Shall

A. Uphold the profession's altruistic responsibilities to help ensure the common good.

B. Take responsibility for educating the public and society about the value of occupational therapy services in promoting health and wellness and reducing the impact of disease and disability.

C. Make every effort to promote activities that benefit the health status of the community.

D. Advocate for just and fair treatment for all patients, clients, employees, and colleagues, and encourage employers and colleagues to abide by the highest standards of social justice and the ethical standards set forth by the occupational therapy profession.

E. Make efforts to advocate for recipients of occupational therapy services to obtain needed services through available means.

F. Provide services that reflect an understanding of how occupational therapy service delivery can be affected by factors such as economic status, age, ethnicity, race, geography, disability, marital status, sexual orientation, gender, gender identity, religion, culture, and political affiliation.

G. Consider offering *pro bono* ("for the good") or reduced-fee occupational therapy services for selected individuals when consistent with guidelines of the employer, third-party payer, and/or government agency.

Procedural Justice

Principle 5. Occupational Therapy Personnel Shall Comply with Institutional Rules, Local, State, Federal, and International Laws and AOTA Documents Applicable to the Profession of Occupational Therapy.

Procedural justice is concerned with making and implementing decisions according to fair processes that ensure "fair treatment" (Maiese, 2004). Rules must be impartially followed and consistently applied to generate an unbiased decision. The principle of procedural justice is based on the concept that procedures and processes are organized in a fair manner and that policies, regulations, and laws are followed. While *the law* and *ethics* are not synonymous terms, occupational therapy personnel have an ethical responsibility to uphold current reimbursement regulations and state/territorial laws governing the profession. In addition, occupational therapy personnel are ethically bound to be aware of organizational policies and practice guidelines set forth by regulatory agencies established to protect recipients of service, research participants, and the public.

Occupational Therapy Personnel Shall

A. Be familiar with and apply the Code and Ethics Standards to the work setting, and share them with employers, other employees, colleagues, students, and researchers.

B. Be familiar with and seek to understand and abide by institutional rules, and when those rules conflict with ethical practice, take steps to resolve the conflict.

C. Be familiar with revisions in those laws and AOTA policies that apply to the profession of occupational therapy and inform employers, employees, colleagues, students, and researchers of those changes.

D. Be familiar with established policies and procedures for handling concerns about the Code and Ethics Standards, including familiarity with national, state, local, district, and territorial procedures for handling ethics complaints as well as policies and procedures created by AOTA and certification, licensing, and regulatory agencies.

E. Hold appropriate national, state, or other requisite credentials for the occupational therapy services they provide.

F. Take responsibility for maintaining high standards and continuing competence in practice, education, and research by participating in professional development and educational activities to improve and update knowledge and skills.

G. Ensure that all duties assumed by or assigned to other occupational therapy personnel match credentials, qualifications, experience, and scope of practice.

H. Provide appropriate supervision to individuals for whom they have supervisory responsibility in accordance with AOTA official documents and local, state, and federal or national laws, rules, regulations, policies, procedures, standards, and guidelines.

I. Obtain all necessary approvals prior to initiating research activities.

J. Report all gifts and remuneration from individuals, agencies, or companies in accordance with employer policies as well as state and federal guidelines.

K. Use funds for intended purposes, and avoid misappropriation of funds.

L. Take reasonable steps to ensure that employers are aware of occupational therapy's ethical obligations as set forth in this Code and Ethics Standards and of the implications of those obligations for occupational therapy practice, education, and research.

M. Actively work with employers to prevent discrimination and unfair labor practices, and advocate for employees with disabilities to ensure the provision of reasonable accommodations.

N. Actively participate with employers in the formulation of policies and procedures to ensure legal, regulatory, and ethical compliance.

O. Collect fees legally. Fees shall be fair, reasonable, and commensurate with services delivered. Fee schedules must be available and equitable regardless of actual payer reimbursements/contracts.

P. Maintain the ethical principles and standards of the profession when participating in a business arrangement as owner, stockholder, partner, or employee, and refrain from working for or doing business with organizations that engage in illegal or unethical business practices (e.g., fraudulent billing, providing occupational therapy services beyond the scope of occupational therapy practice).

Veracity

Principle 6. Occupational Therapy Personnel Shall Provide Comprehensive, Accurate, and Objective Information When Representing the Profession.

Veracity is based on the virtues of truthfulness, candor, and honesty. The principle of *veracity* in health care refers to comprehensive, accurate, and objective transmission of information and includes fostering the client's understanding of such information (Beauchamp & Childress, 2009). Veracity is based on respect owed to others. In communicating with others, occupational therapy personnel implicitly promise to speak truthfully and not deceive the listener. By entering into a relationship in care or research, the recipient of service or research participant enters into a contract that includes a right to truthful information (Beauchamp & Childress,

2009). In addition, the transmission of information is incomplete without also ensuring that the recipient or participant understands the information provided. Concepts of veracity must be carefully balanced with other potentially competing ethical principles, cultural beliefs, and organizational policies. Veracity ultimately is valued as a means to establish trust and strengthen professional relationships. Therefore, adherence to the principle also requires thoughtful analysis of how full disclosure of information may impact outcomes.

Occupational Therapy Personnel Shall

A. Represent the credentials, qualifications, education, experience, training, roles, duties, competence, views, contributions, and findings accurately in all forms of communication about recipients of service, students, employees, research participants, and colleagues.

B. Refrain from using or participating in the use of any form of communication that contains false, fraudulent, deceptive, misleading, or unfair statements or claims.

C. Record and report in an accurate and timely manner, and in accordance with applicable regulations, all information related to professional activities.

D. Ensure that documentation for reimbursement purposes is done in accordance with applicable laws, guidelines, and regulations.

E. Accept responsibility for any action that reduces the public's trust in occupational therapy.

F. Ensure that all marketing and advertising are truthful, accurate, and carefully presented to avoid misleading recipients of service, students, research participants, or the public.

G. Describe the type and duration of occupational therapy services accurately in professional contracts, including the duties and responsibilities of all involved parties.

H. Be honest, fair, accurate, respectful, and timely in gathering and reporting fact-based information regarding employee job performance and student performance.

I. Give credit and recognition when using the work of others in written, oral, or electronic media.

J. Not plagiarize the work of others.

Fidelity

Principle 7. Occupational Therapy Personnel Shall Treat Colleagues and Other Professionals with Respect, Fairness, Discretion, and Integrity.

The principle of fidelity comes from the Latin root *fidelis* meaning loyal. *Fidelity* refers to being faithful, which includes obligations of loyalty and the keeping of promises and commitments (Veatch & Flack, 1997). In the health professions, fidelity refers to maintaining good-faith relationships between various service providers and recipients. While respecting fidelity requires occupational therapy personnel to meet the client's reasonable expectations (Purtillo, 2005), Principle 7 specifically addresses fidelity as it relates to maintaining collegial and organizational relationships. Professional relationships are greatly influenced by the complexity of the environment in which occupational therapy personnel work. Practitioners, educators, and researchers alike must consistently balance their duties to service recipients, students, research participants, and other professionals as well as to organizations that may influence decision-making and professional practice.

Occupational Therapy Personnel Shall

A. Respect the traditions, practices, competencies, and responsibilities of their own and other professions, as well as those of the institutions and agencies that constitute the working environment.

B. Preserve, respect, and safeguard private information about employees, colleagues, and students unless otherwise mandated by national, state, or local laws or permission to disclose is given by the individual.

C. Take adequate measures to discourage, prevent, expose, and correct any breaches of the Code and Ethics Standards and report any breaches of the former to the appropriate authorities.

D. Attempt to resolve perceived institutional violations of the Code and Ethics Standards by utilizing internal resources first.

E. Avoid conflicts of interest or conflicts of commitment in employment, volunteer roles, or research.

F. Avoid using one's position (employee or volunteer) or knowledge gained from that position in such a manner that gives rise to real or perceived conflict of interest among the person, the employer, other Association members, and/or other organizations.

G. Use conflict resolution and/or alternative dispute resolution resources to resolve organizational and interpersonal conflicts.

H. Be diligent stewards of human, financial, and material resources of their employers, and refrain from exploiting these resources for personal gain.

References

American Occupational Therapy Association: Core values and attitudes of occupational therapy practice, *Am J Occup Ther* 47:1085–1086, 1993.

American Occupational Therapy Association: Occupational therapy code of ethics (2005), *Am J Occup Ther* 59:639–642, 2005.

American Occupational Therapy Association: Guidelines to the occupational therapy code of ethics, *Am J Occup Ther* 60:652–658, 2006.

American Occupational Therapy Association: Policy 5.3.1: definition of occupational therapy practice for state regulation, *Am J Occup Ther* 58:694–695, 2004.

Beauchamp TL, Childress JF: *Principles of Biomedical Ethics*, ed 6, New York, 2009, Oxford University Press.

Braveman B, Bass-Haugen JD: Social justice and health disparities: an evolving discourse in occupational therapy research and intervention, *Am J Occup Ther* 63:7–12, 2009.

Maiese M: *Procedural justice*, 2004. Retrieved July 29, 2009, from http://www.beyondintractability.org/essay/procedural_justice/.

Purtillo R: *Ethical Dimensions in the Health Professions*, ed 4, Philadelphia, 2005, Elsevier/Saunders.

Veatch RM, Flack HE: *Case Studies in Allied Health Ethics*, Upper Saddle River, NJ, 1997, Prentice-Hall.

Authors

Ethics Commission (EC):

Kathlyn Reed, PhD, OTR, FAOTA, MLIS, *Chairperson*

Barbara Hemphill, DMin, OTR, FAOTA, FMOTA, *Chair-Elect*

Ann Moodey Ashe, MHS, OTR/L

Lea C. Brandt, OTD, MA, OTR/L

Joanne Estes, MS, OTR/L

Loretta Jean Foster, MS, COTA/L

Donna F. Homenko, RDH, PhD

Craig R. Jackson, JD, MSW

Deborah Yarett Slater, MS, OT/L, FAOTA, *Staff Liaison*

Adopted by the Representative Assembly 2010CApr17.

Note. This document replaces the following rescinded Ethics documents 2010CApril18: the Occupational Therapy Code of Ethics (2005) (*American Journal of Occupational Therapy*, 59, 639–642); the Guidelines to the Occupational Therapy Code of Ethics (*American Journal of Occupational Therapy*, 60, 652–658); and the Core Values and Attitudes of Occupational Therapy Practice (*American Journal of Occupational Therapy*, 47, 1085–1086).

APPENDIX **B**   Standards of Practice for Occupational Therapy

This document defines minimum standards for the practice of occupational therapy. The practice of occupational therapy means the therapeutic use of everyday life activities (occupations) with individuals, groups, organizations, and populations for the purpose of participation in roles and situations in the home, school, workplace, community, or other settings. Occupational therapy services are provided for the purpose of promoting health and wellness and to those who have or are at risk for developing an illness, injury, disease, disorder, condition, impairment, disability, activity limitation, or participation restriction. Occupational therapy addresses physical, cognitive, psychosocial, sensory, communication, and other areas of performance in various contexts and environments in everyday life activities that affect health, well-being, and quality of life (American Occupational Therapy Association [AOTA], 2004). The overarching goal of occupational therapy is "to support [people's] health and participation in life through engagement in occupations" (AOTAa, 2008, p. 626).

The *Standards of Practice for Occupational Therapy* are requirements for occupational therapists and occupational therapy assistants for the delivery of occupational therapy services. *The Reference Manual of Official Documents of the American Occupational Therapy Association, Inc.* (current version as of press time, AOTA, 2010) contains documents that clarify and support occupational therapy practice, as do various issues of the *American Journal of Occupational Therapy.* These documents are reviewed and updated on an ongoing basis for their applicability.

Education, Examination, and Licensure Requirements

All occupational therapists and occupational therapy assistants must practice under federal and state law. To practice as an occupational therapist, the individual trained in the United States

- Has graduated from an occupational therapy program accredited by the Accreditation Council for Occupational Therapy Education (ACOTE®) or predecessor organizations.
- Has successfully completed a period of supervised fieldwork experience required by the recognized educational institution where the applicant met the academic requirements of an educational program for occupational therapists that is accredited by ACOTE or predecessor organizations.
- Has passed a nationally recognized entry-level examination for occupational therapists.
- Fulfills state requirements for licensure, certification, or registration.

To practice as an occupational therapy assistant, the individual trained in the United States

- Has graduated from an occupational therapy assistant program accredited by ACOTE or predecessor organizations.
- Has successfully completed a period of supervised fieldwork experience required by the recognized educational institution where the applicant met the academic requirements of an educational program for occupational therapy assistants that is accredited by ACOTE or predecessor organizations.
- Has passed a nationally recognized entry-level examination for occupational therapy assistants.
- Fulfills state requirements for licensure, certification, or registration.

Definitions

The following definitions are used in this document:

- **Activity (Activities):** A class of human behaviors that are goal-directed.
- **Assessment:** Specific tools or instruments that are used during the evaluation process.
- **Client:** The entity that receives occupational therapy services. Clients may include (1) individuals and other persons relevant to the individual's life, such as family, caregivers, teachers, employers, and others who also may help or be served indirectly; (2) organizations such as business, industry, or agencies; and (3) populations within a community (Moyers & Dale, 2007).
- **Evaluation:** The process of obtaining and interpreting data necessary for intervention. This includes planning for and documenting the evaluation process and results.
- **Intervention:** The process and skilled actions taken by occupational therapy practitioners in collaboration with the client to facilitate engagement in occupation related to health and participation. The intervention process includes the plan, implementation, and review.

- **Occupation:** "Goal-directed pursuits that typically extend over time, have meaning to their performance, and involve multiple tasks" (Christiansen, Baum, & Bass-Haugen, 2005, p. 548); "all the things that people want, need, or have to do, whether of a physical, mental, social, sexual, political, spiritual, or any other nature, including sleep and rest activities" (Wilcock & Townsend, 2009, p. 193); "activities of everyday life named, organized, and given meaning by individuals and a culture" (Law, Polatajko, Baptiste, & Townsend, 1997, p. 32).

- **Outcomes:** What occupational therapy actually achieves for the client. Changes desired by the client that can focus on any area of the client's occupational performance.

- **Reevaluation:** The process of critical analysis of client response to intervention. This analysis enables the therapist to make any necessary changes to an intervention plan in collaboration with the client.

- **Screening:** Obtaining and reviewing data relevant to a potential client to determine the need for further evaluation and intervention.

- **Transitions:** "Actions coordinated to prepare for or facilitate a change, such as from one functional level to another, from one life [change] to another, from one program to another, or from one environment to another" (AOTA, 1998, p. 866).

Standard I. Professional Standing and Responsibility

1. An occupational therapy practitioner (occupational therapist or occupational therapy assistant) delivers occupational therapy services that reflect the philosophical base of occupational therapy and are consistent with the established principles and concepts of theory and practice.

2. An occupational therapy practitioner is knowledgeable about and delivers occupational therapy services in accordance with AOTA standards, policies, and guidelines and state, federal, and other regulatory and payer requirements relevant to practice and service delivery.

3. An occupational therapy practitioner maintains current licensure, registration, or certification as required by law or regulation.

4. An occupational therapy practitioner abides by the *Occupational Therapy Code of Ethics* (AOTA, 2005a).

5. An occupational therapy practitioner abides by the *Standards for Continuing Competence* (AOTA, 2005b) by establishing, maintaining, and updating professional performance, knowledge, and skills.

6. An occupational therapist is responsible for all aspects of occupational therapy service delivery and is accountable for the safety and effectiveness of the occupational therapy service delivery process (AOTA, 2009).

7. An occupational therapy assistant is responsible for providing safe and effective occupational therapy services under the supervision of and in partnership with the occupational therapist and in accordance with laws or regulations and AOTA documents (AOTA, 2009).

8. An occupational therapy practitioner maintains current knowledge of legislative, political, social, cultural, societal, and reimbursement issues that affect clients and the practice of occupational therapy.

9. An occupational therapy practitioner is knowledgeable about evidence-based research and applies it ethically and appropriately to provide occupational therapy services consistent with best practice approaches.

10. An occupational therapy practitioner respects the client's sociocultural background and provides client-centered and family-centered occupational therapy services.

Standard II. Screening, Evaluation, and Reevaluation

1. An occupational therapist is responsible for all aspects of the screening, evaluation, and reevaluation process.

2. An occupational therapist accepts and responds to referrals in compliance with state or federal laws, other regulatory and payer requirements, and AOTA documents.

3. An occupational therapist, in collaboration with the client, evaluates the client's ability to participate in daily life by considering the client's history, goals, capacities, and needs; the activities and occupations the client wants and needs to perform; and the environments and context in which these activities and occupations occur.

4. An occupational therapist initiates and directs the screening, evaluation, and reevaluation process and analyzes and interprets the data in accordance with federal and state law, other regulatory and payer requirements, and AOTA documents.

5. An occupational therapy assistant contributes to the screening, evaluation, and reevaluation process by implementing delegated assessments and by providing verbal and written reports of observations and client capacities to the occupational therapist in accordance with federal and state laws, other regulatory and payer requirements, and AOTA documents.

6. An occupational therapy practitioner uses current assessments and assessment procedures and follows defined protocols of standardized assessments during the screening, evaluation, and reevaluation process.

7. An occupational therapist completes and documents occupational therapy evaluation results. An occupational therapy assistant contributes to the documentation of evaluation results. An occupational therapy practitioner abides by the time frames, formats, and standards established by practice settings, federal and state law, other regulatory and payer requirements, external accreditation programs, and AOTA documents.

8. An occupational therapy practitioner communicates screening, evaluation, and reevaluation results within the boundaries of client confidentiality and privacy regulations to the appropriate person, group, organization, or population.

9. An occupational therapist recommends additional consultations or refers clients to appropriate resources when the needs of the client can best be served by the expertise of other professionals or services.

10. An occupational therapy practitioner educates current and potential referral sources about the scope of occupational therapy services and the process of initiating occupational therapy services.

Standard III. Intervention

1. An occupational therapist has overall responsibility for the development, documentation, and implementation of the occupational therapy intervention based on the evaluation, client goals, best available evidence, and professional and clinical reasoning.
2. An occupational therapist ensures that the intervention plan is documented within the time frames, formats, and standards established by the practice settings, agencies, external accreditation programs, state and federal law, and other regulatory and payer requirements.
3. An occupational therapy practitioner collaborates with the client to develop and implement the intervention plan, on the basis of the client's needs and priorities, safety issues, and relative benefits and risks of the interventions.
4. An occupational therapy practitioner coordinates the development and implementation of the occupational therapy intervention with the intervention provided by other professionals, when appropriate.
5. An occupational therapy practitioner uses professional and clinical reasoning to select the most appropriate types of interventions, including therapeutic use of self, therapeutic use of occupations and activities, consultation, education, and advocacy.
6. An occupational therapy assistant selects, implements, and makes modifications to therapeutic interventions that are consistent with the occupational therapy assistant's demonstrated competency and delegated responsibilities, the intervention plan, and requirements of the practice setting.
7. An occupational therapist modifies the intervention plan throughout the intervention process and documents changes in the client's needs, goals, and performance.
8. An occupational therapy assistant contributes to the modification of the intervention plan by exchanging information with and providing documentation to the occupational therapist about the client's responses to and communications throughout the intervention.
9. An occupational therapy practitioner documents the occupational therapy services provided within the time frames, formats, and standards established by the practice settings, agencies, external accreditation programs, federal and state laws, other regulatory and payer requirements, and AOTA documents.

Standard IV. Outcomes

1. An occupational therapist is responsible for selecting, measuring, documenting, and interpreting expected or achieved outcomes that are related to the client's ability to engage in occupations.

2. An occupational therapist is responsible for documenting changes in the client's performance and capacities and for transitioning the client to other types or intensity of service or discontinuing services when the client has achieved identified goals, reached maximum benefit, or does not desire to continue services.
3. An occupational therapist prepares and implements a transition or discontinuation plan based on the client's needs, goals, performance, and appropriate follow-up resources.
4. An occupational therapy assistant contributes to the transition or discontinuation plan by providing information and documentation to the supervising occupational therapist related to the client's needs, goals, performance, and appropriate follow-up resources.
5. An occupational therapy practitioner facilitates the transition or discharge process in collaboration with the client, family members, significant others, other professionals (e.g., medical, educational, or social services), and community resources, when appropriate.
6. An occupational therapist is responsible for evaluating the safety and effectiveness of the occupational therapy processes and interventions within the practice setting.
7. An occupational therapy assistant contributes to evaluating the safety and effectiveness of the occupational therapy processes and interventions within the practice setting.

References

American Occupational Therapy Association: Standards of practice, *Am J Occup Ther* 52:866–869, 1998.

American Occupational Therapy Association: Policy 5.3.1: definition of occupational therapy practice for state regulation, *Am J Occup Ther* 58:694–695, 2004.

American Occupational Therapy Association: Occupational therapy code of ethics (2005), *Am J Occup Ther* 59:639–642, 2005a.

American Occupational Therapy Association: Standards for continuing competence, *Am J Occup Ther* 59:661–662, 2005b.

American Occupational Therapy Association: Occupational therapy practice framework: domain and process, ed 2, *Am J Occup Ther* 62:625–683, 2008.

American Occupational Therapy Association: Guidelines for supervision, roles, and responsibilities during the delivery of occupational therapy services, *Am J Occup Ther* 63:173–179, 2009.

American Occupational Therapy Association: *The Reference Manual of the Official Documents of the American Occupational Therapy Association, Inc.*, ed 15, Bethesda, MD, 2010, AOTA Press.

Christiansen C, Baum MC, Bass-Haugen J, editors: *Occupational Therapy: Performance, Participation, and Well-Being*, Thorofare, NJ, 2005, Slack.

Law M, Polatajko H, Baptiste W, et al: Core concepts of occupational therapy. In Townsend E, editor: *Enabling Occupation: An Occupational Therapy Perspective*, Ottawa, ON, 1997, Canadian Association of Occupational Therapists, pp 29–56.

Moyers PA, Dale LM: *The Guide to Occupational Therapy Practice*, ed 2, Bethesda, MD, 2007, AOTA Press.

Wilcock AA, Townsend EA: Occupational justice. In Crepeau E, Cohn E, Schell B, editors: *Willard and Spackman's Occupational Therapy*, ed 11, Philadelphia, 2009, Lippincott Williams & Wilkins, pp 192–215.

Authors

The Commission on Practice
  Janet V. DeLany, DEd, OTR/L, FAOTA, *Chairperson*
  Debbie Amini, MEd, OTR/L, CHT
  Ellen Cohn, ScD, OTR/L, FAOTA
  Jennifer Cruz, MAT, MOTS, *ASD Liaison*
  Kimberly Hartmann, PhD, OTR/L, FAOTA, *SISC Liaison*
  Jeanette Justice, COTA/L
  Kathleen Kannenberg, MA, OTR/L, CCM
  Cherylin Lew, OTD, OTR/L
  James Marc-Aurele, MBA, OTR/L
  Mary Jane Youngstrom, MS, OTR, FAOTA
  Deborah Lieberman, MHSA, OTR/L, FAOTA, AOTA *Headquarters Liaison* for The Commission on Practice

The COP wishes to acknowledge the authors of the 2005 edition of this document: Sara Jane Brayman, PhD, OTR/L, FAOTA, *Chairperson;* Susanne Smith Roley, MS, OTR/L, FAOTA, *Chairperson-Elect;* Gloria Frolek Clark, MS, OTR/L, FAOTA; Janet V. DeLany, DEd, MSA, OTR/L, FAOTA; Eileen R. Garza, PhD, OTR, ATP; Mary V. Radomski, MA, OTR/L, FAOTA; Ruth Ramsey, MS, OTR/L; Carol Siebert, MS, OTR/L; Kristi Voelkerding, BS, COTA/L; Lenna Aird, COTA/L, *ASD Liaison;* Patricia D. LaVesser, PhD, OTR/L, *SIS Liaison;* and Deborah Lieberman, MHSA, OTR/L, FAOTA, *AOTA Headquarters Liaison.*

Adopted by the Representative Assembly Coordinating Council (RACC) for the Representative Assembly

Revised by the Commission on Practice 2010

Note: This revision replaces the 2005 document *Standards of Practice for Occupational Therapy* (previously published and copyrighted in 2005 by the American Occupational Therapy Association in the *American Journal of Occupational Therapy,* 59, 663–665).

Note. These standards are intended as recommended guidelines to assist occupational therapy practitioners in the provision of occupational therapy services. These standards serve as a minimum standard for occupational therapy practice and are applicable to all individual populations and the programs in which these individuals are served.

From American Occupational Therapy Association: Standards of practice for occupational therapy, *Am J Occup Ther* 64, 2010.

APPENDIX C Key Information from the Occupational Therapy Practice Framework

All aspects of the domain transact to support engagement, participation, and health. This figure does not imply a hierarchy.

Figure C-1 Aspects of Occupational Therapy's Domain

Areas of Occupations	Client Factors	Performance Skills	Performance Patterns	Context and Environment	Activity Demands
Activities of Daily Living (ADL)*	Values, Beliefs, and Spirituality	Sensory Perceptual Skills	Habits	Cultural	Objects Used and their Properties
Instrumental Activities of Daily Living (IADL)	Body Functions	Motor and Praxis Skills	Routines	Personal	Space Demands
Rest and Sleep	Body Structures	Emotional Regulation Skills	Roles	Physical	Social Demands
Education		Cognitive Skills	Rituals	Social	Sequencing and Timing
Work		Communication and Social Skills		Temporal	Required Actions
Play				Virtual	Required Body Functions
Leisure					Required Body Structures
Social Participation					

*Also referred to as basic activities of daily living (BADL) or personal activities of daily living (PADL).

Table C-1 Areas of Occupation

Areas of Occupation	Examples
Activities of daily living (ADL)	Bathing, showering Bowel and bladder management Dressing Eating Feeding Functional mobility Personal device care Personal hygiene and grooming Sexual activity Toilet hygiene
Instrumental activities of daily living (IADL)	Care of others (including selecting and supervising caregivers) Care of pets Child rearing Communication management Community mobility Financial management Health management and maintenance Home establishment and management Meal preparation and cleanup Religious observance Safety procedures and emergency response Shopping

Table C-1 Areas of Occupation—Cont'd

Areas of Occupation	Examples
Rest and sleep	Rest Sleep Sleep participation Sleep preparation
Education	Formal education participation Informal personal educational needs or interests exploration (beyond formal education) Informal personal education participation
Work	Employment interests and pursuits Employment seeking and acquisition Job performance Retirement preparation and adjustment Volunteer exploration Volunteer participation
Play	Play exploration Play participation
Leisure	Leisure exploration Leisure participation
Social participation	Community Family Peer, friend

Table C-2 Performance Skills

Skill	Definition	Examples
Motor and praxis skills	Motor: Actions or behaviors a client uses to move and physically interact with tasks, objects, contexts, and environments (adapted from Fisher, 2006). Includes planning, sequencing, and executing new and novel movements. Praxis: Skilled purposeful movements (Heilman & Rothi, 1993). Ability to carry out sequential motor acts as part of an overall plan rather than individual acts (Liepmann, 1920). Ability to carry out learned motor activity, including following through on a verbal command, visual-spatial construction, ocular and oral-motor skills, imitation of a person or an object, and sequencing actions (Ayres, 1985; Filley, 2001). Organization of temporal sequences of actions within the spatial context which form meaningful occupations (Blanche & Parham, 2002).	• *Bending* and reaching for a toy or tool in a storage bin • *Pacing* tempo of movements to clean the room • *Coordinating* body movements to complete a job task • *Maintaining* balance while walking on an uneven surface or while showering • *Anticipating* or adjusting posture and body position in response to environmental circumstances, such as obstacles • *Manipulating* keys or lock to open the door
Sensory-perceptual skills	Actions or behaviors a client uses to locate, identify, and respond to sensations and to select, interpret, associate, organize, and remember sensory events based on discriminating experiences through a variety of sensations that include visual, auditory, proprioceptive, tactile, olfactory, gustatory, and vestibular.	• *Positioning the body* in exact location for a safe jump • *Hearing and locating* the voice of your child in a crowd • *Visually determining* the correct size of a storage container for leftover soup • *Locating* keys by touch from many objects in a pocket or purse (i.e., stereognosis) • *Timing* the appropriate moment to cross the street safely by determining one's own position and speed relative to the speed of traffic • *Discerning* distinct flavors within foods or beverages

(Continued)

Table C-2 Performance Skills—Cont'd

Skill	Definition	Examples
Emotional regulation skills	Actions or behaviors a client uses to identify, manage, and express feelings while engaging in activities or interacting with others	• *Responding* to the feelings of others by acknowledgment or showing support • *Persisting* in a task despite frustrations • *Controlling* anger toward others and reducing aggressive acts • *Recovering* from a hurt or disappointment without lashing out at others • *Displaying* the emotions that are appropriate for the situation • *Utilizing* relaxation strategies to cope with stressful events
Cognitive skills	Actions or behaviors a client uses to plan and manage the performance of an activity	• *Judging* the importance of appropriateness of clothes for the circumstance • *Selecting* tools and supplies needed to clean the bathroom • *Sequencing* tasks needed for a school project • *Organizing* activities within the time required to meet a deadline • *Prioritizing* steps and identifying solutions to access transportation • *Creating* different activities with friends that are fun, novel, and enjoyable • *Multitasking*–doing more than one thing at a time, necessary for tasks such as work, driving, and household management
Communication and social skills	Actions or behaviors a person uses to communicate and interact with others in an interactive environment (Fisher, 2006)	• *Looking* where someone else is pointing or gazing • *Gesturing* to emphasize intentions • *Maintaining* acceptable physical space during conversation • *Initiating* and answering questions with relevant information • *Taking turns* during an interchange with another person verbally and physically • *Acknowledging* another person's perspective during an interchange

Table C-3 Performance Patterns

Person	Examples
HABITS—"Automatic behavior that is integrated into more complex patterns that enable people to function on a day-to-day basis" (Neistadt & Crepeau, 1998, p. 869). Habits can be useful, dominating, or impoverished and either support or interfere with performance in areas of occupation.	• Automatically puts car keys in the same place • Spontaneously looks both ways before crossing the street • Repeatedly rocks back and forth when asked to initiate a task • Repeatedly activates and deactivates the alarm system before entering the home • Maintains the exact distance between all hangers when hanging clothes in a closet

Table C-3 Performance Patterns—Cont'd

Person	Examples
ROUTINES—Patterns of behavior that are observable, regular, repetitive, and that provide structure for daily life. They can be satisfying, promoting, or damaging. Routines require momentary time commitment and are embedded in cultural and ecological contexts (Fiese et al., 2002; Segal, 2004).	• Follows the morning sequence to complete toileting, bathing, hygiene, and dressing • Follows the sequence of steps involved in meal preparation
RITUALS—Symbolic actions with spiritual, cultural, or social meaning, contributing to the client's identity and reinforcing values and beliefs. Rituals have a strong affective component and represent a collection of events (Fiese et al., 2002; Segal, 2004).	• Uses the inherited antique hairbrush and brushes hair with 100 strokes nightly as her mother had done • Prepares the holiday meals with favorite or traditional accoutrements, using designated dishware • Kisses a sacred book before opening pages to read
ROLES—A set of behaviors expected by society, shaped by culture, and may be further conceptualized and defined by the client.	• Mother of an adolescent with developmental disabilities • Student with learning disability studying computer technology • Corporate executive returning to work after experiencing a stroke

Organization

ROUTINES—Patterns of behavior that are observable, regular, repetitive, and that provide structure for daily life. They can be satisfying, promoting, or damaging. Routines require momentary time commitment and are embedded in cultural and ecological contexts (Fiese et al., 2002; Segal, 2004).	• Holds regularly scheduled meetings for staff, directors, executive boards • Follows documentation practices for annual reports, timecards, and strategic plans • Turns in documentation on a scheduled basis • Follows the chain of command • Follows safety and security routine (e.g., signing in/out, using pass codes) • Maintains dress codes (e.g., casual Fridays) • Socializes during breaks, lunch, at the water cooler • Follows beginning or ending routines (e.g., opening/closing the facility) • Offers activities to meet performance expectations or standards
RITUALS—Symbolic actions that have meaning, contributing to the organization's identity and reinforcing values and beliefs (adapted from Fiese et al., 2002; Segal, 2004).	• Holds holiday parties, company picnics • Conducts induction, recognition, and retirement ceremonies • Organizes annual retreats or conferences • Maintains fundraising activities for organization to support local charities
ROLES—A set of behaviors by the organization expected by society, shaped by culture, and may be further conceptualized and defined by the client.	• Nonprofit organization provides housing for persons living with mental illness • Humanitarian organization distributes food and clothing donations to refugees • University educates and provides service to the surrounding community

Population

ROUTINES—Patterns of behavior that are observable, regular, repetitive, and that provide structure for daily life. They can be satisfying, promoting, or damaging. Routines require momentary time commitment and are embedded in cultural and ecological contexts (Fiese et al., 2002; Segal, 2004).	• Follows health practices, such as scheduled immunizations for children and yearly health screenings for adults • Follows business practices, such as provision of services for the disadvantaged populations (e.g., loans to underrepresented groups) • Follows legislative procedures, such as those associated with IDEA and Medicare • Follows social customs for greeting
RITUALS—Rituals are shared social actions with traditional, emotional, purposive, and technological meaning, contributing to values and beliefs within the population.	• Holds cultural celebrations • Has parades or demonstrations • Shows national affiliations/allegiances • Follows religious, spiritual, and cultural practices, such as touching the mezuzah or using holy water when leaving/entering, praying to Mecca
ROLES	• See description of these areas for individuals within the population.

Table C-4 **Activity Demands**

Activity Demand Aspects	Definition	Examples
Objects and their properties	Tools, materials, and equipment used in the process of carrying out the activity	• Tools (e.g., scissors, dishes, shoes, volleyball) • Materials (e.g., paints, milk, lipstick) • Equipment (e.g., workbench, stove, basketball hoop) • Inherent properties (e.g., heavy, rough, sharp, colorful, loud, bitter tasting)
Space demands (relates to physical context)	Physical environmental requirements of the activity (e.g., size, arrangement, surface, lighting, temperature, noise, humidity, ventilation)	• Large, open space outdoors required for a baseball game • Bathroom door and stall width to accommodate wheelchair • Noise, lighting, and temperature controls for a library
Social demands (relates to social environment and cultural contexts)	Social environment and cultural contexts that may be required by the activity	• Rules of game • Expectations of other participants in activity (e.g., sharing supplies, using language appropriate for the meeting)
Sequence and timing	Process used to carry out the activity (e.g., specific steps, sequence, timing requirements)	• *Steps to make tea*: Gather cup and tea bag, heat water, pour water into cup, and so forth. • *Sequence*: Heat water before placing tea bag in water. • *Timing*: Leave tea bag to steep for 2 minutes. • *Steps to conduct a meeting*: Establish goals for meeting, arrange time and location for meeting, prepare meeting agenda, call meeting to order. • *Sequence*: Have people introduce themselves before beginning discussion of topic. • *Timing*: Allot sufficient time for discussion of topic and determination of action items.
Required actions and performance skills	The usual skills that would be required by any performer to carry out the activity. Sensory, perceptual, motor, praxis, emotional, cognitive, communication, and social performance skills should each be considered. The performance skills demanded by an activity will be correlated with the demands of the other activity aspects (e.g., objects, space)	• Feeling the heat of the stove • Gripping handlebar • Choosing the ceremonial clothes • Determining how to move limbs to control the car • Adjusting the tone of voice • Answering a question
Required body functions	"[P]hysiological functions of body systems (including psychological functions)" (WHO, 2001, p. 10) that are required to support the actions used to perform the activity	• Mobility of joints • Level of consciousness
Required body structures	"Anatomical parts of the body such as organs, limbs, and their components [that support body function]" (WHO, 2001, p. 10) that are required to perform the activity	• Number of hands • Number of eyes

Client factors include (1) values, beliefs, and spirituality; (2) body functions; and (3) body structures that reside within the client and may affect performance in areas of occupation.

Values, Beliefs, and Spirituality

Table C-5 Client Factors

Category and Definition	Examples
Values: Principles, standards, or qualities considered worthwhile or desirable by the client who holds them.	Person 1. Honesty with self and with others 2. Personal religious convictions 3. Commitment to family Organization 1. Obligation to serve the community 2. Fairness Population 1. Freedom of speech 2. Equal opportunities for all 3. Tolerance toward others
Beliefs: Cognitive content held as true.	Person 1. He or she is powerless to influence others 2. Hard work pays off Organization 1. Profits are more important than people 2. Achieving the mission of providing service can effect positive change in the world Population 1. People can influence government by voting 2. Accessibility is a right, not a privilege
Spirituality: The "personal quest for understanding answers to ultimate questions about life, about meaning, and the sacred" (Moyers & Dale, 2007, p. 28).	Person 1. Daily search for purpose and meaning in one's life 2. Guiding actions from a sense of value beyond the personal acquisition of wealth or fame Organization and Population (see "Person" examples related to individuals within an organization and population)

Body Functions

"[T]he physiological functions of body systems (including psychological functions)" (WHO, 2001, p. 10). The "Body Functions" section of the table below is organized according to the International Classification of Functioning, Disability, and Health (ICF) classifications. For fuller descriptions and definitions, refer to WHO (2001).

Categories	Body Functions Commonly Considered by Occupational Therapy Practitioners (Not Intended to Be an All-Inclusive List)
Mental functions (affective, cognitive, perceptual) *Specific mental functions* • Higher-level cognitive • Attention • Memory • Perception • Thought • Mental functions of sequencing complex movement • Emotional • Experience of self and time	Specific mental functions Judgment, concept formation, metacognition, cognitive flexibility, insight, attention, awareness Sustained, selective, and divided attention Short-term, long-term, and working memory Discrimination of sensations (e.g., auditory, tactile, visual, olfactory, gustatory, vestibular-proprioception), including multi-sensory processing, sensory memory, spatial, and temporal relationships (Calvert, Spence, & Stein, 2004) Recognition, categorization, generalization, awareness of reality, logical/coherent thought, and appropriate thought content Execution of learned movement patterns Coping and behavioral regulation (Schell, Cohn, & Crepeau, 2008) Body image, self-concept, self-esteem

(Continued)

Categories	Body Functions Commonly Considered by Occupational Therapy Practitioners (Not Intended to Be an All-Inclusive List)
Global mental functions	Global mental functions
• Consciousness	Level of arousal, level of consciousness
• Orientation	Orientation to person, place, time, self, and others
• Temperament and personality	Emotional stability
• Energy and drive	Motivation, impulse control, and appetite
• Sleep (physiological process)	
Sensory functions and pain	Sensory functions and pain
• Seeing and related functions, including visual acuity, visual stability, visual field functions	Detection/registration, modulation, and integration of sensations from the body and environment
	Visual awareness of environment at various distances
• Hearing functions	Tolerance of ambient sounds; awareness of location and distance of sounds such as an approaching car
• Vestibular functions	Sensation of securely moving against gravity
• Taste functions	Association of taste
• Smell functions	Association of smell
• Proprioceptive functions	Awareness of body position and space
• Touch functions	Comfort with the feeling of being touched by others or touching various textures such as food
• Pain (e.g., diffuse, dull, sharp, phantom)	Localizing pain
• Temperature and pressure	Thermal awareness
Neuromusculoskeletal and movement-related functions	Neuromusculoskeletal and movement-related functions
• Functions of joints and bones	Joint range of motion
• Joint mobility	Postural alignment (this refers to the physiological stability of the joint related to its structural integrity as compared to the motor skill of aligning the body while moving in relations to task objects)
• Joint stability	
• Muscle power	Strength
• Muscle tone	Degree of muscle tone (e.g., flaccidity, spasticity, fluctuating)
• Muscle endurance	Endurance
• Motor reflexes	Stretch, asymmetrical tonic neck, symmetrical tonic neck
• Involuntary movement reactions	Righting and supporting
• Control of voluntary movement	Eye-hand/foot coordination, bilateral integration, crossing the midline, fine- and gross-motor control, and oculomotor (e.g., saccades, pursuits, accommodation, binocularity)
• Gait patterns	Walking patterns and impairments such as asymmetric gait, stiff gait (*Note*: Gait patterns are considered in relation to how they affect ability to engage in occupations in daily life activities.)
Cardiovascular, hematological, immunological, and respiratory system function	Cardiovascular, hematological, immunological, and respiratory system function
• Cardiovascular system function	Blood pressure functions (hypertension, hypotension, postural hypotension), and heart rate
• Hematological and immunological system function	(Note: Occupational therapy practitioners have knowledge of these body functions and understand broadly the interaction that occurs between these functions to support health and participation in life through engagement in occupation. Some therapists may specialize in evaluating and intervening with a specific function as it is related to supporting performance and engagement in occupations and activities targeted for intervention.)
• Respiratory system function	
• Additional functions and sensations of the cardiovascular and respiratory systems	Rate, rhythm, and depth of respiration
	Physical endurance, aerobic capacity, stamina, and fatigability
Voice and speech functions	
• Voice functions	(Note: Occupational therapy practitioners have knowledge of these body functions and understand broadly the interaction that occurs between these functions to support health and participation in life through engagement in occupation. Some therapists may specialize in evaluating and intervening with a specific function, such as incontinence and pelvic floor disorders, as it is related to supporting performance and engagement in occupations and activities targeted for intervention.)
• Fluency and rhythm	
• Alternative vocalization functions	

Categories	Body Functions Commonly Considered by Occupational Therapy Practitioners (Not Intended to Be an All-Inclusive List)
Digestive, metabolic, and endocrine system function • Digestive system function • Metabolic system and endocrine system function	
Genitourinary and reproductive functions • Urinary functions • Genital and reproductive functions	
Skin and related-structure functions	Skin and related-structure functions
• Skin functions • Hair and nail functions	Protective functions of the skin—presence or absence of wounds, cuts, or abrasions Repair function of the skin—wound healing (Note: Occupational therapy practitioners have knowledge of these body functions and understand broadly the interaction that occurs between these functions to support health and participation in life through engagement in occupation. Some therapists may specialize in evaluating and intervening with a specific function as it is related to supporting performance and engagement in occupations and activities targeted for intervention.)

Body Structures

Body structures are "anatomical parts of the body, such as organs, limbs, and their components [that support body function]" (WHO, 2001, p. 10). The "Body Structures" section of the table below is organized according to the *ICF* classifications. For fuller descriptions and definitions, refer to WHO (2001).

Categories	Examples Are Not Delineated in the "Body Structure" Section of This Table
• Structure of the nervous system • Eyes, ear, and related structures • Structures involved in voice and speech • Structures of the cardiovascular, immunological, and respiratory systems • Structures related to the digestive, metabolic, and endocrine systems • Structure related to the genitourinary and reproductive systems • Structures related to movement • Skin and related structures	(*Note*: Occupational therapy practitioners have knowledge of body structures and understand broadly the interaction that occurs between these structures to support health and participation in life through engagement in occupation. Some therapists may specialize in evaluating and intervening with a specific structure as it is related to supporting performance and engagement in occupation and activities targeted for intervention.)

ICF, International Classification of Function, Disability and Health; OT, occupational therapist; *OTA,* occupational therapy assistant.
Note. Some data adapted from the ICF (WHO, 2001).

Table C-6 **Occupational Therapy Intervention Approaches**

Approach	Focus of Intervention	Examples
Create, promote (health promotion)[a]—An intervention approach that does not assume a disability is present or that any factors would interfere with performance. This approach is designed to provide enriched contextual and activity experiences that will enhance performance for all persons in the natural contexts of life (adapted from Dunn, McClain, Brown, & Youngstrom, 1998, p. 534).	Performance skills	• Create a parenting class to help first-time parents engage their children in developmentally appropriate play
	Performance patterns	• Promote effective handling of stress by creating time use routines with healthy clients
	Context or contexts or physical environments	• Promote a diversity of sensory play experiences by recommending a variety of equipment for playgrounds and other play areas
	Activity demands	• Serve food family style in the congregate dining area to increase the opportunities for socialization
	Client factors (body functions, body structures)	• Promote increased endurance by recommending year-round daily outdoor recess for all school children • Design a dance program for senior citizens that will enhance strength and flexibility
Establish, restore (remediation, restoration)[a]—An intervention approach designed to change client variables to establish a skill or ability that has not yet developed or to restore a skill or ability that has been impaired (adapted from Dunn et al., 1998, p. 533)	Performance skills	• Provide adjustable desk chairs to improve client sitting posture • Work with senior community centers to offer driving educational programs targeted at improving driving skills for persons ages 65 or older
	Performance patterns	• Collaborate with clients to help them establish morning routines needed to arrive at school or work on time • Provide classes in fatigue management for cancer patients and their families • Collaborate with clients to help them establish healthy sleep-wake patterns • Develop walking programs at the local mall for employees and community members
	Client factors (body functions, body structures)	• Support daily physical education classes for entire population of children in a school aimed at improving physical strength and endurance • Collaborate with schools and businesses to establish universal-design models in their buildings, classrooms, and so forth • Gradually increase time required to complete a computer game to increase client's attention span

Table C-6 Occupational Therapy Intervention Approaches—Cont'd

Approach	Focus of Intervention	Examples
Maintain—An intervention approach designed to provide the support that will allow clients to preserve the performance capabilities they have regained, that continue to meet their occupational needs, or both. The assumption is that, without continued maintenance intervention, occupational needs would not be met, or both, thereby affecting health and quality of life.	Performance skills	• Maintain the ability of the client to organize tools by providing a tool outline painted on a pegboard • Develop a refresher safety program for industrial organizations to remind workers of need to continue to use safety skills on the job • Provide a program for community-dwelling older adults to maintain motor and praxis skills
	Performance patterns	• Enable client to maintain appropriate medication schedule by providing a timer to aid with memory • Establish occupational performance patterns to maintain a healthy lifestyle after significant weight loss
	Context or contexts or physical environments	• Maintain safe and independent access for persons with low vision by recommending increased hallway lighting • During a natural disaster, work with facilities identified as "shelters" to provide play and leisure activities for displaced people to allow a constructive outlet and semblance of normalcy • Incorporate principles of universal design in homes to allow people to age in place
	Activity demands	• Maintain independent gardening for persons with arthritic hands by recommending tools with modified grips, long-handled tools, seating alternatives, raised gardens, and so forth
	Client factors (body functions, body structures)	• Provide multisensory activities in which nursing-home residents may participate to maintain alertness • Provide hand-based thumb splint for client use during periods of stressful or prolonged intensive activity to maintain pain-free joints
Modify (compensation, adaptation)[a]— An intervention approach directed at "finding ways to revise the current context or activity demands to support performance in the natural setting, [including] compensatory techniques, [such as]…enhancing some features to provide cues or reducing other features to reduce distractibility" (Dunn et al., 1998, p. 533).	Performance patterns	• Provide a visual schedule to help a student follow routines and transition easily between activities at home and school • Simplify task sequence to help a person with cognitive issues complete a morning self-care routine
	Context or contexts or physical environments	• Assist a family in determining requirements for building a ramp at home for a family member who is returning home after physical rehabilitation • Consult with builders in designing homes that will allow families the ability to provide living space for aging parents (e.g., bedroom and full bath on the main floor of a multilevel dwelling) • Modify the number of people in a room to decrease client's distractibility

(Continued)

Table C-6 Occupational Therapy Intervention Approaches—Cont'd

Approach	Focus of Intervention	Examples
	Activity demands	• Adapt writing surface used in classroom by fourth grader by adding adjustable incline board • Assist a patient with a terminal illness and his or her family in modifying tasks to maintain engagement • Consult with school teams on placement of switches to increase students' access to computers, augmentative communication devices, environmental devices, and so forth • Provide a seat at the assembly station to allow a client with decreased standing tolerance to be able to continue to perform
Prevent (disability prevention)[a]—An intervention approach designed to address clients with or without a disability who are at risk for occupational performance problems. This approach is designed to prevent the occurrence or evolution of barriers to performance in context. Interventions may be directed at client, context, or activity variables (adapted from Dunn et al., 1998, p. 534)	Performance skills	• Prevent poor posture when sitting for prolonged periods by providing a chair with proper back support
	Performance patterns	• Aid in the prevention of illicit chemical substance use by introducing self-initiated routine strategies that support drug-free behavior
	Context or contexts or physical environments	• Prevent social isolation of employees by promoting participation in after-work group activities • Reduce risk of falls by modifying the environment and removing known hazards in the home (e.g., throw rugs)
	Activity demands	• Prevent back injury by providing instruction in proper lifting techniques
	Client factors (body functions, body structures)	• Prevent repetitive stress injury by suggesting that clients wear a wrist support splint when typing • Consult with hotel chain to provide an ergonomics educational program designed to prevent back injuries in housekeepers

[a]Parallel language used in Moyers & Dale, 2007, p. 34.

Therapeutic Use of Self—An occupational therapy practitioner's planned use of his or her personality, insights, perceptions, and judgments as part of the therapeutic process (adapted from Punwar & Peloquin, 2000, p. 285).

   Therapeutic Use of Occupations and Activities[a]—Occupations and activities selected for specific clients that meet therapeutic goals. To use occupations/activities therapeutically, context or contexts, activity demands, and client factors all should be considered in relation to the client's therapeutic goals. Use of assistive technologies, application of universal-design principles, and environmental modifications support the ability of clients to engage in their occupations.

Table C-7 Types of Occupational Therapy Interventions

Occupation-based intervention	*Purpose*: Client engages in client-directed occupations that match identified goals. *Examples*: • Completes morning dressing and hygiene using adaptive devices • Purchases groceries and prepares a meal • Utilizes the transportation system • Applies for a job • Plays on playground and community recreation equipment • Participates in a community festival • Establishes a pattern of self-care and relaxation activities in preparation for sleep
Purposeful activity	*Purpose*: Client engages in specifically selected activities that allow the client to develop skills that enhance occupational engagement. *Examples*: • Practices how to select clothing and manipulate clothing fasteners • Practices safe ways to get in and out of a bathtub • Practices how to prepare a food list and rehearses how to use cooking appliances • Practices how to use a map and transportation schedule • Rehearses how to write answers on an application form • Practices how to get on and off playground and recreation equipment • Role plays when to greet people and initiates conversation • Practices how to use adaptive switches to operate home environmental control system
Preparatory methods	*Purpose*: Practitioner selects directed methods and techniques that prepare the client for occupational performance. Used in preparation for or concurrently with purposeful and occupation-based activities. *Examples*: • Provides sensory enrichment to promote alertness • Administers physical agent modalities to prepare muscles for movement • Provides instruction in visual imagery and rhythmic breathing to promote rest and relaxation • Issues orthotics/splints to provide support and facilitate movement • Suggests a home-based conditioning regimen using Pilates and yoga • Provides hand-strengthening exercises using therapy putty and Thera-Band • Provides instruction in assertiveness to prepare for self-advocacy

   Consultation Process—A type of intervention in which occupational therapy practitioners use their knowledge and expertise to collaborate with the client. The collaborative process involves identifying the problem, creating possible solutions, trying solutions, and altering them as necessary for greater effectiveness. When providing consultation, the practitioner is not directly responsible for the outcome of the intervention (Dunn, 2000a, p. 113).

Person	• Advises a family about architectural options • Advises family how to create pre-sleep nighttime routines for their children
Organization	• Recommends work pattern modifications and ergonomically designed workstations for a company • Recommends disaster evacuation strategies for a residential community related to accessibility and reduced environmental barriers
Population	• Advises senior citizens on older driver initiatives

Education Process—An intervention process that involves imparting knowledge and information about occupation, health, and participation and that does not result in the actual performance of the occupation/activity.

Person	• Instructs a classroom teacher on sensory regulation strategies
Organization	• Teaches staff at a homeless shelter how to structure daily living, play, and leisure activities for shelter members
Population	• Instructs town officials about the value of and strategies for making walking and biking paths accessible for all community members

Advocacy—Efforts directed toward promoting occupational justice and empowering clients to seek and obtain resources to fully participate in their daily life occupations.

Person	• Collaborates with a person to procure reasonable accommodations at worksite
Organization	• Serves on policy board of an organization to procure supportive housing accommodations for persons with disabilities
Population	• Collaborates with adults with serious mental illness to raise public awareness of the impact of this stigma
	• Collaborates with and educates federal funding sources for the disabled population to include cancer patients prior to their full remission

[a]Information adapted from Pedretti & Early, 2001.

The examples listed specify how the broad outcome of engagement in occupation may be operationalized. The examples are not intended to be all-inclusive.

Table C-8 Types of Outcomes

Outcome	Description
Occupational performance	The act of doing and accomplishing a selected activity or occupation that results from the dynamic transaction among the client, the context, and the activity. Improving or enabling skills and patterns in occupational performance leads to engagement in occupations or activites (adapted in part from Law et al., 1996, p. 16).
	• Improvement—Used when a performance limitation is present. These outcomes document increased occupational performance for the person, organization, or population. Outcome examples may include (1) the ability of a child with autism to play interactively with a peer (person); (2) the ability of an older adult to return to the home from a skilled-nursing facility (person); (3) decreased incidence of back strain in nursing personnel as a result of an in-service education program in body mechanics for carrying out job duties that require bending, lifting, and so forth (organizations); and (4) construction of accessible playground facilities for all children in local city parks (populations).
	• Enhancement—Used when a performance limitation is not currently present. These outcomes document the development of performance skills and performance patterns that augment existing performance or prevent potential problems from developing in life occupations. Outcome examples may include (1) increased confidence and competence of teenage mothers to parent their children as a result of structured social groups and child development classes (person); (2) increased membership of the local senior citizen center as a result of diverse social wellness and exercise programs (organization); (3) increased ability by school staff to address and manage school-age youth violence as a result of conflict resolution training to address "bullying" (organizations); and (4) increased opportunities for seniors to participate in community activities due to ride share programs (populations).
Adaptation	A change in response approach that the client makes when encountering an occupational challenge. "This change is implemented when the [client's] customary response approaches are found inadequate for producing some degree of mastery over the challenge" (adapted from Schultz & Schkade, 1997, p. 474). Examples of adaptation outcomes include (1) clients modifying their behaviors to earn privileges at an adolescent treatment facility (person); (2) a company redesigning the daily schedule to allow for an even workflow and to decrease times of high stress (organizations); and (3) a community making available accessible public transportation and erecting public and "reserved" benches for older adults to socialize and rest (populations).

Table C-8 Types of Outcomes—Cont'd

Outcome	Description
Health and wellness	Health is a resource for everyday life, not the objective of living. For individuals, it is a state of physical, mental, and social well-being, as well as a positive concept emphasizing social and personal resources and physical capacities (WHO, 1986). Health of organizations and populations includes these individual aspects but also includes social responsibility of members to society as a whole. Wellness is "[a]n active process through which individuals [organizations or populations] become aware of and make choices toward a more successful existence" (Hettler, 1984, p. 1170). Wellness is more than a lack of disease symptoms; it is a state of mental and physical balance and fitness (adapted from Taber's Cyclopedic Medical Dictionary, 1997, p. 2110). Outcome examples may include (1) participation in community outings by a client with schizophrenia in a group home (person); (2) implementation of a company-wide program to identify problems and solutions for balance among work, leisure, and family life (organizations); and (3) decreased incidence of childhood obesity (populations).
Participation	Engagement in desired occupations in ways that are personally satisfying and congruent with expectations within the culture.
Prevention	"[H]ealth promotion is equally and essentially concerned with creating the conditions necessary for health at individual, structural, social, and environmental levels through an understanding of the determinants of health: peace, shelter, education, food, income, a stable ecosystem, sustainable resources, social justice, and equity" (Kronenberg, Algado, & Pollard, 2005, p. 441). Occupational therapy promotes a healthy lifestyle at the individual, group, organizational, community (societal), and governmental or policy level (adapted from Brownson & Scaffa, 2001). Outcome examples may include (1) appropriate seating and play area for a child with orthopedic impairments (person); (2) implementation of a program of leisure and educational activities for a drop-in center for adults with severe mental illness (organizations); and (3) access to occupational therapy services in underserved areas regardless of cultural or ethnic backgrounds (populations).
Quality of life	The dynamic appraisal of the client's life satisfaction (perceptions of progress toward one's goals), hope (the real or perceived belief that one can move toward a goal through selected pathways), self-concept (the composite of beliefs and feelings about oneself), health and functioning (including health status, self-care capabilities, and socioeconomic factors, e.g., vocation, education, income; adapted from Radomski, 1995; Zhan, 1992). Outcomes may include (1) full and active participation of a deaf child from a hearing family during a recreational activity (person); (2) residents being able to prepare for outings and travel independently as a result of independent-living skills training for care providers of a group (organization); and (3) formation of a lobby to support opportunities for social networking, advocacy activities, and sharing scientific information for stroke survivors and their families (population).
Role competence	The ability to effectively meet the demands of roles in which the client engages.
Self-advocacy	Actively promoting or supporting oneself or others (individuals, organizations, or populations); requires an understanding of strengths and needs, identification of goals, knowledge of legal rights and responsibilities, and communicating these aspects to others (adapted from Dawson, 2007). Outcomes may include (1) a student with a learning disability requesting and receiving reasonable accommodations such as textbooks on tape (person); (2) a grassroots employee committee requesting and procuring ergonomically designed keyboards for their computers at work (organization); and (3) people with disabilities advocating for universal design with all public and private construction (population).
Occupational justice	Access to and participation in the full range of meaningful and enriching occupations afforded to others. Includes opportunities for social inclusion and the resources to participate in occupations to satisfy personal, health, and societal needs (adapted from Townsend & Wilcock, 2004). Outcomes may include (1) people with intellectual disabilities serving on an advisory board to establish programs offered by a community recreation center (person); (2) workers who have enough break time to have lunch with their young children at day care centers (organization); (3) people with persistent mental illness welcomed by community recreation center due to anti-stigma campaign (organization); and (4) alternative adapted housing options for older adult to "age in place" (populations).

Table C-9 Operationalizing the Occupational Therapy Process

Evaluation		Intervention			Outcomes
Occupational Profile ◄—►	*Analysis of Occupational Performance*	*Intervention Plan*	*Intervention Implementation*	*Intervention Review*	*Engagement in Occupation to Support Participation*
Identify: Who is the client? Why is the client seeking services? What occupations and activities are successful or are causing problems? What contexts support or inhibit desired outcomes? What is the client's occupational history? What are the client's priorities and targeted outcomes?	Synthesize information from the occupational profile. Observe client's performance in desired occupation/activity. Note the effectiveness of performance skills and patterns, and select assessments to identify factors (context or contexts, activity demands, client factors) that may be influencing performance skills and patterns. Interpret assessment data to identify facilitators and barriers to performance. Develop and refine hypotheses about client's occupational performance strengths and weaknesses. Collaborate with client to create goals that address targeted outcomes. Delineate areas for intervention, based on best practice and evidence.	Develop plan that includes objective and measurable goals with time frame, occupational therapy intervention approach based on theory and evidence, and mechanisms for service delivery. Consider discharge needs and plan. Select outcome measures. Make recommendation or referral to others as needed.	Determine types of occupational therapy interventions to be used, and carry them out. Monitor client's response according to ongoing assessment and reassessment.	Reevaluate plan relative to achieving targeted outcomes. Modify plan as needed. Determine need for continuation, discontinuation, or referral.	Focus on outcomes as they relate to engagement in occupation to support participation. Select outcome measures. Measure and use outcomes.

————— Continue to renegotiate intervention plans and targeted outcomes. —————

————— Ongoing interaction among evaluation, intervention, and outcomes occurs throughout the process. —————

All text and tables are adapted from American Occupational Therapy Association: Occupational therapy practice framework: domain and process, ed 2, *Am J Occup Ther* 62, 625–683, 2008.

References

Ayres AJ: *Developmental dyspraxia and adult onset apraxia*, Torrance, CA, 1985, Sensory Integration International.

Blanche EI, Parham LD: Praxis and organization of behavior in time and space. In Smith Roley S, Blanche EI, Schaaf RC, editors: *Understanding the Nature of Sensory Integration with Diverse Populations*, San Antonio, TX, 2002, Therapy Skill Builders, pp 183–200.

Brownson CA, Scaffa ME: Occupational therapy in the promotion of health and the prevention of disease and disability, *Am J Occup Ther* 55:656–660, 2001.

Calvert G, Spence C, Stein BE, editors: *The Handbook of Multisensory Processes*, Cambridge, MA, 2004, MIT Press.

Dawson J: *Self-advocacy: a valuable skill for your teenager*, 2007. Retrieved January 20, 2007 from http://www.schwablearning.org.

Dunn W: *Best Practice in Occupational Therapy in Community Service with Children and Families*, Thorofare, NJ, 2000a, Slack.

Dunn W, McClain LH, Brown C, et al: The ecology of human performance. In Neistadt ME, Crepeau EB, editors: *Willard and Spackman's Occupational Therapy*, ed 9, Philadelphia, 1998, Lippincott Williams & Wilkins, pp 525–535.

Fiese BH, Tomcho TJ, Douglas M, et al: A review of 50 years of research on naturally occurring family routines and rituals: cause for celebration? *J Fam Psychol* 16:381–390, 2002.

Filley CM: *Neurobehavioral Anatomy*, Boulder, CO, 2001, University Press of Colorado.

Fisher A: Overview of performance skills and client factors. In Pendleton H, Schultz-Krohn W, editors: *Pedretti's Occupational Therapy: Practice Skills for Physical Dysfunction*, St. Louis, MO, 2006, Mosby/Elsevier, pp 372–402.

Heilman KM, Rothi LJG: *Clinical Neuropsychology*, ed 3, New York, 1993, Oxford University Press.

Hettler W: Wellness—the lifetime goal of a university experience. In Matarazzo JD, Weiss SM, Herd JA, et al, editors: *Behavioral Health: A Handbook of Health Enhancement and Disease Prevention*, New York, 1984, Wiley, pp 1117.

Kronenberg F, Algado SS, Pollard N: *Occupational Therapy Without Borders: Learning from the Spirit of Survivors*, Philadelphia, 2005, Elsevier/Churchill Livingstone.

Law M, Cooper B, Strong S, et al: Person–environment–occupation model: a transactive approach to occupational performance, *Can J Occup Ther* 63:9–23, 1996.

Liepmann H: Apraxie, *Ergebnisse der Gesamten Medizin* 1:516–543, 1920.

Moyers PA, Dale LM: *The Guide to Occupational Therapy Practice*, ed 2, Bethesda, MD, 2007, AOTA Press.

Neistadt ME, Crepeau EB, editors: *Willard and Spackman's Occupational Therapy*, ed 9, Philadelphia, 1998, Lippincott Williams & Wilkins.

Pedretti LW, Early MB: Occupational performance and model of practice for physical dysfunction. In Pedretti LW, Early MB, editors: *Occupational Therapy Practice Skills for Physical Dysfunction*, St. Louis, MO, 2001, Mosby, pp 7–9.

Punwar AJ, Peloquin SM: *Occupational Therapy Principles and Practice*, ed 3, Philadelphia, 2000, Lippincott Williams & Wilkins.

Radomski MV: There is more to life than putting on your pants, *Am J Occup Ther* 49:487–490, 1995.

Schell BAB, Cohn ES, Crepeau EB: Overview of personal factors affecting performance. In Crepeau EB, Cohn ES, Schell BAB, editors: *Willard and Spackman's Occupational Therapy*, ed 11, Baltimore, 2008, Lippincott Williams & Wilkins, pp 650–657.

Schultz S, Schkade J: Adaptation. In Christiansen C, Baum MC, editors: *Occupational Therapy: Enabling Function and Well-Being*, Thorofare, NJ, 1997, Slack, p 474.

Segal R: Family routines and rituals: a context for occupational therapy interventions, *Am J Occup Ther* 58:499–508, 2004.

Taber's Cyclopedic Medical Dictionary, Philadelphia, 1997, FA Davis.

Townsend EA, Wilcock AA: Occupational justice. In Christiansen CH, Townsend EA, editors: *Introduction to Occupation: The Art and Science of Living*, Upper Saddle River, NJ, 2004, Prentice-Hall, pp 243–273.

World Health Organization: November 21. *The Ottawa Charter for Health Promotion*, 1986, First International Conference on Health Promotion, Ottawa. Retrieved February 4, 2008, from http://www.who.int/healthpromotion/conferences/previous/ottawa/en/print.html.

World Health Organization: *International Classification of Functioning, Disability, and Health (ICF)*, Geneva, 2001, Author.

Zhan L: Quality of life: conceptual and measurement issues, *J Adv Nurs* 17:795–800, 1992. Bibliography Accreditation Council for Occupational Therapy.

APPENDIX **D** Resources

Professional Organizations, Foundations, and Certification

American Occupational Therapy Association, Inc. (AOTA)
4720 Montgomery Lane
PO Box 31220
Bethesda, MD 20824-1220
Phone: 301-652-2682
TDD: 1-800-377-8555
Fax: 301-652-7711
Website: www.aota.org

American Occupational Therapy Foundation (AOTF)
4720 Montgomery Lane
PO Box 31220
Bethesda, MD 20824-1220
Phone: 301-652-6611, Ext. 2550
AOTA members: 1-800-SAY-AOTA
Fax: 301-656-3620
E-mail: aotf@aotf.org
Website: www.aotf.org

Australian Association of Occupational Therapists
OT AUSTRALIA National
PO Box 41479
CASUARINA, NT 08 11
Phone: 0408 448 080
E-mail: nt@ausot.com.au
Website: www.ausot.com.au

Canadian Association of Occupational Therapists (CAOT)
CTTC Building, Suite 3400
1125 Colonel By Drive
Ottawa, ON K1S 5R1
Canada
Phone: 613-523-CAOT (2268)
Toll-free: 800-434-CAOT (2268)
Fax: 613-523-2552
Website: www.caot.ca

National Board for Certification in Occupational Therapy, Inc. (NBCOT®)
12 South Summit Avenue
Suite 100
Gaithersburg, MD 20877-4150
Phone: 301-990-7979

Fax: 301-869-8492
Website: www.nbcot.org

World Federation of Occupational Therapists (WFOT)
PO Box 30
Forrestfield
Western Australia
Australia 6058
Fax: 61 8 9453 9746
E-mail: admin@wfot.org.au
Website: www.wfot.org

Research and Education

American Association of Retired Persons (AARP)
601 E Street NW
Washington, DC 20049
Phone: 1-888-687-2277
Website: www.aarp.org

Centers for Disease Control and Prevention (CDC)
1600 Clifton Road, NE
Atlanta, GA 30333 USA
Phone: 800-232-4636
E-mail: cdcinfo@cdc.gov
Website: www.cdc.gov

Centers for Medicare & Medicaid Services
7500 Security Boulevard
Baltimore, MD 21244
Phone: 410-786-3000
Toll-free: 877-267-2323
Website: www.cms.gov

Department of Education
400 Maryland Avenue, SW
Washington, DC 20202
Toll-free: 1-800-872-5327
Website: www.ed.gov

Department of Health and Human Services
200 Independence Avenue, SW
Washington, DC 20201
Toll-free: 1-877-696-6775
Website: www.hhs.gov

Glossary

A

Accreditation A form of regulation that determines whether an organization or program meets a prescribed standard

Accreditation Council for Occupational Therapy Education (ACOTE) The national organization that regulates entry-level education for occupational therapists and for occupational therapy assistants

Active being The view of humans as actively involved in controlling and determining their own behavior

Active listening A manner of communication in which the receiver paraphrases the speaker's words to ensure that he or she understands the intended meaning

Activities of daily living (ADL) Activities involved in taking care of one's own body, including such things as dressing, bathing, grooming, eating, feeding, personal device care, toileting, sexual activity, and sleep/rest

Activity State or condition of being involved (participant); a general class of human actions that is goal-directed

Activity analysis The process in which the steps of an activity and its components are examined to determine the demands on the client

Activity demands The aspects of an activity needed to carry out that activity, such as objects used and their properties, space demands, social demands, sequencing and timing, required actions, required body functions, and required body structures

Activity director The practitioner responsible for planning, implementing, and documenting an ongoing program of activities that meet the needs of the residents

Activity synthesis The process of identifying gaps in performance and bridging those gaps by grading or adapting the activity or the environment in order to provide the "just right challenge" for the client

Acute care The first level on the continuum of care in which a client has a sudden and short-term need for services and is typically seen in a hospital

Adaptation A change in function that promotes survival and self-actualization

Adolescence The period of development between 12 and 20 years of age

Adolf Meyer A Swiss physician committed to a holistic perspective; developed the psychobiological approach to mental illness

Adulthood The period of development after 20 years of age; broken into a young stage (20–40 years of age), middle (40–65 years of age), and late (over 65 years of age)

Advanced beginner A practitioner who is learning to recognize additional cues and beginning to see the client as an individual; still does not see the whole picture

Aging The unique changes that occur over time, such as sensory and physical declines

Aging in place The trend of more elderly people staying at home and living independently or with minimal assistance

Altruism The unselfish concern for the welfare of others

Americans with Disabilities Act of 1990 Legislation that provides civil rights to all individuals with disabilities

American Journal of Occupational Therapy (AJOT) The American Occupational Therapy Association's (AOTA's) official publication that traditionally has served as the main source of research and resource information for the profession

American Occupational Therapy Association (AOTA) Formerly called the National Society for the Promotion of Occupational Therapy; the nationally recognized professional association for occupational therapy practitioners

American Occupational Therapy Foundation (AOTF) A national organization designed to advance the science of occupational therapy and to increase public understanding of the value of occupational therapy

American Occupational Therapy Political Action Committee (AOTPAC) The organization that furthers the legislative aims of the profession by attempting to influence the selection, nomination, election, or appointment of persons to public office

American Student Committee of the Occupational Therapy Association (ASCOTA) Student representatives from all accredited schools who participate in the American Occupational Therapy Association by meeting regularly and providing feedback to the organization

Areas of occupation Various life activities including activities of daily living (ADL), instrumental activities of daily living (IADL), education, work, play, leisure, and social participation

Artistic element The element of clinical reasoning in which the occupational therapy practitioner guides the treatment process and selects the "right action" in the face of uncertainties inherent in the clinical process

Arts and Crafts Movement A late nineteenth-century movement born in reaction to the Industrial Revolution; emphasized craftsmanship and design

Assessment instruments Standardized or nonstandardized measurements used to obtain information about clients

Assessment procedures The clinical techniques and instruments used to determine the strengths and weaknesses of a client for therapeutic purposes

Assistive devices Low- or high-technology aids to improve a person's function

Assistive technology Devices that aid a person in his or her daily life as necessary

Autonomy The freedom to decide and the freedom to act

Axiology component The part of philosophy that is concerned with the study of values

B

Balanced Budget Act (BBA) of 1997 Legislation intended to reduce Medicare spending, create incentives for development of managed care plans, encourage enrollment in managed care plans, and limit fee-for-service payment and programs

Beneficence A principle that requires that the occupational therapy practitioner contribute to the good health and welfare of the client

Benjamin Rush An American Quaker who was the first physician to institute Moral Treatment practices

Biological sphere Sphere of practice in which clients have medical problems caused by disease, disorder, or trauma

Biomechanical frame of reference A frame of reference derived from theories in kinetics and kinematics; used with individuals who have deficits in the peripheral nervous, musculoskeletal, integumentary (e.g., skin), or cardiopulmonary system

Board certification Certification for the occupational therapist or occupational therapy assistant that incorporates more generalized areas of practice that have an established knowledge base in occupational therapy

Brain plasticity The phenomenon that the brain is capable of change and that through activity one may get improved neurological synapses, improved dendritic growth, or additional pathways

C

Canadian Model of Occupational Performance A model of practice that emphasizes client-centered care and spirituality

Career development The process of advancing within the service delivery path or transitioning into a role outside of service delivery

Cerebral palsy (CP) A disorder caused by an insult to the brain before during or soon after birth, which manifests in motor abnormalities

Certification The acknowledgement that an individual has the qualifications to be an entry-level practitioner

Childhood Spans early childhood (1–6 years) and later childhood (6–12 years)

Civilian Vocational Rehabilitation Act Act that provided federal funds to states to provide vocational rehabilitation services to civilians with disabilities

Clarification An active listening technique in which the client's thoughts and feelings are summarized or simplified

Client Person served by occupational therapy in a health facility or training center

Client-centered approach An approach in which the client, family, and significant others are active participants throughout the therapeutic process

Client factors Components of activities consisting of body functions and body structures; used to assess functioning, disability, and health

Client-related tasks Routine tasks in which the aide may interact with the client but not as the primary service provider of occupational therapy

Client satisfaction A measure of the client's perception of the process and the benefits received from occupational therapy services

Clinical reasoning The thought process that therapists use to design and carry out intervention; involves complex cognitive and affective skills

Close supervision The need for direct, daily contact with the supervisee

Code of ethics Professional guidelines for making correct or proper choices and decisions for health care practice in the field

Cognitive disability frame of reference A frame of reference based on the premise that cognitive disorders in those with mental health disabilities are caused by neurobiologic defects or deficits related to the biologic functioning of the brain

Competent practitioner A level of clinical reasoning skills in which the practitioner is able to see more facts and to determine the importance of these facts and observations; has a broader understanding of the client's problems and is more likely to individualize treatment; however, flexibility and creativity are still lacking

Concepts Ideas that represent something in the mind of the individual

Conditional reasoning The clinical reasoning strategy in which the occupational therapy practitioner implements intervention and cognitively checks along the way to compare the client's progress in treatment and goals for the future

Confidentiality The expectation that information shared by the client with the occupational therapy practitioner will be kept private and shared only with those directly involved with the intervention

Consultation A type of intervention in which practitioners use their knowledge and expertise to collaborate with the client, caregivers, significant others, or other providers

Context The setting in which the occupation occurs; includes cultural, physical, social, personal, spiritual, temporal, and virtual conditions within and surrounding the client that influence performance

Continuing competence A process in which the occupational therapy practitioner develops and maintains knowledge, performance skills, interpersonal abilities, critical reasoning skills, and ethical reasoning skills necessary to perform his or her professional responsibilities

Continuum of care A way of characterizing health care settings by the level of care required by the client, including the whole spectrum of needs

D

Developmental delays The general slowing of skills

Developmental frame of reference A frame of reference that postulates that practice in a skill set will enhance brain development and help the child progress through the stages

Diagnosis codes Billing codes that are based on the client's medical condition or the medical justification for needing services

Diagnosis-related groups (DRGs) Groupings of disease categories that Medicare and other third-party payers use as a basis for hospital payment schedules

Dignity The quality or state of being worthy, honored, or esteemed

Direct supervision The supervising occupational therapist is on site and available to provide immediate assistance to the client or supervisee if needed.

Discharge plan The plan developed and implemented to address the resources and supports that may be required upon discontinuation of services

Doctor of Occupational Therapy (OTD) Clinical or practice-based doctoral degree; focuses on practice rather than research

Documentation The process of keeping records on all the aspects of service delivery

Driver rehabilitation specialist An occupational therapy practitioner who evaluates and intervenes in physical, social, cognitive, and psychosocial aspects of functioning that affect driving skills

E

Education The process of gaining knowledge and information

Education for All Handicapped Children Act of 1975 (PL 94–142) Act that established the right of all children to a free and appropriate education, regardless of handicapping condition

Eleanor Clarke Slagle Known as the mother of occupational therapy; developed the area of habit training and organized the first professional school for occupational therapy practitioners

Emergency procedures Actions to follow in case of an injury or accident in the clinic

Empathy The ability of the occupational therapy practitioner to place himself or herself in the client's position and to understand what he or she is experiencing

Entry-level practitioner A practitioner who is still developing his or her skills and is expected to be held responsible for and accountable in professional activities related to the role

Epistemology component The part of philosophy that investigates critically the nature, origin, and limits of human knowledge

Equality The treatment of all individuals with an attitude of fairness and impartiality and the respecting of each individual's beliefs, values, and lifestyles

Ergonomics The science of fitting jobs to people

Ethical dilemma A situation in which two or more ethical principles collide with one another, making it difficult to determine the best action

Ethical distress Situations that challenge how a practitioner maintains his or her integrity or the integrity of the profession along with the integrity of the profession and examining the "right" behaviors or proper choices and decisions

Ethical element The element of clinical reasoning that takes into account the client's perspective and his or her goals for intervention

Ethics The study and philosophy of human conduct

Evaluation The process of obtaining and interpreting data necessary to understand the individual and design appropriate treatment

Evidence-based practice Basing practice on the best available research evidence

Expert A practitioner who has the clinical reasoning skills to recognize and understand rules of practice, use intuition to know what to do next, and use conditional reasoning

F

Family-centered care Care that involves working with the family members of the child on goals that are considered important to them

Fidelity Faithfulness

Fieldwork Practical experience applying classroom knowledge to a clinical setting; categorized as Level I (may be observational) or Level II (development of entry-level skills)

Frame of reference (FOR) A system that applies theory and puts principles into practice, providing practitioners with specifics on how to treat specific clients

Freedom An individual's right to exercise choice

Function Action for which a person is fit; the ability to perform

G

General supervision At least monthly face-to-face contact with the supervisee

George Edward Barton An architect who opened Consolation House for convalescent patients, where occupation was used as a method of treatment

Goal End toward which effort is directed

Grading Changing the process, environment, tools, or materials of the activity to increase or decrease the performance demands on the client

Group More than two people interacting with a common purpose

Group dynamics Refers to the interactions among individuals and how they work together

H

Habit training A re-education program dedicated to restoring and maintaining health by directing activity to construct new habits and discard ineffective ones

Handicapped Infants and Toddlers Act of 1986 An amendment to the Education for All Handicapped Children Act; includes children from 3 to 5 years of age and initiates new early intervention programs for children from birth to 3 years of age

Health The state of physical, mental, and social well-being

Herbert Hall A physician who adapted the Arts and Crafts Movement for medical purposes

Holistic An approach that deems that each individual should be seen as a complete and unified whole rather than a series of parts or problems to be managed

Hospice Care and services provided to help the client be comfortable during the last stages of a terminal illness

Humanism The belief that the client should be treated as a person, not an object

I

Ideal self What an individual would like to be if free of the demands of mundane reality

Independence State or condition of being independent (self-reliant)

Individualized education plan (IEP) A plan that charts the problems, goals, and interventions necessary for the child to have success in school

Individuals with Disabilities Education Act (IDEA) of 1991 Legislation that requires school districts to educate students with disabilities in the least restrictive environment

Infancy The period from birth through 1 year of age

Informed consent The knowledgeable and voluntary agreement by which a client undergoes intervention that is in accord with his or her values and preferences

Instrumental activities of daily living (IADLs) Activities, such as meal preparation, money management, care of others, which involve interacting with the environment; often complex; may be considered optional

Interactive reasoning A strategy used by the occupational therapy practitioner when he or she wants to understand the client as a person

Interdisciplinary team A mix of practitioners from different disciplines who maintain their own professional roles and use a cooperative approach that is very interactive and centered on a common problem to solve

Intermediate-level practitioner A practitioner who has increased responsibility and typically pursues specialization in a particular area of practice

Interrater reliability A measure of the likelihood that test scores will be the same no matter who is the examiner

Intervention An approach that involves working with the client through therapy to reach client goals

Interview The primary mechanism for gathering information for the occupational profile; achieved by the occupational therapy practitioner asking the client and significant others questions

J

Justice The need for all occupational therapy practitioners to abide by the laws that govern the practice and the legal rights of the client

L

Later adulthood The period of development after 65 years of age

Learned helplessness The phenomenon of less activity and independence in functioning among elderly people that results when older persons are not allowed to engage in activities or when others do everything for them

Least restrictive environment The classroom most similar to a regular classroom in which the student can be successful

Licensure The process by which permission is granted to an individual to engage in a given occupation upon finding that the applicant has attained the minimal degree of competence required to ensure that the public health, safety, and welfare will be reasonably protected

Locus of authority Situations that require a decision about who should be the primary decision maker

Long-term care The level of care needed for clients who are medically stable but have a chronic condition requiring services over time, potentially throughout their lives

M

Mechanistic The view that sees the human as passive in nature and controlled by the environment in which he or she lives

Media The means by which therapeutic effects are transmitted

Medicare Enacted in 1965; legislation that provides health care assistance for individuals 65 years or older or those who are permanently and totally disabled

Metaphysical component One part of philosophy that addresses questions such as "What is the nature of humankind?"

Methods The steps, sequences, and approaches used to activate the therapeutic effect of a medium

Modality The media and methods used in occupational therapy intervention

Model of Human Occupation A model of practice that views occupation in terms of volition, habituation, performance, and environment

Model of practice A way of organizing that takes the philosophical base of the profession and provides terms to describe practice, tools for evaluation, and a guide for intervention

Morals A view of right and wrong developed as a result of background, values, religious beliefs, and the society in which a person lives

Moral Treatment A movement grounded in the philosophy that all people, even the most challenged, are entitled to consideration and human compassion

Multidisciplinary team A mix of practitioners from multiple disciplines who work together in a common setting but without an interactive relationship

N

Narrative reasoning The type of clinical reasoning in which storytelling and story creation are used

National Board for Certification in Occupational Therapy (NBCOT®) The organization responsible for administering the national certification examination

National Society for the Promotion of Occupational Therapy Formed on March 15, 1917; marked the birth of the profession of occupational therapy

Non–client-related tasks The preparation of the work area and equipment, clerical tasks, and maintenance activities

Nonmaleficence A principle that instructs the practitioner to not inflict harm to the client

Non-standardized tests Tests that do not provide specific guidelines based upon a normative sample; do not require standardized procedures

Nonverbal communication Communication that includes facial expressions, eye contact, tone of voice, touch, and body language

Normative data Information collected from a representative sample that can then be used by the examiner to make comparisons with his or her clients

Novice A practitioner who is learning the procedural skills (e.g., assessment, diagnostic, and treatment planning procedures) necessary to practice

O

Observation The means of gathering information about a person or an environment by watching and noticing

Occupation Activity in which one engages that is meaningful and central to one's identity

Occupation as a means The use of a specific occupation to bring about a change in the client's performance

Occupation as an end The desired outcome or product of intervention

Occupation-based activity The performance of occupation-related activities by the client, including activities of daily living, instrumental activities of daily living, work and school tasks, and play or leisure tasks

Occupational adaptation A model of practice that proposes that occupational therapy practitioners examine how they may change the person, environment, or task so the client may engage in occupations

Occupational performance The ability to carry out activities in the areas of occupation

Occupational therapist (OT) An allied health professional who uses occupation, purposeful activity, simulated activities, and preparatory methods to maximize the independence and health of any client who is limited by physical injury or illness, cognitive impairment, psychosocial dysfunction, mental illness, or a developmental or learning disability

Occupational therapy A goal-directed activity that promotes independence in function; the practice of using meaningful occupations and purposeful activities to promote function and participation in life activities

Occupational therapy aide A person who provides services under the supervision of an occupational therapist to clients and therapists and helps maintain the work space

Occupational therapy assistant (OTA) An allied health paraprofessional who, under the direction of an occupational therapist, directs an individual's participation in selected tasks to restore, reinforce, and enhance performance, and promote and maintain health

Occupational therapy practitioner Refers to two different levels of clinicians, an occupational therapist (OT) or an occupational therapy assistant (OTA)

Occupational therapy process The interaction between two active agents involved in the process—the practitioner and the client

Organismic The view that a person's behaviors influence the physical and social environment and that, in turn, the person is affected by changes in the environment

Orthotic device An apparatus used to support, align, prevent, or correct deformities or to improve the function of movable parts of the body

Outcome measures An aspect of program evaluation that evaluates the results of the intervention after the service has been provided

P

Participatory research Involves the clinician, client, and faculty member in the research process

Patient Person served in a hospital or rehabilitation setting

Perceived self The aspect that others see; what they perceive without the benefit of knowing a person's intentions, motivations, and limitations

Performance patterns The client's habits, routines, and roles

Performance skills Small units of observable action that are linked together in the process of executing a daily life task performance

Person-Environment-Occupation-Performance A model of practice that provides definitions and describes the interactive nature of human beings

Phenomenological That which is determined by the experience of individuals

Philippe Pinel French physician who advocated humane treatment for mentally ill patients in the late 1700s

Physical agent modalities (PAMs) Preparatory methods used to bring about a response in soft tissue

Play The spontaneous, enjoyable, free from rules, internally motivated activity in which there is no goal or purpose

Political action committees (PACs) The legally sanctioned vehicles through which organizations can engage in political action

Pragmatic reasoning The type of clinical reasoning that takes into consideration factors in the context of the practice setting and in the personal context of the occupational therapy practitioner that may inhibit or facilitate intervention

Preparatory methods Techniques or activities that address the remediation and restoration of problems associated with client factors and body structure, with the long-term purpose of supporting the client's acquisition of performance skills needed to resume his or her roles and daily occupations

Principles Ideas that explain the relationship between two or more concepts

Private for-profit agencies Organizations owned and operated by individuals or a group of investors

Private not-for-profit agencies Organizations that receive special tax exemptions and typically charge a fee for services and maintain a balanced budget to provide services

Private funding sources Businesses that provide funds for medical procedures

Problem-Oriented Medical Record A format that provides a structure to documentation

Procedural reasoning A clinical reasoning strategy used by the occupational therapy practitioner when he or she focuses on the client's disease or disability and determines what will be the most appropriate modalities to use to improve the functional performance

Procedure codes Billing codes that are based on the specific services performed by health care providers

Professional association An organization that exists to protect and promote the profession it represents by (1) providing a communication network and channel for information, (2) regulating itself through the development and enforcement of standards of conduct and performance, and (3) guarding the interests of those within the profession

Professional development Organizing and personally managing a cumulative series of work experiences to add to one's knowledge, motivation, perspectives, skills, and job performance

Professional philosophy A set of values, beliefs, truths, and principles that guide the practitioner's actions

Proficient practitioner A practitioner who views situations as a whole instead of as isolated parts; practical experience allows the proficient practitioner to develop a direction and vision of where the client should be going; able to easily modify the intervention plan if the initial plan does not work

Program evaluation Measuring effectiveness by determining which programs are achieving their goals and objectives, and modifying programs accordingly

Prudence The ability to demonstrate sound judgment, care, and discretion

Psychological sphere A sphere of practice in which client problems manifest as emotional, cognitive, affective, or personality disorders

Public agencies Health care agencies operated by federal, state, or county governments

Public funding sources Agencies at the federal, state, or local level that provide funds for medical procedures

Purposeful activity An activity used in treatment that is goal directed; individual is an active voluntary participant; has both inherent and therapeutic goals

Quality of life A relative measurement of what is meaningful and what provides satisfaction to an individual

R

Real self A blending of the internal and external worlds involving intention and action plus environmental awareness

Reconstruction aides Civilians who helped rehabilitate soldiers who had been injured in the war so that they could either return to active military duty or be employed in a civilian job

Referral A request for service for a particular client or a change in the degree and direction of service

Reflection A response wherein the purpose is to express in words the feelings and attitudes sensed behind the words of the speaker

Registration The listing of qualified individuals by a professional association or government agency

Regulations Policies describing the implementation and enforcement of laws

Rehabilitation Act of 1973 Act that guaranteed certain rights for people with disabilities, emphasized the need for rehabilitation research, and called for priority service for persons with the most severe disabilities

Rehabilitation Movement The period from 1942 to 1960 in which Veterans Administration hospitals increased in size and number to handle the casualties of war and continued care of veterans

Relationship A connection of different roles to one another

Reliability A measure of how accurately the scores obtained from the test reflect the true performance of the client

Restatement The listener repeats the words of the speaker as they are heard.

Role A pattern of behavior that involves certain rights and duties that an individual is expected, trained, and encouraged to perform in a particular social situation

Role competence The ability to meet the demands of roles

Routine supervision Direct contact at least every 2 weeks with interim supervision as needed

S

Scientific element One of the three elements of clinical reasoning that demands careful and accurate assessments, analysis, and recording

Screening The process by which the occupational therapy practitioner gathers preliminary information about the client and determines whether further evaluation and occupational therapy intervention are warranted

Self-awareness Knowing one's own true nature; the ability to recognize one's own behavior, emotional responses, and effect created on others

Service competency A useful mechanism by which it is determined that two people performing the same or equivalent procedures will obtain the same or equivalent results

Service management functions Functions that include maintaining a safe and efficient workplace, making daily schedules, documenting treatment, integrating research into practice, billing for services, supervising fieldwork students, marketing and public relations, and performing quality assurance activities

SOAP note The format used for writing the progress note, wherein "S" is subjective information, "O" is objective information, "A" is the assessment, and "P" is the plan

Sociological sphere A sphere of practice wherein clients have problems meeting the expectations of society

Soldier's Rehabilitation Act Act that established a program of vocational rehabilitation for soldiers disabled on active duty

Specialty certification A credential for occupational therapists and occupational therapy assistants that indicates advanced knowledge in a particular area of practice

Splint A device for immobilization, restraint, or support of any part of the body

Standards of practice Guidelines for the delivery of occupational therapy services

Statutes Laws that are enacted by the legislative branch of a government

Structured observation The means of gathering information about a person by watching the client perform a predetermined activity

Subacute care The level in which the client still needs care but does not require an intensive level or specialized service

Supervision A cooperative process in which two or more people participate in a joint effort to establish, maintain, and or elevate a level of competence and performance

Susan Cox Johnson Demonstrated that occupation could be morally uplifting and could improve the mental and physical state of patients and inmates in public hospitals and almshouses

Susan Tracy A nurse involved in the Arts and Crafts Movement and in the training of nurses in the use of occupations

T

Technology Related Assistance for Individuals with Disabilities Act of 1988 Act that addressed the availability of assistive technology devices and services to individuals with disabilities

Test-retest reliability A measure of the consistency of the results of a given test from one administration to another

Theory A set of ideas that help explain things and how they work

Therapeutic exercise The scientific supervision of exercise for the purpose of preventing muscular atrophy, restoring joint and muscle function, and improving efficiency of cardiovascular and pulmonary function

Therapeutic relationship The interaction between a practitioner and a client in which the occupational therapy practitioner is responsible for facilitating the healing and rehabilitation process

Therapeutic use of occupations and activity The selection of activities and occupations that will meet the therapeutic goals

Therapeutic use of self The art of relating to clients, which involves being aware of oneself and of the client and being in command of what is communicated

Therapy Treatment of an illness or disability

Thomas Kidner An architect who was influential in establishing a presence for occupational therapy in vocational rehabilitation and tuberculosis treatment

Transdisciplinary team A mix of practitioners from different disciplines in which members cross over professional boundaries and share roles and functions

Transition services The coordination or facilitation of services for the purpose of preparing the client for a change

Truthfulness The value demonstrated through behavior that is accountable, honest, and accurate, and that maintains one's professional competence

U

Universal precautions A set of guidelines designed to prevent the transmission of HIV, HBV, and other blood-borne pathogens to health care providers

Universal stages of loss Stages of death and dying first identified by Elisabeth Kübler-Ross, which include denial, anger, bargaining, depression, and acceptance; can also be applied to individuals experiencing loss due to a disabling condition

V

Validity Having a true measure of what it claims to measure

Veracity The duty of the health care professional to tell the truth

Vision A statement or ethos of a profession or organization that is developed with the members and constituents over time and that clarifies values, creates a future, and focuses the mission

W

Wellness The condition of being in good health

William Rush Dunton, Jr. Considered the father of occupational therapy; introduced a regimen of crafts for his patients

William Tuke An English Quaker who opened the York Retreat, which pioneered new methods of treatment of mentally ill patients

World Federation of Occupational Therapists (WFOT) Organization established in 1952 to help occupational therapy practitioners access international information, engage in international exchange, and promote organizations of occupational therapy in schools in countries where none exists

Young adulthood The ages between 20 and 40 years

Index

Note: Page numbers followed by *b* indicate boxes, *f* indicate figures, and *t* indicate tables.